# Encyclopedia of Wellness

# Encyclopedia of Wellness

## From Açaí Berry to Yo-Yo Dieting

### Volume 3: P–Y

### Sharon Zoumbaris, Editor

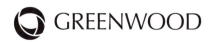

GREENWOOD

AN IMPRINT OF ABC-CLIO, LLC
Santa Barbara, California • Denver, Colorado • Oxford, England

**Library of Congress Cataloging-in-Publication Data**

Encyclopedia of wellness : from açaí berry to yo-yo dieting / Sharon Zoumbaris, editor.
    p. cm.
  Includes index.
  ISBN 978-0-313-39333-4 (hardback) — ISBN 978-0-313-39334-1 (ebook)
1. Health—Encyclopedias.  2. Medicine, Preventive—Encyclopedias.
I. Zoumbaris, Sharon, 1955–
  RA776.E524  2012
  613.03—dc23      2011045406

ISBN: 978-0-313-39333-4
EISBN: 978-0-313-39334-1

16  15  14  13  12    1  2  3  4  5

This book is also available on the World Wide Web as an eBook.
Visit www.abc-clio.com for details.

Greenwood
An Imprint of ABC-CLIO, LLC

ABC-CLIO, LLC
130 Cremona Drive, P.O. Box 1911
Santa Barbara, California 93116-1911

This book is printed on acid-free paper ∞

Manufactured in the United States of America

This book discusses treatments (including types of medication and mental health therapies), diagnostic tests for various symptoms and mental health disorders, and organizations. The authors have made every effort to present accurate and up-to-date information. However, the information in this book is not intended to recommend or endorse particular treatments or organizations, or substitute for the care or medical advice of a qualified health professional, or used to alter any medical therapy without a medical doctor's advice. Specific situations may require specific therapeutic approaches not included in this book. For those reasons, we recommend that readers follow the advice of qualified health care professionals directly involved in their care. Readers who suspect they may have specific medical problems should consult a physician about any suggestions made in this book.

# Contents

# *Alphabetical List of Entries*

# Entries Arranged by Broad Topic

**Alternative Health Care and Complementary Medicine**

Acupuncture
Ayurveda
Biofeedback
Chelation
Dance Therapy
Dietary Supplements
Dream Therapy
Guided Imagery
Homeopathy
Hypnosis
Macrobiotics
Medical Marijuana
Meditation
National Center for Complementary and Alternative Medicine
Naturopathic Medicine
Pauling, Linus
Probiotics
Qigong
Reflexology
Reiki
Rodale, Jerome
Spas, Medical
Tai Chi
Therapeutic Touch
Traditional Chinese Medicine

## Government, Legislation, and Public Policy

Center for Food Safety and Applied Nutrition (CFSAN)
Centers for Disease Control and Prevention (CDC)
Cheeseburger Bill
Comprehensive Smoking Education Act
Dietary Guidelines for Americans
Dietary Reference Intakes (DRI)
Environmental Protection Agency (EPA)
Food and Drug Administration (FDA)
Food Recalls
Head Start and Healthy Start
Human Papillomavirus (HPV)
Institute of Medicine (IOM)
Living Wills and Advance Directives
Medicaid
Medical Power of Attorney
Medicare
MyPlate
National Cancer Institute
National Institutes of Health (NIH)
National Organic Program (NOP)
National School Lunch Program (NSLP)
Nutrition Facts Label
Pandemic
Physical Education
President's Council on Fitness, Sports, and Nutrition
Recommended Dietary Allowance (RDA)
School Meals Initiative
U.S. Department of Agriculture (USDA)
U.S. Department of Health and Human Services (HHS)
Vaccinations
Women's Health Initiative (WHI)
Workplace Wellness
World Health Organization (WHO)

## Health Care

Antibiotics
Bariatric Surgery
Blood Pressure
Cardiopulmonary Resuscitation (CPR)
Dieting, Online Resources
Doctors in the Media
Health and Medical Tourism

**Nutritional Health**

Açaí Berry
Amino Acids
Atkins, Robert C.
Basic Four (Foods)
Blueberries
Caffeine
Calcium
Calories
Carbohydrates
Cholesterol
Daily Value of Nutrients
Dietary Supplements
Dieting
Diets, Fad
Fast Food
Fats
Fiber
Flaxseeds
Free Radicals
Garlic
Ginger
Ginseng
Glycemic Index
Graham, Sylvester
High-Fructose Corn Syrup
Kava
Kellogg, John Harvey
Lactose Intolerance
Minerals (Food)
Nestle, Marion
Nutrients
Nutrigenomics
Nutrition
Organic Food
Ornish, Dean
Pritikin, Nathan
Sodium
Soy
Trans Fats
Vegetables
Vegetarians
Vitamins
Water

Waters, Alice
Yo-Yo Dieting

**Physical Health**

Allergies
Allergies, Food
Antioxidants
Back Pain
Bacteria
Basal Metabolism
Bone Health
Common Cold (Upper Respiratory Viruses)
Dental Health
Deoxyribonucleic Acid (DNA)
Ghrelin
Heart Health
Immune System/Lymphatic System
Metabolism
Resting Metabolic Rate
Sleep
Target Heart Rate
Virus
Weight Control. *See* Dieting

# P

## PANDEMICS

The term *pandemic* has often been thrown around with little regard to a proper definition, especially in popular media and common usage. This is likely due to the fact that traditional definitions have varied. Strictly speaking, a pandemic is any epidemic that has spread into multiple world regions. It is important to distinguish the concept of world regions from countries. For instance, a disease spread between Canada and the United States but not anywhere else would be an epidemic, not a pandemic.

Pandemics typically involve a new infectious disease or reemerging infectious disease that a large proportion of the population has no natural immunity to, otherwise known as immunologically naïve. This lack of immunity causes a much higher rate of infection than would be expected in a given amount of time from the disease. Contrary to the view that is often presented in popular media, a pandemic need not be fast-spreading. In fact, some of the greatest pandemics in history have recurred in waves over the course of hundreds of years, although there is often a single, most devastating wave that is the best-known and remembered.

The World Health Organization (WHO) defines a pandemic (with the above criteria) as a disease with sustained human-to-human transmission in at least two distinct world regions (WHO, 2009). These criteria are also important for recognizing what can or cannot be called a pandemic. For example, human immunodeficiency virus/acquired immune deficiency syndrome (HIV/AIDS) is a current pandemic because it is infectious, with sustained human-to-human transmission in multiple world regions. On the other hand, obesity has sometimes been inaccurately referred to as an epidemic or a pandemic. Although the usage may be useful for attempting to describe the importance or severity of obesity as a public health issue around the world, obesity is not infectious and there is no direct human-to-human transmission, meaning it cannot be considered a pandemic.

**H1N1 Pandemic of 2009**    A recent pandemic beyond HIV/AIDS, which public health officials around the world consider ongoing, which received tremendous media attention, was the novel H1N1 ("swine flu") pandemic from 2009 to 2010.

H1N1 refers to two particular subunits of the influenza virus, hemagglutinin and neurominidase. These supplanted the "normal" seasonal variants of influenza as the dominant flu strain for 2009. The novel H1N1 was dubbed swine flu in the United States because it was a reassortment of human, avian, and swine influenza. First recognized in Mexico in March 2009, it quickly spread around the world and was declared a pandemic by the WHO on June 11, 2009.

There was great initial concern and a strong reaction to the novel H1N1 for several reasons. The first was simply that, other than some individuals over the age of 65, virtually none of the world's population had any immunity against it, meaning the virus had the potential to infect far greater numbers and potentially cause more serious disease than the seasonal flu. Second, novel H1N1 had a different age distribution than seasonal flu. The majority of deaths caused by novel H1N1 occurred among young people, a surprising statistic since a seasonal flu most commonly kills the elderly. It was equally surprising that these deaths occurred among previously healthy young individuals (WHO, 2010).

Third, no vaccine was available at the start of the pandemic to immunize people against the new flu strain even though one was developed during the pandemic. Finally, worries about pandemic influenza were already heightened following the H5N1 scare in the preceding few years. The H5N1 had already demonstrated a high mortality rate.

The public health response worldwide was overwhelming and, in retrospect, most likely overdone. Schools in many regions were shut down, while individuals of virtually all ages, employees, college students, and others alike, were asked to stay home if ill. Although there was no possibility of actually catching novel H1N1 from eating pork products, the nickname of "swine flu" led many individuals to erroneously avoid pork and actually led to the slaughter of pigs in several countries along with import bans in others.

During the actual pandemic, numerous reports came out suggesting that novel H1N1 was more virulent than seasonal strains. This information fueled concerns about the devastating potential that an influenza pandemic could have. Ultimately though, flu cases peaked by late 2009 and rapidly went into decline. The WHO officially announced the end of the pandemic on August 10, 2010. The total number of lab-confirmed deaths worldwide attributed to H1N1 by the end of the pandemic was 18,036.

Unfortunately, since worldwide seasonal flu deaths are estimated statistically to affect 5–15 percent of the population worldwide with 250,000–500,000 deaths per year, it is impossible to directly compare the novel H1N1 number to other seasonal flu numbers, as the total of deaths is undoubtedly much higher. However, a retrospective analysis published in 2010 (Belongia et al., 2010) found that despite initial reports during the pandemic, novel H1N1 actually did not have a higher mortality rate than seasonal flu. Instead there was some evidence that it may have actually had a lower mortality rate.

In the end, the novel H1N1 pandemic did not have the devastating effects that were feared. Certainly, the strong public health response likely helped lessen its impact, but it appears likely that novel H1N1's virulence and pathogenicity were also grossly overestimated. There have been numerous accusations that many advisors to the WHO had conflicts of interest in the form of financial stake in pharmaceutical companies manufacturing vaccines, which may have pushed the WHO to declare pandemic status when it may not have been warranted. The WHO has defended its decision as a choice that was based on clearly defined epidemiological criteria. Investigations by several bodies into the appropriateness of the response to novel H1N1 continue.

**Historical Pandemics** Pandemics have affected humans since recorded history. Although there are certainly many diseases responsible for the pandemics of the past, some of the greatest include the bubonic plague, cholera, influenza, smallpox, measles, tuberculosis, and others. Two of the more well-known pandemics in history include the following.

*Bubonic Plague:* The bubonic plague has recurred throughout history numerous times. Caused by the bacteria *Yersinia pestis,* the first recorded pandemic was the Plague of Justinian (541–750), which was also the first major outbreak of bubonic plague. During this time period, the plague affected almost the entire known world, across Asia, Europe, and Africa. Over its 200-year course, it was believed to have eliminated at least a quarter of Europe's population and killed 25 million worldwide (Benedictow, 2004). Approximately 600 years later, the disease returned in the form of the infamous Black Death (1346–1353). The 14th-century wave of that version of the disease claimed approximately 75–100 million lives in Europe, another quarter of Europe's population at the time. The disease continued to reappear in Europe over the next several hundred years, claiming millions more (Benedictow, 2004).

*Influenza:* Various outbreaks of influenza have been described repeatedly over the course of recorded human history, typically associated with the emergence of a new, especially virulent influenza strain. The greatest influenza pandemic of the 20th century was the Spanish flu (1918–1920), notable not only for the high number of deaths, but also for how quickly it struck and disappeared again. Unlike seasonal influenza, the Spanish flu predominantly killed young, healthy adults. The Spanish flu was the most global of any pandemic in history, spreading into the majority of the world's remote regions. The severity of the pandemic was heightened by World War I, with troop movements during the war putting large numbers of people in tightly confined spaces, traveling long distances around the world. The actual case-fatality rate is not known, but it has been estimated at 10–20 percent, killing approximately 50–100 million people (Taubenberger et al., 2006).

Unlike pandemics caused by other diseases, which often recurred over the course of many years, the Spanish flu quickly disappeared again. One theory suggests that the virus mutated to a less lethal form, although this has never been confirmed. It is worth noting that the name *Spanish flu* is a misnomer and although the origin of the virus has been debated, it most likely originated in the United States or France, not Spain.

**Future Pandemics**   A major concern for any future pandemic is the possibility of an entirely novel disease emerging and spreading rapidly around the world. Of known diseases, scientists suggest the primary candidate for a pandemic outbreak in the near future is influenza. Many of the pandemics of the past, like cholera, bubonic plague, and others, are unlikely to recur due to advances in medical treatment and public health measures. Influenza, on the other hand, has the potential to rapidly mutate into a highly virulent strain before a vaccine can be developed, and spread around the world in a very short period of time, especially with the current level of global travel.

Though influenza is the prime candidate for a pandemic in the near future, there has also been growing concern over diseases, once quickly and readily treatable, which are now developing drug resistance. Examples include multidrug-resistant tuberculosis (MDR-TB) or methicillin-resistant staphylococcus aureus (MRSA).

Finally, there is another, more unusual potential pandemic scenario public health officials around the world have now prepared for, the possibility of an artificial pandemic created as the result of biological warfare. With the scientific advances in the field of genetic engineering, it is virtually impossible to predict what form a weaponized pandemic might take, though public health officials have shared several viral hemorrhagic fevers as potential candidates.

Surveillance is the first and perhaps the most important part of preparing to respond to a pandemic. The WHO, along with other public health officials in countries around the world, continuously monitor and sample influenza viruses, watching for unusual mutations or other signals of a disease outbreak. Similar mechanisms are used in other parts of the world to watch for unusual disease cases or unusual epidemiological patterns of disease.

Surveillance aside, public health officials plan for pandemics by building strong public health infrastructures, including the ability to rapidly distribute vaccinations and/or medication as needed in a pandemic, maintaining strategic stockpiles of important drugs, having the systems in place to mobilize and organize all the necessary elements of a pandemic response (e.g., law enforcement, health care workers, etc.) quickly and effectively, and demonstrating the ability to coordinate such responses with the rest of the country and rest of the world (WHO, 2009). Some of the tools available to officials in the event of an outbreak include isolation/quarantine of suspected cases, closing schools, canceling public gatherings, altering work schedules, and more.

Individuals have an important role to play in helping control the damage pandemics can cause. First and most important, individuals should simply get accustomed to good, basic hygiene, including regular hand-washing. Furthermore, individuals should stay home if they become sick to avoid spreading the disease. Finally, individuals should be ready to cooperate with instructions from public health officials to ensure a coordinated event at the local, national, and international levels.

*David Chen*

*See also* Acquired Immune Deficiency Syndrome (AIDS); Influenza; Methicillin-Resistant Staphylococcus Aureus (MRSA); World Health Organization (WHO).

### References

Belongia, Edward, Stephanie A. Irving, Stephen C. Waring, Laura A. Coleman, Jennifer K. Meece, Mary Vandermause, Stephen Lindstrom, Debra Kempf, and David K. Shay. "Clinical Characteristics and 30-Day Outcomes for Influenza A 2009 (H1N1), 2008–2009 (H1N1), and 2007–2008 (H3N2) Infections." *Journal of the American Medical Association* 304 no. 10 (2010): 1091–98.

Benedictow, Ole J. *The Black Death 1346–1353: The Complete History.* Woodbridge: Boydell Press, 2004.

Byerly, Carol R. *Fever of War: The Influenza Epidemic in the U.S. Army during World War I.* New York: New York University Press, 2005.

Davis, Mike. *The Monster at Our Door: The Global Threat of Avian Flu.* New York: New Press, 2005.

Pendergrast, Mark. *Inside the Outbreaks: The Elite Medical Detectives of the Epidemic Intelligence Service.* Boston: Houghton Mifflin Harcourt, 2010.

Taubenberger, Jeffrey K., and David M. Morens. "1918 Influenza: The Mother of All Pandemics." *Emerging Infectious Diseases* 12, no. 1 (2006): 15–22.

World Health Organization. "Current WHO Phase of Pandemic Alert for Avian Influenza H5N1." 2009. www.who.int/csr/disease/avian_influenza/phase/en/index.html.

World Health Organization. "Pandemic Preparedness." 2009. www.who.int/csr/disease/influenza/pandemic/en/.

World Health Organization. "What Is the Pandemic (H1N1) 2009 Virus?" 2010. www.who.int/csr/disease/swineflu/frequently_asked_questions/about_disease/en/index.html.

## PASTEUR, LOUIS

The French microbiologist and chemist Louis Pasteur is, with German biologist Robert Koch, one of the founders of bacteriology and immunology. Pasteur was born in Dôle, France, and studied in Paris at the École Normale Supérieure, where he showed promise as an artist but soon turned to science. In 1849 he was appointed acting professor of chemistry at the University of Strasbourg. From 1854 to 1857, he was professor of chemistry and dean of sciences at the University of Lille, eventually returning to the École Normale Supérieure as administrator and director of scientific studies. In 1867, the Sorbonne appointed him professor of chemistry. His own microbiological research center, the Pasteur Institute, was inaugurated in Paris in 1888.

From his early work on crystals, such as those of tartaric acid, a product in the fermentation of grapes, Pasteur proceeded to examine the process of fermentation

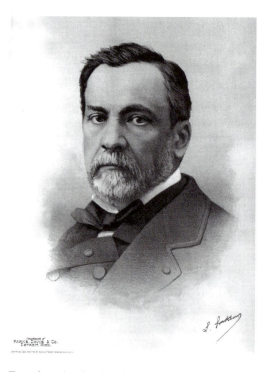

French scientist Louis Pasteur made important contributions to the field of microbiology. (Library of Congress)

itself, a topic that would provide him with important background information and methods for his later research on contagious diseases. Yeast had been thought to be a chemical structure that served as a catalyst in the conversion of sugar into alcohol, but Pasteur discovered that yeast was organic matter, feeding on sugar and thus producing alcohol. When wine soured, it simply indicated the presence of the "wrong" kind of microorganisms. Pasteur conducted numerous experiments to prove his point, also examining the souring of milk. In 1857, he discussed this latter problem in his famous report on lactic acid fermentation. Pasteur's discoveries raised the question of how these microorganisms entered the fluids. There existed at the time a belief in "spontaneous generation," which meant that microorganisms could come into existence without parental organisms. Pasteur proved, however, that nothing would happen with a fermentable fluid when surrounded by sterile air. As soon as "regular" air was brought in contact with the substance, microorganisms began to develop. Hence, he concluded that air contains spores of microbes.

The next step for Pasteur was to examine the problem of contagious diseases that seemed to spread through direct or indirect contact. Could microorganisms possibly cause these as well? There had been germ theories of disease for a long time, yet they could not be proven until Pasteur's day. Pasteur was aware of these theories and in 1857 became convinced that microorganisms might also be responsible for infectious diseases. Though at first it was only a theoretical concept, in the mid-1860s, Pasteur began to work on an actual problem: he was asked to examine a deadly disease of the silkworm, which threatened to ruin the silk industry in France.

By the late 1860s, Pasteur had identified two different silkworm diseases and the microbes that were responsible for them. Even though in the middle of his investigation Pasteur suffered a stroke that left the left half of his body permanently paralyzed, he continued to work. Indeed, already as a young student he had been convinced that it "means a great deal . . . to have will power; for deeds and work always follow the will."

However, his findings did not have an immediate effect, as many physicians did not think that a link existed between the ailments of the silkworm and those of human beings. In 1876 and 1877, however, Pasteur showed that microorganisms were the cause for a disease in higher animals and human beings: anthrax. At about the same time, Robert Koch came to the same conclusion. In 1877, Pasteur published a study on anthrax, a paper that became a significant document in supporting the germ theory of disease.

Pasteur applied the methods he had used in his experiments with fermentation to prove that anthrax bacteria spread the disease. These experiments showed that no matter how often an infected substance was passed from animal to animal, anthrax bacteria continued to multiply and thus remained potentially as deadly as in the blood of the first infected animal.

Since he had established these facts, Pasteur wondered what could be done to protect human beings and higher animals from those often-deadly diseases. He thus became interested in the concept of vaccination that had first been applied by the English physician Edward Jenner. Pasteur realized that a germ can change and consequently can actually be used as a vaccine. He first experimented with the problem of fowl cholera in chickens and found that some cultures of microorganisms did not cause the disease and instead made chickens resistant against virulent cultures in the future.

Pasteur became convinced that it would be possible to produce vaccine in the laboratory. He proceeded to create a vaccine against anthrax, the effectiveness of which he demonstrated in a well-publicized demonstration in 1881. However, his antirabies treatment is usually cited as Pasteur's greatest triumph. In July 1885, he successfully treated the first human being, Joseph Meister, a boy suffering from rabid dog bites.

If Pasteur were alive today, he might be worried that we depend on techniques directed against microorganisms above all. Indeed, Pasteur taught that many other factors might have an effect on the course of an illness, such as the hereditary constitution of a patient, his or her nutritional state, his or her emotional equilibrium, the season of the year, and the climate.

Even before the opening of the Pasteur Institute, Pasteur had many students who would make important contributions to microbiology. Currently, the Pasteur Institute is a private nonprofit foundation with about 20 establishments on five different continents. Research is focused on fighting infectious viral, bacterial, and parasitic diseases such as AIDS. It has produced eight recipients of the Nobel Prize; its distinguished alumni include Alexandre Yersin, a French doctor of Swiss extraction who discovered the bacterium that causes bubonic plague, *Yersinia pestis*, which was named after him.

*Anja Becker*

*See also* Bacteria; Immune System/Lymphatic System.

## References

Debré, Patrice. *Louis Pasteur.* Translated by Elborg Forster. Baltimore: Johns Hopkins University Press, 1998.

Dubos, René. *Pasteur and Modern Science,* new first ed. Madison, WI: Science Tech, 1988.

Geison, Gerald L. *The Private Science of Louis Pasteur.* Princeton, NJ: Princeton University Press, 1995.

Pasteur, Louis, and Joseph Lister. *Collected Writings.* New York: Kaplan, 2008.

Trachtman, Paul. "Hero of Our Time: Challenged to Prove His Germ Theory, Louis Pasteur Shaped the Terrain on Which the Battle against Anthrax Is Being Fought." *Smithsonian* (January 2002): 34.

## PAULING, LINUS

Americans can thank Dr. Linus Pauling, a two-time Nobel Prize–winning scientist for this country's love affair with vitamin C. At age 65, when most people consider retirement, Pauling began his research on the therapeutic effects of vitamin C. He published those findings and his opinions in his 1970 book *Vitamin C and the Common Cold.* In his book he claimed massive amounts of the vitamin would boost the immune system and protect people against a variety of diseases including colds. He also supported the idea that vitamin C would work well in the control of cancers. Pauling personally took 18,000 milligrams of vitamin C each day, which is more than 300 times the recommended daily allowance.

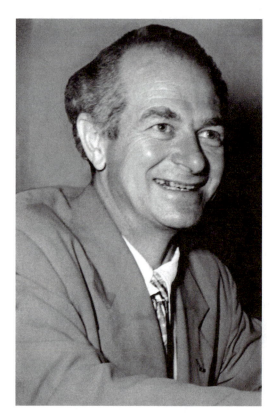

Pauling, a Nobel Prize–winning chemist, remained a strong proponent of the use of vitamin C. (Library of Congress)

Pauling was born in Portland, Oregon, in 1901 to Herman and Lucy Pauling. The family lived a modest existence until 1910 when Pauling's father died. Luckily, Pauling was able to earn a scholarship to study at Oregon State College. He was then accepted into the doctoral program at California Institute of Technology (Cal Tech) and received his degree in 1925. Pauling's early research focused on the use of x-rays to examine the molecular structure of crystals. He later turned his research to the way molecules bond and that research led to the creation of many of the medicines, dyes, plastics, and other synthetic fibers still in use today. From there he studied in Europe under noted physicists Arnold Sommerfield, Erwin Schrodinger, and Niels Bohr. These three top scientists were all working in the new field of quantum mechanics.

After two years in Europe, Pauling returned to Cal Tech as an assistant professor of chemistry. He later was promoted to full professor and eventually to chairman of the chemistry department. He worked at Cal Tech for more than 30 years. In 1954 Pauling was awarded the Nobel Prize for Chemistry for his work on the nature of the chemical bond that holds molecules together, research that led to the discovery of the structure of DNA. His work also led to a new understanding of the disease sickle cell anemia. He won a second Nobel Prize, this one for peace in 1963 for his work toward a nuclear test ban treaty. Pauling is the only person to have won two undivided Nobel prizes.

It was after World War II that Pauling turned his attention to the effects of the atomic bomb and the dangerous health effects of nuclear fallout. He joined Albert Einstein's Emergency Committee of Atomic Scientists along with other pro-peace organizations and protested the development of the hydrogen bomb while he lobbied for a nuclear test ban treaty. The award ceremony for Pauling's peace prize coincided with the signing of a limited nuclear test ban treaty between the United States and the Soviet Union. He worked as a research professor at the Center for the Study of Democratic Institutions in California from 1964 until 1967.

However, it was after Pauling was awarded his second Nobel Prize that he began his story of the role of nutrition in fighting disease. It was then he began his famous work in support of the therapeutic value of ascorbic acid, also known as vitamin C. It was biochemist Irwin Stone who introduced Pauling to the value of vitamin C in preventing colds. Stone had suggested people were only getting about 1 or 2 percent of the amount of ascorbic acid they needed to be healthy. Stone's research was published in 1972, in a book titled *The Healing Factor: Vitamin C against Disease.*

Pauling credited Stone's research for sparking his own ideas and wrote the foreword for Stone's book along with Dr. Albert Szent-Gyorgyi who was the recipient of the 1937 Nobel Prize for his discovery of vitamin C. Szent-Gyorgyi was the first to suggest vitamin C could be used in treating cancer, and at age 80 Szent-Gyorgyi founded the National Foundation for Cancer Research in 1973. The NFCR supports cancer research, along with public education on the prevention, early diagnosis, treatment, and continuing search for a cure for cancer.

Meanwhile, Pauling and several colleagues founded the Institute of Orthomolecular Medicine (IOM), later renamed the Linus Pauling Institute of Science and Medicine, in Palo Alto, California. Pauling is regarded as the founder of the science of orthomolecular medicine, which looks at using natural substances, especially nutrients, for the treatment of illness and for maintenance of good health. Orthomolecular medicine focuses on the use of a whole food diet together with high dosages of vitamins, minerals, and amino acids as a way to prevent or to treat disease.

According to the International Society for Orthomolecular Medicine (ISOM) website, vitamins and supplements are important for good health. The ISOM website describes such orthomolecular treatments as dietary manipulation, nutrition supplementation, herbal remedies, homeopathic treatments, detoxification, and safe forms of megavitamin therapy. Megavitamin therapy dose size is defined in scientific terms as a dose that is 10 times the Recommended Dietary Allowance (RDA) or more.

Although Pauling was recognized for his theories, studies have shown little benefit to vitamin C even when used in large doses. The Women's Health Initiative Study, released in early 2009, reported no difference in cancer or heart disease rates among those participants using vitamins E and C compared to those taking a placebo. At the same time, an editorial in the *Journal of the National Cancer Institute* noted that most trials had shown no cancer benefits from vitamins with a few exceptions. In fact, scientists suspect that eating whole fruits or vegetables rather than taking synthetic vitamins provide the real benefits of a healthful diet (Parker-Pope, 2009).

The federal government chose to recognize Pauling's contribution to science by issuing the Linus Pauling stamp on March 6, 2008, as part of the U.S. Postal Service's new American Scientists stamps. Pauling died in 1994 of cancer at the age of 93. He maintained that his use of vitamin C had delayed the onset of the cancer, possibly for some 20 years. While the medical community remains skeptical of some of Pauling's ideas, the Food and Drug Administration (FDA) in 2007 did approve the first clinical trial in the United States to study whether high doses of intravenous vitamin C would be a safe and effective treatment in the fight against cancer.

Scientific studies have demonstrated that high doses of vitamin C had shown significant anticancer effects in some animal studies. Other early clinical research had also suggested that intravenous doses of vitamin C had in some cases improved symptoms and prolonged survival in terminal cancer patients (Riordan et al., 2001). Researchers are also looking at the effects of taking 500 milligrams of vitamin C twice daily to lessen Alzheimer's stroke or head trauma damage. And a major study in Europe has suggested that blood levels of ascorbic acid above a certain level are associated with a more than 60 percent drop in the chances of getting cataracts (Ordman, 2010).

*Sharon Zoumbaris*

*See also* Cancer; Vitamins.

## References

"Died, Linus Pauling." *Time* (August 29, 1994): 25.

Kaprowski, Gene J. "FDA Approves Trial of Intravenous Vitamin C for Anti-Cancer Therapy." *Life Extension* (May 2007).

"Linus Pauling." In *Biology,* edited by Richard Robinson. New York: Macmillan References USA, 2009. Gale Biography in Context. http://ic.galegroup.com/ic/bic1/Reference

DetailsPage/ReferenceDetailsWindow?displayGroupName=K12-Reference&prodid= BIC1&action=e&windowstate=normal&catId=&documented=Gale%7CK2642110016& mode=view&userGroupName=va0054_0009&jsid=b4e577923612814324f7775399 eb5e37.

Ordman, Alfred Roc. "Vitamin C Twice a Day Enhances Health." *Health* 2, no. 8 (August 2010): 819–24.

Parker-Pope, Tara. "Vitamin Pills: A False Hope?" *New York Times,* February 17, 2009, D1.

Pauling, Linus, Clifford Mead, and Thomas Hager. *Linus Pauling: Scientist and Peacemaker.* Corvallis: Oregon State University Press, 2008.

Riordan, N.H., H.D. Riordan, J.A. Jackson, and J.P. Casciari. "Clinical and Experimental Experiences with Intravenous Vitamin C." *Journal of Orthomolecular Medicine* 15, no. 4 (2001): 201–13.

## PERSONAL TRAINER

A personal trainer is a fitness professional who traditionally works one-on-one with clients who are seeking support to reach their fitness goals. They may own a workout studio, work independently in a client's home, or be employed by a fitness club. Personal trainers provide fitness screening and testing, design individualized exercise programs, and coach clients through exercise sessions. Personal trainers do not diagnose, prescribe, treat, or counsel their clients; unless specifically licensed in these disciplines, these skills are considered outside the personal trainer's scope of practice.

The Certified Personal Trainer (CPT) obtains his skill set by independent study or by attending college classes or specialized training courses that offer certification preparation. Certification is received by passing a comprehensive written test. After becoming certified, the CPT must complete a certain number of continuing education courses to maintain certification. According to the American Council on Exercise, in 2005, there were more than 300 fitness-testing organizations worldwide offering to certify prospective personal trainers. Because of the wide variability in competency levels required by some organizations, there was concern within the fitness industry that the public was not adequately protected from unqualified or ineffective practitioners. In response, the more stringent certification organizations have sought accreditation through independent examination quality assurance groups, such as the National Commission for Certifying Agencies (NCCA) and the American National Standards Institute (ANSI). This change has served to establish comprehensive, effective certification testing, standardize continuing education course requirements, and increase awareness that CPTs are competent, knowledgeable professionals.

Qualified personal trainers will be well versed in the basics of human physiology, anatomy, biomechanics, and kinesiology and are trained to effectively screen and test new clients. Screening clients includes understanding the various health conditions that might affect physical activity, as well as knowing which medications can alter biochemistry and affect the body's response to exercise. Screening also involves helping clients set realistic and measurable fitness goals, so a basic grasp of behavior change psychology is useful knowledge. Fitness assessment testing provides trainer and client with baseline scores and a periodic measurement of changing fitness levels. Fitness testing requires the personal trainer to understand the specific physical testing protocols, formulas, and apparatus used to evaluate physical functioning. Examples include the sphygmomanometer for blood pressure measurement, the Ross Submaximal Treadmill Protocol to test oxygen uptake, or skinfold calipers that measure body mass index (BMI).

As personal trainers begin to design individualized client exercise programs, they incorporate their knowledge of how the human body responds and adapts to various exercises, including but not limited to cardiovascular training, strength training, and flexibility training. Personal trainers help prevent training injuries by developing programs that provide a correct balance in musculature. Mind-body exercises have become popular within the last 10 years, so today's personal trainers are learning to incorporate elements of yoga, tai chi, and qigong into training sessions. Injury prevention and first aid are important skills for all fitness professionals, and current cardiopulmonary resuscitation (CPR) and automated external defibrillator (AED) training are usually required to maintain certification and employment. Above all, the qualified personal trainer will have an understanding of human behavior that enhances his ability to motivate clients toward successfully meeting their fitness goals.

*Janice H. Hoffman*

*See also* Cardiopulmonary Resuscitation (CPR); Exercise; Qigong; Tai Chi; Weight Training; Yoga.

### References

American College of Sports Medicine. *ACSM's Guidelines for Exercise Testing and Prescription.* 7th ed. Philadelphia: Lippincott Williams & Wilkins, 2006.

American Council on Exercise. "What Every Fitness Professional Needs to Know about the Accreditation of Certification Programs." *ACE Certified News* (August/September 2005): 20–21. www.acefitness.org/aboutace/accreditation.aspx.

Bryant, Cedric X., and Daniel J. Green, eds. *ACE Personal Trainer Manual: The Ultimate Resource for Fitness Professionals.* 3rd ed. San Diego, CA: American Council on Exercise, 2003.

## PHYSICAL EDUCATION

Formal physical education instruction has traditionally played a fundamental role in bringing health information to students throughout the world. This is based on the long-standing recognition that health is important to learning and that schools can play an important role in educating youth about healthy living. The roles that schools have played in health education are well documented. We must never forget that because public school education reaches a huge number of youth throughout the world, schools and their curricula, including physical education and formal health classes—reinforced by other curricula—will always serve as an important vehicle for providing health information to youth.

And there is increasing evidence that students who meet fitness criteria also do better on standardized tests than classmates who are not as fit. A 2006 study of fifth- through ninth-grade students in California found those who matched six fitness criteria, including aerobic capacity to healthy body mass index, scored more than 40 percent higher on math and reading tests than their less-fit classmates (Schachter, 2010). Still, shrinking school budgets are prompting school boards and administrators to cut physical education along with art and music. According to recent figures, only 3.8 percent of elementary schools, 7.9 percent of middle schools, and 2.1 percent of U.S. high schools offer daily PE classes or the equivalent (CDC, 2006).

**Physical Education History**  Society generally recognizes that among the first cultures to institutionalize sports were the ancient Greeks. The first Olympiad of the ancient Greek world was held in 776 BCE. Not only were physical games and competition a part of ancient Greek society, but they surrounded all elements of that society (at least for the privileged classes), including philosophy, religion, medicine, and views of mental health. The ideas of health rested on these basic concepts: "balance, harmony, proportion, equilibrium, regularity and proper mixture of blending (temperament)" (Von Staden, 2006).

In Greek life, health resided at the top of a hierarchy of values, followed by prosperity, pleasure, and owing no debts. Health was viewed as necessary so that all other important aspects of life could be enjoyed, including family and children. Moderation and moral behavior in all parts of life were also a part of the Greeks' ideas about good health behaviors (Von Staden, 2006). Some of these values still affect our modern views of health and life.

The 19th century witnessed an expansion of physical education into schools, especially in Europe. In 1814, Denmark started to require physical education. By 1820, some American schools had begun to integrate physical education into their curricula. Generally, these included games and exercises. In 1866, California became the first American state to require physical education in its schools (Mechikoff, 2009).

Charles Beck was the first physical education teacher in the United States. He modeled his program on the German system that emphasized gymnastics. Dio Lewis, deploring the health of Americans of the day, advanced physical education and its instructional pedagogy when he established the Normal Institute of Physical Education in Boston in 1861 (Welch, 1994). Today, many school systems throughout the world require some degree of formal physical education, including colleges and universities ("Physical Education," 2009). Almost all governments are involved to some extent in health education in schools.

In 1984, the Centers for Disease Control and Prevention (CDC) in the United States conducted an extensive study of 30,000 students in fourth through seventh grades in 1,071 classrooms in 20 states to determine the effectiveness of formal health and fitness programs. Data indicated that students in formal health education increased their knowledge of health issues, developed better attitudes about health, acquired better health behaviors and skills, and were able to better perform those than students who did not receive similar instruction. According to the data, time exposed to health instruction plays a significant role in instructional effectiveness. The study reported that 50 hours of instruction is required to reach a stable level of health information (CDC, 2006).

In recent years in the United States, the CDC, through its Healthy Youth! Program, has become active in promoting compressive health and physical education (CDC, 2006). In 1999, the New Jersey State Department of Education moved to support a "comprehensive health education and physical education" based on CDC principles. The New Jersey program design reflects these values:

- *Empower* students to make informed decisions about issues that impact their present health, the health of their family and friends, and the health of society at large.
- *Enable* students to enact health-enhancing behaviors before damaging patterns have become firmly established.
- *Enhance* students' ability to become cautious and competent consumers.
- *Strengthen* students' ability to recognize, analyze, and react to unhealthy or dangerous situations in a safe and appropriate manner.
- *Strengthen* students' ability to focus on learning, academic achievement, and preparation for the world of work.
- *Empower* students to navigate through and around conflicting messages, risky behaviors, and mounting pressures and to develop dependable support systems.
- *Assist* students to recognize, understand, and address immediate or chronic health problems in order to prevent long-term health problems.
- *Empower* students to choose lifetime physical activities that they enjoy and in which they have confidence.
- *Enable* students to participate in lifetime activities that promote, support, and maintain wellness (New Jersey Department of Education, 1999).

The department stated the rationale for these values as: "Good health is necessary for effective learning. Feeling physically and mentally healthy is essential as students face intense competition, peer and media pressure, and the stresses of daily physical, emotional, social, intellectual, and work-related activities" (New Jersey Department of Education, 1998). The relationship with health and physical education is well developed in New Jersey's Comprehensive Health and Physical Education curriculum. The curriculum standards for Grade 8 illustrate this relationship. Along with major attention given to health issues, the curriculum addresses these physical education issues: motor skills; movement concepts; strategy (offensive, defensive, and cooperative strategies and their appropriate applications); sportsmanship, rules, and safety; sport psychology; fitness and physical activity; training; and achieving and assessing fitness.

**Value of Physical Education**   Current values of physical education in connection with health education reflect many of the CDC principles, in their evolution over the years. This value is again seen in physical education moving away from large group instruction to small groups supported with adequate equipment to promote participation. Good programs now encourage the success of all students in activities, lessening the role of the athletic leader. Modern approaches reduce the role of competition and grades in favor of teachers as guides, promoting cooperation among participants, and self-improvement.

Physical education has had its detractors over the years. Often, these negatives attacks are attached to claims that the programs take time away from academic subjects and that instructional programs are elitist, as they encourage high attainment of athletic skills. The counterargument is that physical education promotes teamwork, excitement, and good health and other intrinsic and extrinsic gains.

Like most areas in modern society, comprehensive physical education and health instruction are concerned with gender and race discrimination, individual lifestyles, family lifestyles and compositions, athletes as role models (and the means that mass media uses to present these models to youth), aggression and violence in society, and the role that athletics plays in endorsing these actions.

Social and political issues also are a part of modern physical education. These include environmental issues: health and injury, affordable health care, ethnicity, sporting conduct and ethical behaviors, social mobility, life changes for individuals, social planning that ensures safe participating areas for sports, and the political and economic use of sports in modern life. Comprehensive health and physical education programs often face problems (e.g., the filtering and/or censorship of information is a common problem). Sexual health is an important aspect of compressive health and physical education, and cultural conflicts often play a role in how sexual health information is delivered.

Science, including mathematics, has contributed greatly to the advancement of physical education in the 20th and 21st centuries. Based on the training provided to teachers of physical education, we can easily see the influence of science on the modern curriculum. Biology provides an understanding of human structure and functions as well as human growth and development and how to adapt to different human circumstances.

Kinesiology provides insight into the mechanics and anatomy in relation to human movement. Nutrition and its relationship to both sports performance and general health promote a healthier society. Microbiology, cell biology, immunology, and genetic studies offer the physical education curriculum and programs important for preventing disease. For example, using a microscope, Joseph J. Kinyoun—in the Laboratory of Hygiene, which he established as part of the United States Marine Hospital Service (USMHS)—isolated the organism that caused cholera. This laboratory later became the National Institute of Health.

Mathematics and statistics are important means of measuring the many components of health and physical education, including food intake, drug dosages, weight measurements, temperature measurement, and blood pressure readings. Sports medicine relies on mathematics and statistics to provide diagnostics and treatment for a wide array of injuries encountered on playgrounds, gyms, and sports arenas.

The use of technology in physical education classes is also being expanded, in some areas thanks to government dollars. The U.S. Department of Education (DOE) has awarded millions of dollars in grants to schools and community-based organizations for its Physical Education Program (PEP). This federally funded initiative helps grant recipients improve PE classes so they focus more on lifestyle education. Grant funds have been used to purchase heart rate monitors, Wii Fit equipment, elliptical machines, pedometers, and other equipment, allowing students to learn how their bodies work and how different activities would impact their fitness. For example, students use the heart rate monitors to calculate their target heart rate zone following an activity, integrating math into their PE class.

*W. Bernard Lukenbill and Barbara Froling Immroth*

*See also* Aerobic Exercise; Body Mass Index; Heart Health; Nutrition; Weight Training.

### References

Centers for Disease Control and Prevention. "Healthy Youth! Coordinated School Health Program." www.cdc.gov/healthyyouth/CSHP.

Centers for Disease Control and Prevention. "Physical Education: School Health Policies and Programs Study 2006." www.cdc.gov/HealthyYouth/shpps/2006/factsheets/pdf/FS_physicaleducation_SHPPS2006pdf.

Dakss, Brian. "Obesity Up, Phys Ed Down." *CBS News,* February 11, 2009. www.cbs.news.com/stories/2005/01/27/earlyshow/contributors/debbyturner/main669760.shtml.

"History of Physical Education: Now and Then." people.dbq.edu/students/jveach/images/PEPP%20pack/History%20of%20Physical%20Education.ppt.

Mechikoff, Robert A. *A History and Philosophy of Sport and Physical Education: From Ancient Civilizations to the Modern World.* New York: McGraw-Hill, 2009.

New Jersey State Department of Education. "Comprehensive Health Education and Physical Education Curriculum Framework." Summer 1999. www.state.nj.us/education/frameworks/chpe.

New Jersey State Department of Education. Quoting E. Marx, S. Wooley, and D. Northrup. *Health Is Academic: A Guide to Coordinated School Health.* New York: Columbia University, Teachers College Press, 1998. University of Texas Health Science Center at San Antonio. www.state.nj.us/education/frameworks/chpe.

"Physical Education." Psychology.wikia.com/wiki/Physical education. 2009.

Schachter, Ron. "Sports for Life: Physical Education Classes Incorporate Alternative Activities for Students to Lead Healthier Lives." *District Administration* 46, no. 4 (April 2010): 30 (5).

Von Staden, Heinrich. "Health." In *Encyclopedia of Ancient Greece,* edited by Nigel Guy Wilson. New York: Routledge, 2006.

Welch, Paula. "Dio Lewis Normal Institute for Physical Education." *The Journal of Physical Education, Recreation and Dance* 65 (March 1, 1994): 29 (3).

## PHYSICAL ENDURANCE

Physical endurance can be defined as the time span between the beginning of a physical activity and the termination of that activity because of exhaustion. Endurance activity mainly utilizes the body's cardiovascular system, including the heart, lungs, and blood vessels, to deliver the oxygen necessary to help fuel and sustain repeated muscular contractions.

**Early Endurance**   Endurance was first necessary to mankind as a survival skill. Most predators in the animal kingdom are covered with fur and cannot sweat efficiently; instead they rely on panting for thermoregulation. Because of this, predators must use their strength and speed alone to catch prey. If they do not capture their prey within 10 to 15 minutes they risk becoming overheated and are forced to rest. They also do not hunt during high heat for the same reason.

By comparison scientists theorize that early humans, with their comparatively hairless bodies, were able to meet their food source needs by what has been termed persistence hunting. Persistence hunting calls for great endurance on the part of the hunter and utilizes to best advantage the capacity of humans to regulate body temperature by sweat evaporation. The modern-day Bushmen of the Kalahari offer some insight into how scientists think our ancestors hunted. They do not need to use distance weapons such as the bow and arrow or the atlatl. Instead, they typically begin a hunt in the high heat of midday while their prey is at rest. After selecting a target, a marathon begins. Their strategy is to outlast and run their prey to exhaustion by never providing it a chance to completely cool down. The hunt lasts many hours, with the animal attempting to rest unsuccessfully, until it is finally immobilized by heat stroke and may then be slaughtered at close quarters.

So we see the ability to physically endure is very different from strength and power. Physical power involves activities that require maximal effort set within a minimal period of time. Power and strength work is essentially anaerobic (without oxygen) because the body is using its energy at a faster rate than it can be reproduced. In comparison, physical endurance requires submaximal effort, yet sustains that lesser effort over a maximal period of time. It is considered aerobic (with oxygen) as the body works to keep energy expenditure and energy production rates at synchronized levels. It does this by stabilizing body temperature and waste products removal, and constantly replenishing muscle fuel sources.

**Modern Endurance Needs**   While modern humans may no longer need to hunt food for survival, physical endurance is still an important factor in modern life. The objective of athletic endurance training is to develop the body's energy production systems so they can meet the demands of activity for as long as they are required. Endurance training has a positive impact on overall health. It is often recommended for optimal functioning of

664 | PHYSICAL ENDURANCE

the heart, improving blood circulation and keeping cardiovascular diseases at bay. Endurance training also improves the flexibility and stability of joints by strengthening the muscles and ligaments that surround the joint, making them more resistant to injury. Increased mental alertness and the ability to concentrate for longer periods of time are an added benefit to endurance training. The respiratory system benefits as well by adapting to increased demands with a greater supply of oxygen to working muscle. Finally, endurance workouts alter metabolism and so encourage a decrease in excess body fat.

Some examples of modern-day endurance sports include 5k and 10k races, marathons, triathlons, ironman competitions, century bike rides, and cross-country skiing. Superior performance in any of these sports is determined by many factors. Genetic makeup plays a part, along with respiratory, cardiovascular, musculoskeletal, and metabolic systems adaption to endurance-specific training. In fact, a large heart is a hallmark characteristic of great endurance athletes. The left ventricle of the heart in particular increases in size over time. The larger the left ventricle, the more blood it can capture, and the more blood it can capture, the more blood it can pump. The volume of blood pumped with each contraction by the heart's ventricles is known as stroke volume. Stroke volume and heart rate in turn are important determinants of overall cardiac output, and adjust the volume of blood going out to the working muscles. The amount of blood received in the muscles depends on several more factors: the amount of resistance in the blood vessels, adequate blood vessel dilation, red blood cell volume for good oxygen capacity, and the amount of capillaries found in the muscle fiber.

**Economy and Intensity**   There are marked differences in the amount of oxygen different people use when doing identical endurance tasks; athletes with a high exercise economy are able to expend less energy and consume less oxygen. In the 1930s researchers Dill, Talbot, and Edwards (1930) studied differences in exercise economy and concluded it was a major factor in endurance performance. Their pioneering research led to our knowledge of what constitutes good exercise economy. $VO_2$max is the maximum volume of oxygen that muscles are capable of utilizing per minute. Surprisingly, $VO_2$max is not a good predictor of endurance performance. More significant is the speed at which an athlete can perform at $VO_2$max. For example, two marathon runners may have the same level of aerobic power, but one reaches $VO_2$max at a running speed of 19 km/hr while the other reaches $VO_2$max at 21 km/hr. So $VO_2$max provides an indicator of aerobic potential, but it does not show how much of that potential is being tapped. In fact, other markers such as lactate threshold (LT) are actually better indicators of performance outcome. Genetically, men are at an advantage to women when it comes to cardiac endurance. They have greater stroke volume and cardiac output and so can transport more blood and oxygen to their muscles. However, women have a greater capacity to metabolize energy sources, which provides an advantage the longer a physical endurance demand is extended.

The metabolic factors that influence physical endurance include adequate lactate removal and the avoidance of metabolic acidosis. The lactate threshold (LT) indicates the highest exercise intensity that can be sustained for a long time period. It is also the exercise intensity at which lactate starts to accumulate in the bloodstream. When exercise intensity stays below the lactate threshold, lactate produced by the muscles is utilized by the body without excess buildup. But when exercising without oxygen at higher intensities and there is a higher reliance on glycolysis as an energy source, the body's metabolic system begins to encounter a lag between lactate production and lactate removal.

Additionally, hydrogen ions ($H_3O^+$) begin to accumulate, leading to metabolic acidosis and muscle fatigue. The point at which lactate is produced faster than it can be metabolized it is referred to as the anaerobic threshold (AT). Accurately measuring the lactate threshold involves taking small blood samples during performance testing where the exercise intensity is progressively increased. Measuring the threshold can also be performed noninvasively using respiratory gas-exchange equipment that measures air inspired and expired.

When the muscle fibers receive oxygenated blood from the heart, it is used by mitochondria in the muscles to generate energy. The mitochondria are often called cellular "power plants" because they generate adenosine triphosphate (ATP), a source of chemical energy that contracts and moves skeletal muscle. The density of mitochondria is an important determinant of physical endurance, since mitochondria control the rate at which ATP is produced.

Regarding muscle fiber, slow-twitch (Type 1) fibers are very efficient at using oxygen and can generate more fuel (ATP). They fire more slowly than fast-twitch fibers and can provide continuous muscle contractions over an extended time. Great endurance athletes tend to have a higher proportion of slow-twitch fibers.

The overall factors affecting the endurance performance include genetics, age, gender, exercise economy, and specificity of training. Heredity accounts for between 25 and 50 percent of the variance in $VO_2$max values, and research suggests heredity also plays a role in individual exercise economy, with responders who show larger improvements versus nonresponders who have less improvement with identical training. A higher proportion of slow-twitch skeletal muscle is another genetic gift that increases endurance performance. Age-related decreases in $VO_2$max are generally accepted to be about 1 percent per year or 10 percent per decade after the age of 25. Gender plays a smaller role in the $VO_2$max values of male and female endurance athletes, about a 10 percent difference. Training for endurance must be specific to be of value. Power-based anaerobic training will not engender the same physical changes needed for good endurance performance.

From the beginning of recorded history, we see that the human race has shown great interest in promoting physical stamina and endurance. From early human survival via persistence hunting, to Pheidippides, a Greek runner who reportedly covered 150 miles in two days in 490 BC, and the first Olympians whose distance races helped build battle endurance, until today's venerated Tour de France athletes, feats of remarkable physical endurance have indicated an apex of human health and well-being.

*Janice H. Hoffman*

*See also* Aerobic Exercise; Anaerobic Exercise; Basal Metabolism.

### References

Costill, D.L., and E.L. Fox. "Energetics in Marathon Running." *Medicine and Science in Sports* 1 (1969): 81–86.

Coyle, E.F. "Physical Activity as a Metabolic Stressor." *American Journal of Clinical Nutrition* 72, no. 2 (2000): 5125–205.

Dill, D.B., J.H. Talbot, and H.T. Edwards. "Studies in Muscular Activity VI: Response of Several Individuals to a Fixed Task." *Journal of Physiology* 69, no. 3 (1930): 267–305.

Lieberman, H.R., C.M. Falco, and S.S. Slade. "Carbohydrate Administration during a Day of Sustained Aerobic Activity Improves Vigilance, as Assessed by a Novel Ambulatory Monitoring Device, and Mood." *American Journal of Clinical Nutrition* 76 (2002): 120–27.

Naylor, L.H., K. George, G. O'Driscoll, D.J. Green, et al. "The Athlete's Heart: A Contemporary Appraisal of the 'Morganroth Hypothesis.'" *Sports Medicine* 38, no. 1 (2008): 69–90.

NOVA Series (PBS). *Becoming Human: Unearthing Our Earliest Ancestors*. Especially episode 2, *Birth of Humanity*. DVD. WGBH Educational Foundation for NOVA, 2009.

Tarnopolsky, M.A. *Gender Differences in Metabolism: Practical and Nutritional Implications*. Boca Raton, FL: CRC Press, 1998.

## PILATES

Pilates (pronounced puh-LAH-teez) is an exercise method developed by Joseph Pilates to promote well-being. The exercises he designed incorporate specific breathing patterns, focused muscle contractions, torso stabilization, proper body mechanics, and good support of the spine for better body alignment. Pilates believed a well-aligned body would, in turn, provide a fluidity and economy of all body movement. For many years his method was called "Contrology," which he defined as the complete coordination of mind, body, and spirit.

Joseph Hubertus Pilates (1880–1967) was a German national working in England before the start of World War 1. As a German, he became a political prisoner of war, and was placed in a British internment camp on the Isle of Man. At the camp he and his fellow prisoners found it difficult to adequately exercise and stay fit. To keep himself strong and flexible, Pilates developed a unique fitness routine that could be accomplished in a small space.

He trained some of his fellow inmates in his new technique as well, and when the great flu pandemic of 1918 arrived at the camp, the British military observed that inmates who had exercised with Pilates had a high survival rate. Assuming their survival was a direct result of Pilates's fitness routine, the military, within a short time, moved Pilates to a rehabilitation hospital to work with ill and injured men. To assist patients who were supposed to remain on their backs in bed,

Pilates refitted some hospital beds by removing the springs and attaching them to the bedposts to create a resistance system. This new apparatus allowed a patient to work on his strength and flexibility while still on bed rest. Much of today's Pilates exercise equipment, including the Universal Reformer, the Cadillac, and the Wunda Chair, are built with spring resistance and a sliding carriage, and are considered refined versions of his original hospital bed prototype. After the war, Pilates moved back to Germany for several years, and then to the United States in 1925.

He and his new wife, Clara, set up a New York City Body Contrology studio located in the same building as several ballet rehearsal studios and before long, dancers who needed help with injuries were visiting Pilates's studio. Even New York City Ballet dancers without injuries found his unique approach beneficial and soon filled his studio. Admirers included the well-known dance choreographers George Balanchine, Jerome Robbins, and Martha Graham. As Joseph Pilates wrote in *Return to Life through Contrology* (new edition 2001), "Physical fitness is the first requisite of happiness. Our interpretation of physical fitness is the attainment and maintenance of a uniformly developed body with a sound mind fully capable of naturally, easily, and satisfactorily performing our many and varied daily tasks with spontaneous zest and pleasure."

Today we call the ability to accomplish ADLs (activities of daily living) with ease and vigor a necessary component for wellness. In 1945 Pilates wrote a book

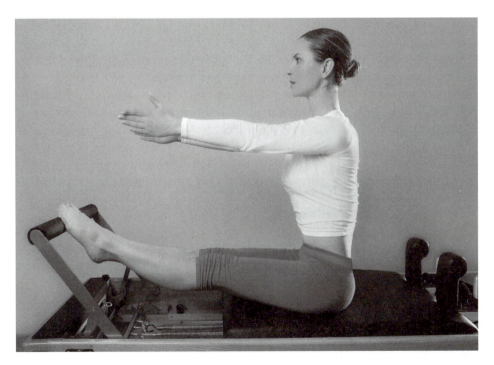

A woman practices pilates on a modern version of the Reformer developed by Joseph Pilates. (Lunamarina/Dreamstime.com)

titled *Return to Life through Contrology,* which described his philosophy, explained the health benefits of his method, and delivered 34 movement progressions plus six guiding principles. Pilates wrote his six principles because he was convinced that a fusion of mind and body during Contrology training was vitally important. His reasoning behind incorporating mind-body fusion was simple: It would eliminate the need to think about movement before actually moving, thereby creating an optimal physical dynamic that was economic, graceful, and balanced. This fusion would then provide a reserve of energy for sports, for recreation, and for life's emergencies.

### Pilates Six Guiding Principles

*Breath*  Pilates thought of the lungs as bellows and advocated using full breaths to completely pump air in and out of the body. He advised his practitioners to "squeeze every atom of air from your lungs until they are almost as free of air as a vacuum." This was done to keep the blood circulating, oxygenate the muscles, energize cells, and carry away waste products that could cause fatigue. His original 34 Contrology exercises worked in coordination with specific breath flow patterns and these patterns have remained an integral part of Pilates exercise today.

*Centering*  To Pilates, centering included body alignment, placement, and positioning. He referred to the abdomen, lower back, hips, and gluteals as the body's "powerhouse." He proposed that, when performing Pilates, all energy should originate from the powerhouse and flow out to coordinate movement of the extremities.

*Concentration*  Intense focus is used to guide all movement in Pilates. Pilates said that only by bringing full attention and commitment to each exercise could maximum value for effort be obtained. He said that mastering movements to the point of automatic, subconscious reaction would create grace and balance.

*Control*  Joseph Pilates believed muscle control was essential to maintain good postural alignment. All his exercises call for slow, controlled motion performed at constant speed throughout. He stated, "A few well-designed movements, properly performed in a balanced sequence, are worth hours of doing sloppy calisthenics or forced contortion."

*Precision*  Every movement in Pilates has a purpose and is considered intrinsically important to mastering the exercises. Each exercise requires exact movement of each part of the body. Pilates believed that repeatedly performing in a precise manner would, in time, lead to economy of movement.

*Flow*  Once the precision required is mastered, Pilates is performed in a continuous manner with transitions that flow with grace and ease into one another. These transitions were designed by Pilates to help build stamina. The transitions from one exercise to another are considered just as important as the exercises themselves.

Today Pilates is done as a series of movements on a thick mat or on Pilates-specific resistance apparatus, such as the Universal Reformer or the Pilates

Cadillac. Equipment like the Reformer and the Cadillac use coils or trapeze arms with springs to provide progressive resistance as they are lengthened. Each individual exerciser's weight is used to create the needed resistance. This is different from traditional weight training that uses heavy objects moved against gravity, which Joseph Pilates believed could be harmful.

Pilates movements are performed in order, with low repetitions, and at a prescribed speed. Breathing during Pilates exercise is done with awareness, deeply filling the back and sides of the ribcage on inhalation, and focusing on an engagement of abdominal and pelvic floor muscles while exhaling and inhaling. Practitioners believe correct breathing not only sends oxygen to the muscles but will also reduce upper neck tension. Joseph Pilates said, "Even if you follow no other instructions, learn to breathe correctly."

To get the best out of each exercise, correct postural alignment is considered crucial during Pilates exercise. Optimal alignment places the pelvis, ribcage, shoulders, and head in "neutral position," and uses the body's natural stabilizer muscles to maintain that alignment. Alignment is also used to guide extremity range of motion and keep joints free from strain. The effectiveness of Pilates in preventing or reducing back pain has not been scientifically proven to date, although it should be noted that many Pilates exercises are very similar to common physical therapy rehabilitation exercises used to treat low-back pain.

A study conducted at Florida Atlantic University found that Pilates reduced back pain in 22 subjects who followed a 12-week Pilates program. And while there have been claims that Pilates creates long, lean muscles, Michele Olson, PhD, FACSM, a researcher at Auburn University states, "People made these assumptions some 80 years ago because dancers often practiced Pilates, and they often have long, lean bodies. Back then, the physiology research wasn't available compared to what we have now. Muscles cannot grow longer, but you can improve your flexibility from the exercises. Muscles are lean anyway; they are non-fat structures in our body. You can increase your lean tissue, but what you're doing is actually putting on muscle. So you are actually increasing muscle, which is a good thing, but not narrowing the muscles."

While advocates believe that, when done correctly, Pilates is a suitable form of exercise for all persons and regardless of age, there are possible risks. EMG (electromyography) results indicate that "The Teaser," a mat exercise where the body forms a "V" position, creates such a strong contraction in the hip flexors that it can place unsafe pressure on lumbar disks. Other classic Pilates exercises like the Roll-Over and the Jack-Knife, where the upper back rolls off the floor and places a great deal of body weight on the cervical vertebrae, are suspect. In vulnerable individuals this pressure could block blood flow from the jugular veins, or even cause cervical disks to rupture. Similar body positions have been declared high-risk and were removed from general fitness classes more than a decade ago. There are divergent schools of thought on correct Pilates instruction today. Classical Pilates teachers choose to preserve Joseph Pilates's methods as he developed them, adapting only within the framework of his traditional exercises; other Pilates advocates have sought to expand and change his exercise method, and have begun to create new Pilates-based exercises designed to suit their modern client base.

*Janice H. Hoffman*

*See also* Back Pain; Exercise; Weight Training; Yoga.

### References

Anders, M. "New Study Puts the Crunch on Ineffective Ab Exercises." *ACE Fitness Matters* (May–June 2001): 9–11.

Crowther, Ann. *Total Pilates: The Step-by-Step Guide to Pilates at Home for Everybody.* New York: Duncan Baird, 2009.

Fiasca, P. *Discovering Pure Classical Pilates.* New York: Pure Classical Pilates, 2009.

Graves, S., Jill V. Quinn, Joseph A. O'Kroy, and Donald J. Torok. "Influence of Pilates-Based Mat Exercise on Chronic Lower Back Pain." *Medicine and Science in Sports and Exercise* (2005).

Herdman, Alan, with Gill Paul. *Pilates Plus.* London: Gaia, 2005.

Olson, M., and C.M. Smith. "Pilates Exercise: Lessons from the Lab." *IDEA Journal* 2, no. 10 (2005): 38–43.

Pilates, J.H., R. Kryzanowska, and J.M. Miller. *The Complete Writings of Joseph H. Pilates: Return to Life through Contrology, and Your Health—The Authorized Editions.* Philadelphia: Bainbridge Books, 2001.

Silere, Brooke. *Your Ultimate Pilates Body Challenge: At the Gym, On the Mat, and On the Move.* New York: Broadway Books, 2006.

## POLYCYSTIC OVARY SYNDROME (PCOS)

Polycystic ovary syndrome is a common hormonal disorder believed to affect some 10 percent of American women of childbearing age. Often young women go undiagnosed until they try to become pregnant and cannot. There are a host of associated symptoms but except for infertility, most are easily dismissed for years by the women rather than seen as pieces in a frustrating health problem.

While no two women have the same symptoms, the characteristics include gaining weight, especially around the waist; an inability to lose weight; menstrual irregularities; acne; excess facial hair; anxiety and/or depression; fatigue; sleep apnea; male-pattern baldness or thinning hair; food cravings; ovarian cysts.

PCOS is an endocrine or hormonal disorder and while the exact cause is unknown, experts believe genetics do play a role. Women with PCOS likely have a mother, sister, or other female relative who also has PCOS. Symptoms often appear in adolescence but in some women they do not appear until their 20s.

The major problem with PCOS is the hormonal imbalance that develops. The ovaries of affected women make more androgens than normal. Androgens are male hormones such as testosterone. Even though females make some androgens, in a woman with PCOS that level of testosterone is disproportionately high.

High levels of testosterone then impact the women's ability to release eggs during ovulation.

The change in hormones can seriously affect insulin, which controls the change of sugar, starches, and other food into energy the body can either use or store. Women with PCOS frequently develop insulin resistance and their body then produces too much insulin, while at the same time their endocrine system struggles to use the excess insulin that has already been released. Food is no longer changed into energy and instead gets stored as fat, especially around the middle. PCOS causes steady weight gain and often leads to obesity. This can be especially difficult for women since American media vigorously promotes a body image of exceptionally slim women as the ideal. Also, since excess insulin is known to increase production of androgens, a vicious cycle continues; high levels of androgens create too much insulin and the insulin keeps the androgen levels high. Without a diagnosis, many women with PCOS simply think their inability to lose weight is something they are doing wrong and this can intensify their feelings of anxiety or depression as they struggle to control their growing girth.

There is no specific test for PCOS, although there are several exams or tests routinely used to aid in the diagnosis. Blood tests to measure androgen hormone levels and glucose are routinely used. A pelvic exam may be done to determine if ovaries are swollen or enlarged, which would indicate the possibility of cysts. A medical history is needed, including details of menstrual periods, weight gain, or other symptoms. The doctor generally begins the diagnosis with a physical exam to check blood pressure, and to look for other signs of the disease.

PCOS is a chronic condition that cannot be cured. However, there are several treatment options used to improve symptoms. One main goal of treatment is to prevent women with PCOS from developing heart disease or diabetes. Doctors have had some success prescribing Metformin, a prescription drug used to treat Type 2 diabetes for women with PCOS. Although Metformin has not specifically been approved by the Food and Drug Administration (FDA) for PCOS treatment, it has shown some improvement in controlling insulin levels, which then lowers testosterone production. Because of excess testosterone and insulin resistance, losing weight will remain especially challenging for PCOS patients. But weight loss can decrease excess insulin, which can lower testosterone levels and break that cycle.

Doctors can also prescribe medications that stimulate ovulation, which help women who wish to become pregnant. Women with PCOS are also encouraged to pay close attention to their nutrition, to eat a controlled-carbohydrate diet with small but frequent meals to prevent spikes in blood sugar, which can trigger more insulin production and to limit processed foods with added sugars. It is believed that if a woman can achieve a 10 percent loss in body weight it might be possible that normal menstrual cycles can be restored (U.S. Department of Health and Human Services, 2010).

Birth control pills can also be used by women with PCOS who are not trying to get pregnant to reduce male hormone levels, help control acne, and to control menstrual cycles. Unfortunately, women with PCOS may also have higher-than-average rates of miscarriage if they become pregnant, may experience gestational diabetes or preeclampsia, which is pregnancy-induced high blood pressure, and may also have a higher rate of premature delivery. Studies are now underway to determine if Metformin can be used safely by pregnant women.

There are several serious long-term health problems associated with PCOS, including the increased risk of heart disease and diabetes. In fact, the risk of heart attack is up to seven times higher for women with PCOS (U.S. Department of Health and Human Services, 2010). Women with PCOS are also at greater risk from high levels of cholesterol, from high blood pressure, and have a greater chance of developing diabetes than women without PCOS.

One last difficult aspect of PCOS is the emotional toll it takes on women with the disease. Sufferers often feel responsible for their weight gain and embarrassed by their appearance, especially with the acne and hirsutism or excessive hair growth. There are PCOS support groups available as well as hair removal by electrolysis or laser. Research is continuing into the root causes of the disease as well as new treatments to alleviate symptoms, as researchers hope to offer millions of women relief from a difficult, frustrating condition.

*Sharon Zoumbaris*

*See also* Body Image; Diabetes; Heart Health; Nutrition.

### References

Dilbaz, Berna, Enis Ozkaya, Mehmet Cinar, Evrim Cakir, and Serdar Dilbaz. "Cardiovascular Disease Risk Characteristics of the Main Polycystic Ovary Syndrome Phenotypes." *Endocrine* 39, no. 3 (June 2011): 272 (6).

Dowdy, Diana L. "Development of a Guidebook for Teens with PCOS." *Journal of Obstetric, Gynecologic and Neonatal Nursing* 40 (June 2011): S2.

"New Polycystic Ovarian Syndrome Research Reported from University of Michigan." *Women's Health Weekly,* June 9, 2011, 25.

"Polycystic Ovary Syndrome." MayoClinic.com. December 8, 2009. www.mayoclinic.com/health/polycystic-Ovary-Syndrome.pdf.

"Unraveling the Mysteries of PCOS." *Harvard Health Commentaries.* August 21, 2006. www.harvardhealthcontent.com/66,COL072503.

U.S. Department of Health and Human Services. "Polycystic Ovary Syndrome (PCOS)." Office on Women's Health. March 17, 2010. www.womenshealth.gov/faq/polycystic ovary-syndrome.cfm.

Yasmin, Ephia, and Adam H. Balen. "The Metabolic Apects of Polycystic Ovary Syndrome." *Expert Review of Obstetrics and Gynecology* 6, no. 3 (May 2011): 331 (11).

## PRESIDENT'S COUNCIL ON FITNESS, SPORTS, AND NUTRITION

Childhood obesity, diabetes, and other diseases of excess are at unprecedented levels and have many Americans asking how we can improve the health and fitness of our youth. First Lady Michelle Obama has joined the list of prominent Americans calling for a national focus on the need for healthy eating and more exercise for children. In June 2010 the First Lady unveiled the newest name for the program that promotes fitness and health for all Americans. The updated President's Council on Physical Fitness, Sports and Nutrition now reflects a mandate that coincides with the First Lady's "Let's Move!" initiative to focus on healthy eating and to encourage families to pursue an active lifestyle.

The original President's Council on Physical Fitness and Sports (PCPFS) was founded on July 16, 1956, by President Dwight D. Eisenhower after a study showed American children were less physically fit than children in other countries. Originally named the President's Council on Youth Fitness, the agency name was changed to the PCPF four years later in 1960 by President John F. Kennedy. The Kennedy administration wanted to reflect an expanded mandate to serve Americans of all ages. And in 1968 President Lyndon B. Johnson added the word *sports* to the council title in a move to emphasize the importance of participation in sports. Johnson also began the tradition of presenting Presidential Physical Fitness Awards in 1966; the Presidential Sports Award program was created in 1972.

The Obama administration expanded the focus and changed the name to the Presidents Council on Fitness, Sports, and Nutrition (PCFSN) to help combat childhood obesity. According to U.S. Department of Health and Human Services Secretary Kathleen Sebelius, nearly one in three American kids is overweight or obese, which then puts them at a much greater risk of diabetes, heart disease, and cancer (HHS, 2010). The PCFSN is made up of 25 volunteer citizens appointed by the president to serve as advisors and to promote healthy lifestyles through fitness, sports, and nutrition programs that educate, empower, and engage Americans of all ages, backgrounds, and abilities.

Assisted by the U.S. Public Health Service, the PCFSN provides guidance to the president and to the secretary of health and human services on how to encourage more Americans to be physically fit. In its efforts to educate Americans about the benefits of physical fitness, the Council develops and distributes publications and pamphlets, and works with individual citizens, civic groups, private enterprise, community organizations, and others to promote fitness for all Americans. The PCFSN encourages and supports the development of community recreation and sports programs and works with business, industry, government, and labor organizations to set up workplace physical fitness programs. The Council also partners with agencies to encourage research in sports medicine, physical fitness, and sports performance.

In addition, the Council promotes and maintains the President's Challenge Physical Activity and Fitness Awards program, which encourages all Americans to include up to 30 minutes of physical activity each day for adults and up to 60 minutes each day for children. Under the umbrella of the challenge program are youth physical fitness tests, adult fitness tests, two school recognition programs and two physical activity award programs, the Presidential Active Lifestyle Award (PALA), and the Presidential Champions Award. The PALA is an important

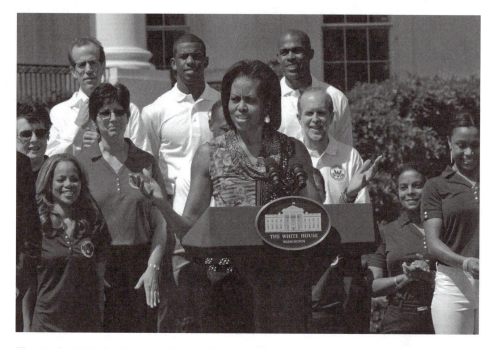

First Lady Michelle Obama joined military families and members of the president's council for a day of fitness activities. (President's Council on Fitness, Sports and Nutrition)

component of the "Let's Move!" initiative and is available for free on the PCFSN website.

*Marjolijn Bijlefeld and Sharon Zoumbaris*

*See also* Exercise; Nutrition; Obesity; Physical Education.

## References

Keller, Susan Jo. "Obama Expands Fitness Council's Mission." *New York Times,* June 23, 2010, www.nytimes.com.

"President's Council on Fitness, Sports and Nutrition" (PCFSN). www.presidentschallenge.org.

"Secretary Sebelius and President's Council on Fitness, Sports and Nutrition Announce the Million PALA Challenge to Get Americans Moving." *HHS News*, U.S. Department of Health and Human Services. September 14, 2010. www.fitness.gov.

"State Indicator Report on Physical Activity 2010." Centers for Disease Control and Prevention. www.cdc.gov/physicalactivity/professionals/reports/index.html.

## PRIMARY CARE PHYSICIANS

A primary care physician (PCP) is another name for a physician or doctor who is the basic, first contact in the medical care system. Physicians, no matter what area of medicine they specialize in, must first complete medical school. To become primary care physicians, graduates from medical school take postgraduate training in primary care programs, including general medicine or family medicine or internal medicine. Some HMOs consider pediatricians and gynecologists as PCPs. In other instances insurance companies also allow allergists caring for people with asthma and nephrologists who treat patients on kidney dialysis to act as PCPs.

## Preventive Care Checklist for Adults

Preventive care is an important cornerstone of wellness. These dozen exams, services, and screenings should be standard for all adults, with specific tests recommended for women and pregnant women.

### Adults

1. Alcohol screening and, if needed, cessation program
2. Blood pressure measurement, every two years for most adults, more frequently depending on risk factors
3. Cholesterol screening, beginning at age 35, younger for smokers, those with high blood pressure or those at high risk
4. Colorectal cancer, beginning at age 50, younger based on physician recommendation or for those at high risk
5. Dental exam, at least yearly or every six months for evaluation and cleaning
6. Depression screening
7. Diabetes screening, especially important for those with high blood pressure
8. Eye exam, for everyone, especially anyone with a change in vision or eye problem
9. Glaucoma screening, for everyone over 65, earlier if at high risk or for those with a family history
10. Influenza vaccine, for everyone, especially those over 65 or with compromised immune systems
11. Obesity screening
12. Prostate cancer screening for men, at age 50, younger based on physician recommendation or for those at high risk

### Adult Women

1. Mammography, every one to two years after age 40 with a baseline film at age 35
2. Breast cancer check, yearly and repeated self-examination

*(Continued)*

3. Pap test, ages 21 to 65 every 1 to 3 years depending on physician recommendation
4. Chlamydia screening
5. Osteoporosis screening for women age 40, younger for those at high risk

**Pregnant Women**

1. Anemia screening
2. Breast-feeding counseling
3. Folic acid screening
4. Genetic testing
5. Hepatitis B screening
6. RH compatibility screening
7. Tobacco use screening and cessation program
8. Urinary tract infection screening

*—Sharon Zoumbaris*

The PCP set of skills includes basic diagnosis and nonsurgical treatment of common illnesses and medical conditions. Diagnosis is based on interviews, information about symptoms, prior medical history, health details, and a basic physical examination. Primary care physicians are also trained in the use of and interpretation of medical test results, including blood and other patient samples, electrocardiograms, and x-rays. If more complex tests are needed those are usually obtained through referrals to specialists. In many managed health care insurance programs the primary care physician must see patients before they can be referred to a specialist. That places a demand on PCPs, who see conditions ranging from uncomplicated upper respiratory infections to coronary heart disease, depression, arthritis, and other chronic conditions.

Studies have found that when the knowledge base and quality of care provided by PCPs versus specialists are compared, the specialists are more knowledgeable in their domain. However, it was also found that in the area of preventive health care, primary care physicians performed best for patients ("Summaries for Patients," 2002).

Unfortunately, shortages of primary care physicians are an increasing problem in the United States as well as in other countries. The World Health Organization (WHO) has identified worsening trends in access to PCPs in developed and developing nations ("World Health Report," 2006). At the same time, primary care positions in the United States are increasingly being filled by foreign medical graduates as fewer American medical students are choosing careers in primary care (Bodenheimer, 2006).

One reason medical school graduates are turning away from primary care careers is the difference in income between specialists and primary care physicians, a gap that is widening. In 2004 the median income of specialists was almost twice that of primary care physicians. Data from the Medical Group Management Association indicate that while income for PCPs increased another 2.8 percent in 2009, specialists such as dermatologists saw a 12 percent increase that same year (Baginski, 2010). Another reason that medical students may choose not to become primary care physicians are more on-call hours.

A system of primary-based health care has the potential to reduce rising health costs while maintaining quality when the PCP acts as a type of gatekeeper to regulate access to more costly procedures or specialists. The primary care physician also advocates on behalf of the patient and her specific medical needs by helping her coordinate care with other medical providers such as rehabilitation clinics or hospitals. As the number of seniors in the U.S. population grows in the next few decades, the need for PCPs will increase. An aging population brings with it increases in the prevalence of chronic health conditions, most of which would ideally be handled in the primary care setting. Supporters of a primary health care system suggest it is time for a national primary care policy that will work to increase the number of medical school graduates entering the field and at the same time support those PCPs already in the workplace.

*Sharon Zoumbaris*

*See also* Health Insurance; World Health Organization (WHO).

### References

Anderson, Jane. "Access Doesn't Guarantee Care." *Family Practice News* 40, no. 17 (October 15, 2010): 67.

Baginski, Caren. "Highlights of MGMA's 2010 Physician Compensation Survey." Medical Group Management Association. http://blog.mgma.com/blog/bid/34089/Highlights-of-MGMA-s-2010-physician-compensation-survey.

Bodenheimer, Thomas. "Primary Care: Will It Survive?" *New England Journal of Medicine* 355 (August 2006): 861–64.

"Summaries for Patients. Comparing the Quality of Diabetes Care by Generalists and Specialists." *Annals of Internal Medicine* 136, no. 2 (2002): I42. www.ncbi.nlm.nih.gov/pubmed/11928735.

"World Health Report—2006." World Health Organization (WHO). www.who.int.whr/2006/overview/en.

## PRITIKIN, NATHAN

Nathan Pritikin (born August 29, 1915, in Chicago; died February 21, 1985, in Albany, New York) was a self-taught nutritionist and an inventor who championed the concept that a low-fat, high-fiber diet of natural foods like fruits, vegetables, and whole grains, combined with regular aerobic exercise, could prevent and reverse heart disease and other diseases of affluent society.

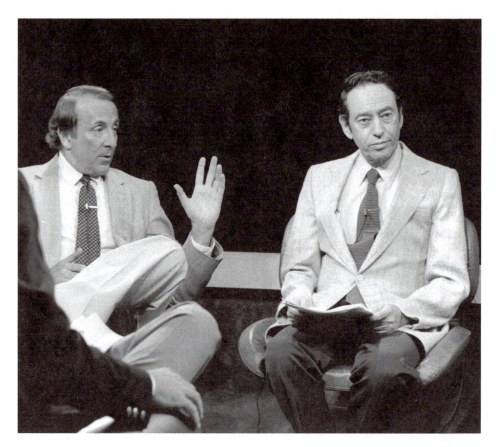

Dr. Robert Atkins, center, speaks during a discussion with nutritionist Nathan Pritikin, right, on WNBC-TV's *Live at Five* in New York City on June 24, 1981. (AP/Wide World Photos)

The Pritikin program, introduced in 1977 when Pritikin and his cardiologist, Dr. David Lehr, appeared on *60 Minutes* to explain what they described as a new way to treat heart disease, led to Pritikin's career as an inventor and author as well as the 1975 establishment of the Pritikin Longevity Center and Spa in California.

Now based in Florida, the center offers health and weight-loss programs to individuals as well as families. Several years ago the spa introduced a family program to encourage youngsters and their parents to visit the facility together to address nutritional and obesity-related health problems. Plans were also announced in January 2010 for the Pritikin Center to explore a partnership with the Indian company VLCC to set up medical spas in India and other overseas locations, modeled on the Pritikin program.

Pritikin wrote six books, including the first, *Live Longer Now* (1974) and his best-selling *Pritikin Program for Diet and Exercise* (1979). Other titles included *The Pritikin Permanent Weight-Loss Manual* (1982), *The Pritikin Promise: 28 Days to a*

*Longer, Healthier Life* (1983), *The Official Pritikin Guide to Restaurant Eating,* co-authored with wife Ilene (1985), and *Diet for Runners* (1985). Newer titles authored by Nathan Pritikin's son Robert Pritikin include *The New Pritikin Instinct* (1998) and *The Pritikin Principle: The Calorie Density Solution* (2000).

Published in 2007, *The Pritikin Edge: 10 Essential Ingredients for a Long and Delicious Life* continued promoting Pritikin's program of changes in lifestyle and diet as a way to treat heart disease. The book, written by Paul Tager Lehr, son of Pritikin's cardiologist, and Dr. Robert Vogel, the cardiologist and chief medical officer of the Pritikin Center, also examines the rising rate of obesity in children and adults, as well as the continued growth in high blood pressure and Type 2 diabetes in the United States.

Although Pritikin received little formal education (he dropped out of the University of Chicago), he began his lifelong study of human anatomy and physiology as a youth. During World War II, Pritikin began to develop his theory concerning the causes and cures of heart disease. Scientific thinking at that time held that heart disease was caused, in large part, by stress. Yet in looking over statistics on the civilian populations of Europe, he noticed that death rates due to heart attack had fallen during the stress-filled war years. In a 1991 interview in *Vegetarian Times,* Pritikin's son Robert said that his father had also noticed that while stress was high, rationing during the war meant people were eating very little meat and few dairy products. After the war, when rationing ended but stress subsided, Pritikin noted that the rates of heart disease went right back up.

Pritikin's years of research were put to the test in 1956 when he had his own cholesterol checked. It was over 300. He then underwent a stress electrocardiogram, which showed coronary insufficiency. A second cardiologist and second testing confirmed that Pritikin's arteries were clogging up. He was diagnosed with substantial coronary heart disease. He was 41 years old. A prestigious team of cardiologists gave him the standard prescription of the day: stop all exercise, stop climbing stairs, take it easy, and take naps in the afternoon. But Pritikin's readings of population studies had convinced him that dangerous arterial plaque would form at any cholesterol level over 160. If he could get his cholesterol level down with dietary measures, he figured he might have a chance of surviving. By April 1958, he had become a vegetarian. He had also started running three to four miles daily. By May, his cholesterol had fallen to 162. By January 1960, his cholesterol had dropped to 120, and a new electrocardiogram showed his coronary insufficiency had disappeared.

Encouraged by the results of his diet and exercise program, Pritikin launched several research projects over the next 25 years that validated the efficacy of his program. But the medical establishment was slow at first to accept Pritikin's theory that heart disease could be cured through dietary changes and exercise. Groups like the American Heart Association and the American Medical Association initially dismissed his claims and criticized the diet, saying it did not show lasting benefits and it was too restrictive as a lifelong program. Pritikin ignored the criticism. His studies on heart disease, diabetes, hypertension, and nutrition were published in several key medical journals, including the *New England Journal of Medicine, Journal of the American Medical Association,* and *Circulation.* Pritikin's theories and practices are similar to the low-fat, high-fiber diet recommended by Dr. Dean Ornish, a physician whose medical studies have also shown significant reduction in heart disease when patients are treated through diet, exercise, and stress reduction. Dr. John McDougall is another physician who developed an eating program sharing the common theme of low-fat and high-fiber foods. Like Pritikin and Ornish, McDougall also established his own health facility, the St. Helena Health Center.

The Pritikin diet calls for a menu rich in natural foods: fruits, vegetables, whole grains, all varieties of legumes (such as pinto beans, black beans, and lentils), moderate amounts of nonfat dairy products like nonfat milk and nonfat yogurt, and small amounts of poultry, lean meat, and seafood. Limited, too, are salt, sugar, and other refined carbohydrates like white flour. On a typical day an individual following the Pritikin diet would eat three meals and three snacks consisting of many different foods, such as hot oatmeal with banana and strawberries for breakfast; fresh fruit and yogurt for a midmorning snack; pasta with marinara sauce, fruit, and steamed vegetables for lunch; soups such as minestrone, lentil, or gazpacho for an afternoon snack; for dinner, broiled seafood, a large green salad, steamed asparagus, and a baked potato; and for dessert or an evening snack, popcorn or frozen yogurt.

Pritikin went public with his program through lectures, his presentations to medical communities, and the establishment of his Pritikin Longevity Center in Santa Barbara, California, an in-residence program of nutrition, exercise, and lifestyle education that has attracted people from all over the world. The Pritikin Longevity Center in Florida continues to operate as both a lifestyle-training program and a research center, with a laboratory that works to investigate the relationship between diet, exercise, and disease prevention. Movie producer and documentary filmmaker Michael Moore stayed at the Florida center after the release of his movie *Sicko.*

Pritikin also established the Pritikin Research Foundation, a nonprofit organization that both conducts and funds research examining the relationship between diet and disease. Robert Pritikin, Nathan's son, was named director of the Pritikin Program in 1985. In 1984, shortly before Nathan Pritikin's death, the National Heart, Lung, and Blood Institute announced that lowering blood cholesterol reduced the risks of heart attacks and coronary disease, vindicating Pritikin's earlier dietary recommendations.

Years before Pritikin first learned of his heart disease, he had been diagnosed with leukemia, an illness that would eventually lead to his death. Pritikin suspected that radiation he had been exposed to during World War II had contributed to his contracting leukemia. For decades, the leukemia was in remission. In 1984 the cancer reappeared. Pritikin suffered complications caused by his cancer treatments and grew increasingly weak.

Even though his health was failing, Pritikin continued to work on new technology designed to remove fats from the blood without the use of drugs. Pritikin held more than two dozen patents in physics, chemistry, and electrical engineering, and marketed his inventions to companies including Honeywell, General Electric, Bendix, and Corning. Following his death in 1985, Pritikin's autopsy published in the *New England Journal of Medicine* showed a heart and arteries that were in extraordinarily healthy condition, "like that of a 16-year-old," noted the supervising pathologist. Nathan Pritikin was buried in Santa Monica, California.

*Marjolijn Bijlefeld and Sharon Zoumbaris*

*See also* Ornish, Dean; Spas, Medical; Vegetarians.

## References

Barnard, Neal D. "The Pritikin Legacy." *Vegetarian Times,* May 1991, 64–73.

Hoover, Eleanor. "When His Health Deserted Him, Diet and Fitness Guru Nathan Pritikin Turned to Suicide." *People Weekly,* March 11, 1985, 57–59.

Pritikin, Nathan. *The Pritikin Program for Diet and Exercise.* New York: Grosset and Dunlap, 1979.

"Pritikin, Nathan." *Almanac of Famous People.* 6th ed. Farmington Hills, MI: Gale Research, 1998.

"Pritikin, Nathan." *Scribner Encyclopedia of American Lives.* Vol. 1: 1981–85. Farmington Hills, MI: Gale Group, 1998.

Rudeen, Jan Craig. "Fresh Look at Pritikin Famous Heart-Healthy Lifestyle Pitched at New Generation of Overeaters." *Denver Post,* June 14, 2009, E-13.

Shute, Nancy. "A Childhood without Twinkies: Young Pritikin Modifies His Father's Draconian Fat-Free Message." *U.S. News & World Report,* January 12, 1998, 62.

## PROBIOTICS

A *probiotic* is an expansive term referring to bacteria and other microorganisms that can be found in a number of food products and have generally been considered to be beneficial to human health. Knowledge of the functions of probiotics goes back several hundreds of years, as people used them to create and preserve foods such as dairy products, meats, and baked goods.

In the early 1900s, more scrutiny was directed at the microbes in human bodies. Researchers determined that benign and helpful microbes could be introduced into the body through eating. They worked with the research of Bulgarian scientist Stamen Grigorov, which indicated that Bulgarian yogurt was fermented with the help of the starter culture *Bacillus bulgaricus*. They determined that the bacteria found in that particular yogurt and sour milk were not to be found naturally in the human intestinal tract. Researchers also observed that there were an extraordinary number of Bulgarians who were more than 100 years old compared with people in other countries studied. They concluded that the consumption of the yogurt, with its special bacterial composition, was linked to the longevity of Bulgarians. The microbe was renamed *Lactobacillus bulgaricus*.

Fellow Institute scientist Henry Tissier was studying the presence of bacteria in children at the same time, and his research indicated that those children who were breast-fed by their mothers had higher levels of the bacteria *Bifidobacterium bifidum* than children who were not breast-fed. When he also discovered that sick children's stool contained fewer numbers of the *Bifidobacterium* than healthy children's, he suggested that treatment start with the administration of these bacteria.

The work of these scientists indicated that specific microbes could be digested to improve the health of the intestines. It soon became apparent that it was almost commercially impossible at the time to create an ingestible bacteria formula that would help cure intestinal problems. Research continued through animals and occasionally people, but it did not take off particularly well until renewed studies in the United States indicated their benefits.

Nutritionist Werner Kollath seems to have coined the word *probiotic* in 1953 as he discussed the benefits of foods that contained helpful bacteria as opposed to harmful antibiotics. After that, the definition has been debated and hashed out, resulting in medical, pharmaceutical, and alimentary probiotics. Alimentary probiotics are used in food production and fermentation. The two strains first promoted by Elie Metchnikoff and Henry Tissier, *Lactobaccillus* and *Bifidobacterium*, have been most used to produce food and supplements that are probiotic.

There are many health claims for probiotic supplements and foods—from helping inflammatory bowel disease to diarrhea, eczema symptoms, bad breath, and respiratory problems. However, the lack of regulation in the claims of these products is beginning to become a problem as illness caused by food-borne microorganisms becomes more common.

The World Health Organization and the Food and Agriculture Organization of the United Nations convened in 2001 to examine the health claims of probiotic foods and to determine what was accurate and appropriate for mass consumption. Following the study, the organizations determined that there should be a standard to judge and evaluate any product that claims to have beneficial probiotics. The groups formed a set of guidelines that addressed the basic problems.

Basically, the probiotic had to be specifically identified, tested thoroughly, and labeled with information such as proper storage, minimum bacteria count left at the expiration date, and exactly what manufacturers claimed it would do. Even with these guidelines, there is no legal regulation regarding the labeling of probiotics in the United States.

Health officials are addressing the lack of regulation, and organizations are meeting to craft Food and Drug Administration (FDA) requirements for proper labeling, description, and evaluation of health claims. The number of ways that probiotics can be consumed means that the FDA will have to consider each possibility in a different category: food, drugs, and supplements. It introduced a regulation for "Dietary Supplement Current Good Manufacturing Practices and Interim Final Rule" in 2007 that required dietary supplements to be produced in a clean and consistent manner to maintain proper quality of the supplement. Probiotics have shown that they have promise to help with a variety of human health complaints, but further research and regulation seem to be necessary to monitor their quality and effects.

*Kelsey Parris*

*See also* Antibiotics; Bacteria; Food and Drug Administration (FDA).

### References

FAO/World Heath Organization. "Probiotics in Food." ftp://ftp.fao.org/docrep/fao/009/a0512e/a0512e00.pdf.

Rusch, Volker. "Probiotics and Definitions: A Short Overview." www.old-herborn-university.de/literature/books/OHUni_book_15_article_1.pdf.

Sonal, Sekhar P. "Probiotics: Friendly Microbes for Better Health." www.ispub.com/journal/the_internet_journal_of_nutrition_and_wellness/volume_6.

## PSYCHOSOMATIC HEALTH CARE

Psychosomatic health care or psychosomatic medicine is a multidisciplinary field focusing on the often-complex interactions between psychological, social, and behavioral elements that impact individuals' health. A variety of health care providers contribute to the practice of psychosomatic medicine in both inpatient and outpatient medical settings, including physicians, psychologists, psychiatrists, and neurologists, among others. A team comprising a mixture of these providers works together during the onset, duration, and/or resolution of medical and psychological issues to assure that both areas are addressed equally and satisfactorily. In this way, the person is treated as a unified whole, rather than addressed via isolated aspects of health. Psychosomatic medicine may also be referred to as consultation-liaison psychiatry, medical-surgical psychiatry, psychological medicine, and psychological care of the complex medically ill (Levenson, 2007).

**History**  The word *psychosomatic* was first used in 1818, and *psychosomatic medicine* was first introduced in 1922 (Gitlin, Levenson, & Lyketsos, 2004, p. 5). The term *psychosomatic* comes from the combination of *psyche,* meaning mind, and *soma,* meaning body. Therefore, the name *psychosomatic medicine* recognizes the interaction of mind and body as an important consideration in wellness and the treatment of disease. Although the interaction between mind and body may now be taken as common knowledge, this was not always the case.

In the 17th century, René Descartes promoted and popularized mind-body, or Cartesian, dualism (Decartes, 1984). This line of thought asserted that the nonphysical mind and the physical body were separate entities on parallel tracks that could only have limited interactions with each other through the pineal gland. Descartes's identification of mind and body as distinct entities as a point of view remained popular in medical science until the mid- to late 1900s, although traces of this view can still be seen in the modern medical system.

Over time, more and more individuals began to embrace the idea that the mind and body were more intimately intertwined. Rather than being separate entities, the mind and body are enmeshed in a fluid, reciprocal relationship. Determining where mind begins and body ends, or what affects the mind versus the body, is virtually impossible. The practice of psychosomatic health care operates under the premise that they constantly affect each other. Thus, barriers to both physical and mental health must be addressed in order to promote overall well-being.

Interdisciplinary treatment teams practicing psychosomatic medicine were first present in hospitals in the 1930s (Gitlin, Levenson, & Lyketsos, 2004, p. 5). However, psychosomatic medicine did not become a formal clinical discipline until many decades later. It was recognized in 2003 as an official subfield by the American Board of Medicine. As recognition of the links between mind and body grow, so does the number of health care professionals who achieve board certification in these disciplines. In 1991 the American Board of Professional Psychology began board certification in Clinical Health Psychology.

**Mind-Body Research**   Currently, more than one in four acutely medically ill patients meet criteria for a psychological illness, and some estimates of prevalence for specific disorders (e.g., depression) are even higher (e.g., Silverstone, 1996). A broad range of issues has been tackled by health care providers practicing psychosomatic medicine. Some of these issues are more general, such as the link between stress and health, and others are more disease-specific (e.g., anxiety and cancer).

It has long been believed that high levels of acute and chronic stress increase risks for disease, and research in the past few decades has supported this. Doctors now suggest our bodies adapt when confronted with stress by producing behavioral, cardiovascular, metabolic, and immune changes (i.e., the "fight-or-flight" response). When these responses occur in the absence of a real (e.g., immediately life-threatening) experience or continue to occur even after the threat has passed, it means these "fight-or-flight" responses are overactive. During overactive reactions, medical problems are more likely to develop, such as chronic inflammatory disease (e.g., arthritis), infectious disease (e.g., influenza), and cancer (e.g., Kemeny & Schedlowski, 2007).

In the modern Western world, stresses often are psychological instead of physical. In other words, we perceive and react to social situations, job problems, and so forth as stressors when there is no actual physical threat to our physical well-being. In turn, the onset or worsening of disease can increase stress further, which may then contribute to disease progression. This is one way in which psychological and physical problems interact with each other.

Beyond general stress, evidence indicates that psychological disorders affect medical disease as well. For example, studies have shown that depression contributes to an array of medical illnesses and mortality (e.g., Stover, Fenton, Rosenfeld, & Insel, 2003). Another example is the well-documented association between anxiety and medical disorders (e.g., Sareen, Jacobi, Cox, Belik, Clara, & Stein, 2006). These related medical conditions include, but are not limited to, cardiovascular disease, thyroid disease, respiratory disease, gastrointestinal disease, and migraine headaches. Although depression and anxiety are two of the most thoroughly researched psychological conditions, evidence also supports the detrimental effects of most other psychological illnesses on physical well-being to varying extents.

**Assessment**  Within psychosomatic medicine, several types of assessment are used to identify any negative influences that psychological illness may be having on a patient's physical illness and vice versa. Psychosomatic medicine is unique in its combination of both medically and psychologically oriented tests.

An array of psychologically based testing may be used. A measure of mental status is almost always included in this array to determine if the patient's memory and attention are intact. For example, a cognitive disorder may involve memory difficulties. If a patient has a cognitive disorder, the psychosomatic treatment providers will test for memory deficits. The patient's medical condition may be getting worse because the patient is forgetting to take his or her prescribed medications. Additional neuropsychological screeners that are more specific to different types of memory problems, information-processing speed, and other related domains may be used to address similar problems as well.

Diagnostic interviews and/or screeners for particular psychological disorders may be used in addition to cognitive testing if a disorder is suspected to be present and contributory to the patient's medical problems. For instance, a patient with increasingly poor liver function due to alcohol dependence may use alcohol to self-medicate for anxiety symptoms. If it becomes apparent when speaking with the patient that he or she identifies traumatic and intrusive memories as a reason for drinking, following up with an assessment for posttraumatic stress disorder would be appropriate. An affirmative assessment could then lead to treatment, which may result in reduced drinking and liver damage.

Several medical tests are utilized by practitioners in psychosomatic health care as well. Brain imaging may be used to clarify the interaction between psychological and physical problems. For instance, if a patient survived a brain injury but sustained damage to an area of the brain that plays a large role in attention, the patient may have difficulty listening to a treatment provider explain a complex medical regimen and thus experience problems with medication adherence or appointment attendance.

Electrophysiological tests that measure brainwaves, heart activity, and other bodily processes can be very informative as well. To illustrate, electroencephalography (EEG) can be used to examine brainwaves and determine the presence of unhealthy sleep patterns. It may be the case that an individual has deficient sleep, which could lower his or her risk for infectious disease as well as create depressed mood and exacerbate general stress levels.

Finally, lab tests that use blood, urine, and so forth could show that certain substances in the body are abnormal and are contributing to medical and/or psychological symptoms. For example, high levels of thyroid stimulating hormone (TSH) suggests poor thyroid functioning, which can mimic the symptoms of depression (e.g., fatigue, poor concentration). If a medically ill patient's lab results show high levels of TSH, and he or she is showing symptoms of depression, poor thyroid functioning should be considered as a possible contributing factor for the depression symptoms and cotreated with medication and psychotherapy.

These are only a few examples of domains of testing that are covered in the field of psychosomatic medicine that can clarify the ways in which physical and psychological states may affect each other. Multiple methods are often used to increase confidence that these interactions are well understood so that proper treatment can occur to increase patients' well-being both medically and psychologically.

**Treatment**   Psychosomatic health care involves treatment catered to each individual patient's issues, as determined through the various assessment methods. Medical and psychological treatment providers interface to provide treatments that will complement each other to achieve the best outcome for the patient both physically and psychosocially. In this way, treatment emerges from a "biopsychosocial" perspective that takes into account the patient as a whole rather than a patient with distinct, and unconnected, medical and psychological difficulties.

The psychosomatic health care practitioner will focus on delivery of treatments that manipulate the psychological and social components of the overall clinical picture, taking into account which approach will best impact the biological components as well. For example, a patient who just suffered a heart attack may not meet diagnostic criteria for a psychological disorder, but it may be apparent through an assessment that he or she has little to no skill in general stress management. Therefore, providing psychoeducation and teaching the patient relaxation and stress reduction skills provides a mechanism for the patient to reduce cardiovascular reactivity to stressors, reduce overall stress, reduce risk for future cardiovascular complications, and improve overall quality of life.

Another patient may have a similar medical event, but it may become apparent through the assessment that he or she does qualify for a diagnosis, such as schizophrenia. Due to the established link between schizophrenia and poorer cardiovascular outcomes, going above and beyond stress management is warranted. For example, beginning a regimen of antipsychotic medication, educating the patient and his or her family on the condition, and referring the patient to an outpatient care facility to manage the newly diagnosed disorder would be warranted.

**Applications to Prevention and Wellness**   Although assessment and treatment is extremely relevant in medical settings where patients are exhibiting mental and physical health issues, the spirit of psychosomatic medicine can be applied in a preventive way to individuals who are relatively healthy physically and psychologically. As discussed earlier, the stress response is a natural response. Everyone experiences it to an extent in their everyday lives. Psychosomatic medicine practices can provide a powerful tool to maintain well-being by helping people recognize the link between stress, psychological health, and physical health.

Once people recognize this critical link, they can begin to identify how areas in their life negatively impact both their mental and physical well-being. This awareness helps individuals begin to prioritize promoting the globally healthy self. It is not unusual for individuals to initiate self-care only when there is evidence of a problem. However, actively identifying areas for improvement and addressing them through self-care may prevent disease and promote wellness. The old saying goes "an ounce of prevention is worth a pound of cure," and a psychosomatic medicine approach that focuses on wellness may decrease the likelihood of problems occurring. A psychosomatic medicine approach can assist individuals in decreasing stress and negative psychological symptoms, such as intermittent sadness or anxiety, before these symptoms expand to exert detrimental influences in the form of a diagnosable medical or psychological illness. Consider the following example:

> Laurie is 31 years old, is married, has two children, and recently was laid off from her job. Because Laurie's husband recently returned to school full time to get an advanced degree and a better job, the plan was for Laurie to be the primary source of income in the household. Laurie feels guilty about losing her job, and she and her husband have started arguing frequently about the issue. Finances are a major stressor in the family. Laurie is experiencing added stress because she has been unsuccessful so far in her ongoing job hunt. She has increased duties in childcare since they can no longer afford daycare, and she has less emotional support from her husband who is attending classes and is out of the house more. She feels frustrated because she does not know how to cope with all of these adjustments. Laurie worries at night about all of these issues and she finds that her sleep is suffering more and more as time goes on, and she also is not eating as healthily because she feels she does not have time to do so.

Beyond the physical strain on her body from multiple sources of stress, Laurie is putting herself at risk for health problems due to decreased sleep and poor eating. Specifically, much of the body's immune responses that fight off infection occur during sleep, and the body needs sufficient nutrition to adequately overcome infections. Deficiency in both of these areas can be particularly detrimental when facing large amounts of stress as in Laurie's situation.

In addition to stress and feelings of guilt, Laurie may begin to experience other symptoms such as decreased energy and weight changes. These changes may further lead to decreased feelings of self-worth and lack of motivation to continue her job search. As these symptoms worsen, Laurie's sleep and eating habits may further decline, creating a negative spiral toward anxiety and depression. It is in this way that Laurie may be putting herself at risk for issues such as insomnia, depression, obesity, and so forth.

However, these long-term outcomes are not inevitable. Building in stress management, social support, and resources for good physical self-care can prevent this sort of downward spiral away from well-being and into disease. Building these psychological and medical wellness skills into everyday life not only decreases risk for medical and psychological illness, but it also improves overall quality of day-to-day life. Daily stress management practices, good sleep habits, physical exercise, and a well-balanced diet are just a few ways individuals can increase their mood, energy, productivity, and so forth—in short, their overall personal well-being. These practices allow individuals to be better psychologically and physically prepared for mental and medical stressors of varying magnitudes that will inevitably surface each day. The premise of psychosomatic medicine allows individuals to arm themselves with the tools to exert control over their well-being, and empower them to make positive changes in their mental and physical health.

**Conclusion**   Psychosomatic health care is an area that recognizes the far-reaching and reciprocal effects of balancing physical and psychological wellness. The intimate enmeshment of body and mind has not always been appreciated (e.g., Cartesian dualism). However, the existence and success of psychosomatic medicine as a distinct field of practice is a testament to the overwhelming importance of considering both physical and mental health domains when optimizing wellness. Whereas psychosomatic medicine is typically practiced in settings where illness has already occurred, its basic foundations may be implemented to ensure that well-being reaches its fullest capacity within each individual who is willing to make the efforts to address both his or her psychological and physical health needs.

*Amanda Wheat and Amy Wachholtz*

*See also* Depression; Psychotherapy; Stress.

**References**

Descartes, René. "Meditations on First Philosophy." In *The Philosophical Writings of René Descartes,* edited by John Cottingham, Robert Stoothoff, and Dugald Murdoch, 1–62. Cambridge: Cambridge University Press, 1984.

Gitlin, David F., James L. Levenson, and Constantine G. Lyketsos. "Psychiatric Medicine: A New Psychiatric Subspecialty." *Academic Psychiatry* 28 (2004): 4–11.

Kemeny, Margaret, and Manfred Schedlowski. "Understanding the Interaction between Psychosocial Stress and Immune-Related Diseases: A Stepwise Progression." *Brain, Behavior, and Immunity* 21 (2007): 1009–18.

Levenson, James L., ed. *Textbook of Psychosomatic Medicine.* Washington, DC: American Psychiatric Publishing, 2007, xix–xxi.

Sareen, Jitender, Frank Jacobi, Brian Cox, Shay-Lee Belik, Ian Clara, and Murray Stein. "Disability and Poor Quality of Life Associated with Comorbid Anxiety Disorders and Physical Conditions." *Archives of Internal Medicine* 166 (2006): 2109–16.

Silverstone, Peter H. "Prevalence of Psychiatric Disorders in Medical Inpatients." *Journal of Nervous and Mental Disease* 184 (1996): 43–51.

Stover, Ellen, Wayne Fenton, Anne Rosenfeld, and Thomas R. Insel. "Depression and Comorbid Medical Illness: The National Institute of Mental Health Perspective." *Biological Psychiatry* 54 (2003): 184–86.

# PSYCHOTHERAPY

Psychotherapy may involve the use of "talk therapy" and other psychological techniques to treat mental disorders or other personal issues. The focus is on changing detrimental behaviors, thoughts, moods, emotions, and perceptions that may be contributing to a person's problems.

Several types of psychotherapy can be beneficial for people with depression, for example. The two with the strongest research support are *cognitive-behavioral therapy* (CBT) and *interpersonal therapy* (IPT). In CBT, individuals work to change habitual patterns of thinking and behaving that are associated with their depression. In IPT, individuals work to address interpersonal triggers for their mental, emotional, and behavioral symptoms. Research has shown that both CBT and IPT can be effective as short-term (12- to 20-week) therapies for depression. For mild to moderate depression, psychotherapy alone is sometimes sufficient. For more severe depression, psychotherapy may not be enough by itself, so it is often combined with *antidepressants.*

Psychotherapy relies heavily on verbal interaction between a patient and a therapist. Although the therapist serves as a guide, the patient plays an active and central role in the treatment process. The best results are achieved when both parties tackle the process with vigor, concentration, and commitment. Therapy sessions typically last 45 to 50 minutes. Homework activities also may be assigned between sessions.

The relationship between patient and therapist is unique. Although it is not a friendship, it is most effective when built upon trust and rapport. Confidentiality is another key element, which is emphasized in the ethical codes published by the American Psychiatric Association, American Psychological Association, and other professional organizations. Both parties have responsibilities. To get the most out of psychotherapy, the patient must be honest and forthright, even when it involves talking about topics that may be embarrassing or uncomfortable. The patient also should be actively engaged in the process, open to new insights, and willing to take steps for change. Meanwhile, the therapist must be willing to listen carefully and respectfully. The therapist also should guide the patient in recognizing and modifying unhealthy patterns.

**Approaches to Psychotherapy**  By some estimates, there are currently more than 400 different therapeutic approaches. However, most boil down to one of three basic orientations.

*Action-Oriented Therapies*  These approaches focus on current patterns of thought and behavior rather than past experiences. A classic example is *behavioral therapy,* which systematically uses the principles of learning to decrease undesirable behaviors and increase desirable ones. The primary goal is to help patients make positive changes, whether or not they understand how their problems started. CBT, an outgrowth of behavioral therapy, falls solidly into this category. IPT, with its stress on changing interpersonal behaviors and learning new social and communication skills, also may be considered an action-oriented therapy.

*Insight-Oriented Therapies*  These approaches focus on self-understanding, based on the assumption that greater insight will lead to better functioning. The best-known example is *psychodynamic therapy,* which emphasizes the role of past events in shaping current experiences as well as the importance of unconscious influences on behavior. Although psychodynamic therapy is frequently used for depression, its effectiveness has not been as well established as that of CBT and

## Table 1. Types of Psychotherapists

Mental health professionals from several disciplines provide psychotherapy. Each field has its own licensure requirements, which vary from state to state. In addition, the disciplines differ in training, credentials, and typical treatment approach.

| | Training and Credentials | Typical Treatment Approach | Can Prescribe Medication? |
|---|---|---|---|
| **Psychiatrist** | Medical school plus at least four years of residency training. Many are board certified by the American Board of Psychiatry and Neurology. | Prescribing and monitoring medication. Some provide psychotherapy as well. Others work closely with therapists from other fields. | Yes |
| **Clinical Psychologist** | Doctoral degree including a clinical internship plus at least one year of postdoctoral experience. Some are board certified by the American Board of Professional Psychology. | Providing psychotherapy and doing psychological testing. Some also provide other psychologically based treatments, such as cognitive rehabilitation and biofeedback. | In New Mexico and Louisiana only, with advanced training. |
| **Psychiatric Nurse** | Licensure as a registered nurse plus additional training in mental health care. Advanced practice registered nurses have a master's degree or above in psychiatric–mental health nursing. | Providing psychotherapy and helping manage medication. Some are supervised by medical doctors, but those with advanced practice credentials may work independently. | In many states, with advanced training. |
| **Clinical Social Worker** | Master's degree or above, usually plus two years of supervised clinical experience. | Providing psychotherapy and helping people overcome social and health problems. Some provide assistance in getting help from government agencies. | No |
| **Marriage and Family Therapist** | Typically master's degree or above plus postdegree experience. A few states do not require licensure or certification, however. | Providing individual, couples, and family therapy. The focus is on mental health problems in the context of close relationships. | No |

*(Continued)*

**Table 1. Types of Psychotherapists (*Continued*)**

| | Training and Credentials | Typical Treatment Approach | Can Prescribe Medication? |
|---|---|---|---|
| **Mental Health Counselor** | Typically master's degree or above plus postdegree experience. California does not require licensure or certification, however. | Providing psychotherapy and advising people on how to cope with problems of everyday living. Therapy often takes a problem-solving approach. | No |
| **Pastoral Counselor** | Training as a mental health professional plus in-depth religious or theological training. Requirements for licensure or certification vary. | Providing psychotherapy in a spiritual context. Both spiritual resources and psychological techniques are utilized for healing and growth. | No |

IPT. In some cases, psychodynamic therapy may not be feasible until the worst symptoms of depression are under control with other treatments.

*Growth-Oriented Therapies* These approaches often are grouped together under the label *humanistic therapy*. They are concerned with fostering personal growth through direct experience. The primary focus is on current feelings, rather than thoughts and behaviors, as well as the potential for future development. Other common themes include taking responsibility for oneself and putting trust in spontaneous feelings and natural processes. *Emotion-focused therapy* is one growth-oriented approach that has been adapted to the treatment of depression.

*Group, Couples, and Family Therapy* Any of these approaches can be used in individual therapy, in which a patient works one-on-one with a therapist. However, the approaches also are sometimes used in situations where more than one person meets with the therapist at the same time. *Group therapy* involves bringing together several patients with similar diagnoses or issues for therapy sessions. The interaction among group members adds an extra dimension to each person's therapy, providing support and perhaps modifying behavior. The therapist can use the interaction to help group members explore shared problems.

*Couples therapy* and *family therapy* are a little different, in that the "patient" is the relationship rather than an individual. Partners or family members may meet with the therapist either separately or at the same time, but the focus remains on how they relate to one another. The assumption is that destructive relationship patterns can contribute to a host of mental, emotional, and behavioral problems, including depression. One person's depression, in turn, can take a heavy toll on a marriage or family. The aim of couples and family therapy is to correct faulty patterns of interaction, improving the relationship as a whole and helping the individuals in it function better.

One downside to medication is the risk of harmful side effects. Psychotherapy is relatively safe by comparison. Nevertheless, it may involve confronting unpleasant situations or disturbing thoughts and feelings. Occasionally, the process may give rise to considerable distress, which is one reason it is crucial that psychotherapy be carried out by a qualified mental health professional.

Appropriate psychotherapy can help people with depression and other issues pinpoint and address factors that may be contributing to their symptoms. Psychotherapy also can help depressed individuals regain a sense of control over their lives and return to activities that were once sources of pleasure and meaning. For those people, as the depression starts to lift, they gradually become able to experience enjoyment and fulfillment in their lives again.

In addition, research suggests that appropriate psychotherapy may reduce the risk of future episodes of depression and other mental illness issues or decrease their severity. Through effective psychotherapy, people with depression and other problems can learn lifelong skills that help them cope more effectively with future problems and avoid unnecessary suffering.

*Linda Wasmer Andrews*

*See also* Addiction; Bipolar Disorder; Depression; Eating Disorders; Psychosomatic Health Care; Suicide.

### References

American Psychiatric Association Work Group on Major Depressive Disorder. *Practice Guideline for the Treatment of Patients with Major Depressive Disorder.* 2nd ed. Washington, DC: American Psychiatric Publishing, 2000.

Bureau of Labor Statistics. *Occupational Outlook Handbook, 2006–07 Edition.* Washington, DC: U.S. Department of Labor, 2005.

*Depression.* National Institute of Mental Health. 2000. www.nimh.nih.gov/health/publica tions/depression/summary.shtml.

Harvard Medical School. *Understanding Depression.* Boston: Harvard Health Publications, 2003.

*How Psychotherapy Helps People Recover from Depression.* American Psychological Association. 2004. http://apahelpcenter.org/articles/article.php?id=49.

*Psychotherapy.* American Psychiatric Association. http://healthyminds.org/psychotherapy. cfm.

*Types of Mental Health Providers.* Mayo Clinic. 2007. www.mayoclinic.com/health/mental-health/MH00074.

U.S. Department of Health and Human Services. *Mental Health: A Report of the Surgeon General.* Rockville, MD: U.S. Department of Health and Human Services, 1999.

# Q

## QIGONG

Its movements are synchronized like ballet and sometimes practitioners mimic the motions of animals. Qigong (pronounced chee-gung) is more than just physical exercise, it's a form of classical Chinese exercise said to help practitioners achieve both optimum mental and physical health. Similar to the ancient Chinese practice of tai chi, qigong emphasizes positions, breathing techniques, and mental focus. Researchers estimate some half million Americans now practice qigong as a way to relax, improve respiration, blood flow, heart rate, and digestion. Studies are also underway to explore possible health effects of qigong for diabetics. According to the Centers for Disease Control and Prevention, some 24 million Americans have some form of diabetes, with Type 2, the most common form, accounting for upward of 90 percent of all U.S. cases.

Researchers at Bastyr University in Seattle launched a pilot study in 2009 to investigate the effects of qigong when compared to other physical exercise or conventional diabetes treatment on glucose control in adults with Type 2 diabetes (Sun, 2009). Researchers say they found participants in the qigong group had significantly lower levels of fasting blood glucose, less insulin resistance, and reduced stress along with weight loss when compared with the other two groups.

Researchers at Arizona State University also examined the advantages of qigong and tai chi and compared these two wellness practices to other exercises or to a sedentary state. The research, published between 1993 and 2007, studied the effects of tai chi and qigong on overall health, physical function, quality of life, immune system functioning, psychological symptoms, and other factors (Jahnke et al., 2010). The Arizona study reported strong evidence that the qigong and tai chi offer help for physical function, bone health, heart improvement, lung function improvement in addition to psychological and quality-of-life benefits. While results are not yet conclusive, qigong has become an accepted treatment in the United States as part of the field of complementary and alternative medicine. It also continues to be used extensively in China in the practice of traditional Chinese medicine.

Qigong dates back as far as the Yellow Emperor (2696 BC to 2598 or 2597 BC) in ancient China according to Chinese history. Although it became a component of traditional Chinese medicine, during the fall of the Qing Dynasty (from the mid-17th century to the early 20th century), there was little done to shape its development. Later, during the rule of Mao Zedong (1949–1976), the Chinese government promoted a socialist view and rejected all ties to traditional Chinese philosophies. However, qigong resurfaced in the 1950s and by the 1970s support for traditional Chinese medicine improved and qigong departments were established within the Chinese universities and hospitals that practiced traditional medicine. Qigong continues to grow in popularity in the United States. TV host and cardiologist Dr. Mehmet Oz showed his enthusiasm for qigong when he advised his audiences "if you want to be healthy and live to be 100, do Qigong" (Li, 2010). He also described it as a miracle exercise for people seeking to avoid drugs, surgery, and expensive doctor bills.

When practiced correctly qigong consists of a series of gentle movements involving the entire body. It is combined with meditation, visualization, and breathing, the combination of which is designed to balance each individual's opposing yin and yang forces and unblocks his or her *qi* or chi, the energy force that flows through the body. There are several types of qigong, which are differentiated by four kinds of training: dynamic, static, meditative, and activities requiring external aids. Dynamic qigong is recognized as a series of choreographed movements designed to increase the flow of chi throughout the body. Tai chi is one well-known type of dynamic qigong. Other examples include the Wild Goose or Dayan qigong, where the practitioner mimics the movements of animals.

Static qigong is performed by holding poses or positions for a period of time, and because of the duration of poses, it resembles the practice of yoga. All types of qigong involve some form of meditation. Additionally, the slowed movements and breathing exercises promote relaxation and reduce stress. As with the meditative form of qigong, many systems of qigong training include the use of external agents such as food and drinks, massage, or other body conditioning.

The practice of qigong is also an important component in Chinese martial arts. The ability to break hard objects is a well-known martial arts activity attributed to qigong training. While Americans routinely equate sweating at the gym with healthy exercise, practitioners of qigong describe it as a healing form of exercise that for some has accomplished what Western medicine has not been able to cure. U.S. qigong instructors, such as Dr. Roger Jahnke, director of the Institute of Integral Qigong and tai Chi (IIQCT), suggested the future for qigong may be as a tool in bringing down rising U.S. health care costs (Jahnke et al., 2010). Jahnke and others associated with qigong suggest its preventative properties can help Americans take control of their health and their wellness. Only time will tell, but qigong supporters are confident time is on their side.

*Sharon Zoumbaris*

*See also* Acupuncture; Diabetes; Tai Chi; Traditional Chinese Medicine.

## References

Doheny, Kathleen. "Tai Chi, Qigong Good for Body, Mind: Studies Find Tai Chi and Qigong Have Physical, Mental Health Benefits." WebMD Health News. July 2, 2010. www.webmd.com/balance/news/20100702.

Jahnke, Roger, Linda Larkey, Carol Rogers, Jennifer Etnier, and Fang Lin. "A Comprehensive Review of Health Benefits of Qigong and Tai Chi." *American Journal of Health Promotion* 24, no. 6 (July/August 2010): E1–25.

Li, Violet. "Managing Stress with Qigong." *Tai Chi Examiner.* September 12, 2010. www.examiner.com.

Palmer, David A. *Qigong Fever: Body, Science and Utopia in China.* New York: Columbia University Press, 2007.

Sun, Guan-Cheng, Jennifer C. Lovejoy, Sara Gillham, Amy Putirl, Masa Sasagawa, and Ryan Bradley. "Effects of Qigong on Glucose Control in Type 2 Diabetes: A Randomized Controlled Pilot Study." *Diabetes Care* 33, no. 1 (December 29, 2009): E8.

# R

## RECOMBINANT BOVINE GROWTH HORMONE (rBGH)

A cold glass of milk is considered by many to be a completely wholesome snack. However, more and more Americans are asking if that milk is rBGH-free. This controversial question comes from the use of bovine growth hormone in dairy cows. Known as recombinant bovine growth hormone (rBGH) or recombinant bovine somatotropin (rBST), its use in U.S. dairy cows was approved by the FDA in 1993 after years of testing and studies. At that time the FDA ruled that milk and meat from cows given rBGH were the same as those from other cows and safe for U.S. consumers.

Critics continue to dispute those findings and warn that rBGH is bad for the health of the cows and may even pose health risks for people. At the same time, a growing consumer demand for dairy products free of rBGH has resulted in more of these products showing up on supermarket shelves in the United States as more and more retailers are moving to rBGH-free products. Internationally, the use of rBGH in dairy cows has already been banned in all of the European Union nations, as well as Canada, Australia, New Zealand, and Japan.

Among critics of the use of rBGH or rBST in dairy cows is the American Nurses Association, which publicly supports the development of national and state laws and policies that would specifically stop the sale and use of rBGH. Other organizations calling for an end to rBGH use in U.S. dairy cows include Health Care without Harm (HCWH), an international coalition of more than 400 organizations in some 50 countries working to raise awareness about food and environmental issues. The group supports buying fresh food locally, purchasing certified organic food, avoiding food with growth hormones and antibiotics, and the need for sustainable food systems in health care facilities.

In answer to consumer concerns, Kraft Foods introduced hormone-free cheeses in 2008. In 2009, General Mills responded to a campaign by groups including HCWH and Breast Cancer Action (BCA) and announced it would stop using rBGH milk as an ingredient in its popular Yoplait yogurt products. General

Mills is among a growing number of manufacturers to heed consumer demands for rBGH-free products. Wal-Mart, Starbucks, and Chipotle Restaurants joined other retailers who have stopped using milk from rBGH-treated cows in their store brand products. Kroger, Safeway Dairy Group, and Publix Super Markets are either partially or completely rBGH-free as well (Sayre, 2008).

The rBGH hormone is a genetic replica of a hormone animals produce naturally, and was one of the first applications of genetic engineering used in American food production. It is injected into the cows after they give birth, and it acts to boost their milk production by up to a gallon per day and keep them making milk longer. It works by altering the gene that sends glucose to the cow's mammary gland, which in turn produces more milk.

The FDA requires a warning label on Posilac, its trademarked name, which lists more than 20 potential side effects of rBGH on cows including cystic ovaries, uterine disorders, decrease in gestation length and birth weight of calves, increased incidence of twins, problems with the placenta after birth, and serious problems with mastiris, an inflammation of the udder.

The increased incidence of multiple births may be shared by dairy cows and women according to a 2000 study in the *Journal of Reproductive Medicine.* That research showed women who drank milk with rBGH were three times more likely to have twins than women who did not (Barone, 2007). The reason appears to be the substance IFG-1 (insulinlike growth factor), which is found in cows' milk and encourages cells to divide. Milk from cows treated with rBGH has three times more IFG-1 than milk from untreated cows.

According to the study's author, Dr. Gary Steinman, an assistant clinical professor of obstetrics, his research showed a relationship between bovine growth hormone in the food supply and the fact that the U.S. rate of twin births has almost tripled in the last 30 years (Barone, 2007). Steinman said the use of assisted reproductive technologies in the United States doesn't fully account for the increase in multiple births in this country. He added that "the rate has gone up twice as fast here in the U.S. as in Britain, where there's been a moratorium on synthetic BGH" (Bakalar, 2006).

Scientific studies have also found that high levels of IFG-1 in the blood have been associated with prostate and breast cancer, although no studies have shown that milk from cows treated with rBGH directly causes cancer (Hankinson, 1998). However, statistics continue to show that cows treated with rBGH, first sold under Monsanto's brand name Posilac, have higher rates of problems including udder infections, uterine disorders, diarrhea, foot problems, and twin births (Kingsnorth, 1998).

Monsanto maintained for years there is no difference in milk or dairy products from cows given rBGH. To support that claim, Monsanto sued the Oakhurst Dairy Company of Portland, Maine, in 2003, when the company printed a pledge on its milk containers saying it did not contain artificial growth hormones. Monsanto complained that since it was the only seller of the hormone for dairy cows in the country, the label must refer to it.

Company officials also suggested that the label was designed to make milk buyers think there was a difference between milk from cows getting the hormone and other cows, and they argued that this was untrue. The suit was settled when Oakhurst agreed to add the words, "FDA states: No significant difference in milk from cows treated with artificial growth hormone."

In recent years more dairy products are carrying rBGH-free statements on their labels, moving the controversy over its use to the state level. In October 2007, the Pennsylvania Department of Agriculture (PDA) declared "rBGH-free milk" labeling was illegal. The department eventually withdrew the ban, but other states have also considered similar action, including New Jersey, Ohio, Kansas, Utah, and Indiana (Sayre, 2008).

In 2008 Monsanto sold Posilac to the Eli Lilly Corporation for $300 million along with a portion of future Posilac sales. Monsanto announced it would focus instead on its GMO seed and crop business. Almost immediately the Lilly Corporation came under criticism by Breast Cancer Action (BCA), a nonprofit education and advocacy organization, which launched a campaign to stop the manufacture of rBGH. According to the organization's website, the campaign, titled "Milking Cancer," is aimed at stopping the pharmaceutical giant from making the hormone. As the sole manufacturer of Posilac, if Lilly stops making rBGH it would no longer be available. The earlier BCA campaign focused on persuading General Mills to discontinue the use of rBGH in Yoplait yogurt. That campaign was successful.

*Sharon Zoumbaris*

*See also* Cancer; Genetically Modified Organisms (GMOs).

## References

Bakalar, Nicholas. "Rise in Rate of Twin Births May be Tied to Dairy Case." *New York Times,* May 30, 2006. www.nytimes.com/2006/05/30/health/30twin.html.

Barone, Jennifer. "Milk Drinkers More Likely to Have Twins." *Discover* 28, no. 1 (January 2007): 48.

"Cancer Advocacy Organization Confronts the Source of rBGH and Demands Eli Lilly Stop Milking Cancer." *US Newswire,* September 22, 2009. http://find.galegroup.com/gtx/infomark.do?&contentSet=IAC-Documents&type=retrieve&tabID=T004&prodId=GRGM&docId=A208191612&source=gale&srcprod=GRGM&userGroupName=va0054_009&version=1.0.

Hankinson, S.E., Walter C. Willett, Graham A. Colditz, David J. Hunter, Dominique S. Michaud, Bonnie Deroo, Bernard Rosner, Frank E. Speizer, and Michael Pollak. "Circulating Concentrations of Insulin-Like Growth Factor 1 and Risk of Breast Cancer." *The Lancet* 351, no. 9113 (May 9, 1998): 1393–96.

"Hospitals and Healthcare Leaders Shift Dairy Market." *US Newswire,* February 9, 2009. General Reference Center Gold.

Kingsnorth, Paul. "Bovine Growth Hormones." *The Ecologist* 28, no. 5 (September–October 1998): 266.

Sayre, Laura. "Protecting Milk from Monsanto." *Mother Earth News* (June–July 2008): 27.

Schneider, K. "Lines Drawn in War over Milk Hormone." *New York Times,* March 9, 1994, A12.

"Thanks to the Work of Breast Cancer Action, Food Product Manufacturer General Mills Has Committed to Making Yogurt without Recombinant Bovine Growth Hormone (rBGH), Which Has Been Linked to Cancer." *Women's Health Activist* 34, no. 4 (July–August 2009): 12.

"Three Things You Should Know about Your Food: Hormones in Milk and Meat from Genetically Engineered Animals." *Consumer Reports* 73, no. 7 (July 2008): 61.

## RECOMMENDED DIETARY ALLOWANCE (RDA)

The first set of Recommended Dietary Allowances (RDAs) was released by the Food and Nutrition Board of the National Academy of Sciences in 1941, thanks in part to the efforts of President Franklin Roosevelt to bring about a national conversation on nutrition. Roosevelt had asked that solid nutritional information come from the National Nutrition Conference for Defense that year. The RDAs were the most specific recommendations by the government to this point calling for specific intakes of calories and nine essential nutrients including protein, iron, calcium, vitamins A and D, thiamin, riboflavin, niacin, and ascorbic acid or vitamin C. The conference was born of the recognized need for nutrition education for U.S. consumers.

The last RDAs were issued in 1989 and were replaced by the Dietary Reference Intakes, DRIs, also created by the Food and Nutrition Board of the Institute of Medicine.

*Sharon Zoumbaris*

*See also* Dietary Reference Intakes (DRI); Nutrition.

### Reference

"Basic 4 Food Guide (1956–1979)." U.S. Department of Agriculture. www.nal.usda.gov/fnic/history/asic4.htm.

## REFLEXOLOGY

Reflexology is a holistic health practice by which pressure is placed on the feet and hands in order to promote health and well-being. In particular, reflexology is used to diagnose illness, reduce stress, and treat illness.

Reflexology proponents maintain that reflexology was practiced in ancient Egypt, Greece, India, China, and Japan, but there is no evidence that when foot therapies were practiced in these cultures, they were related to the modern understanding of reflexology "zones." Reflexology was first practiced in 1913 by a doctor named William Fitzgerald, who called it "zone therapy" and who came up with the idea that the body is broken into zones that correspond to specific areas of the hands and feet. It was promoted by Eunice Ingham, a nurse, in the 1930s and 1940s, but it did not become popular until the 1990s.

According to proponents, by placing pressure on specific areas of the hands and feet, this will affect the corresponding body parts and result in better blood flow to the affected regions. In that sense, reflexology is like acupuncture, which finds that acupuncture points correspond to areas of the body, and by inserting a needle into a particular point, healing will occur.

In reflexology, the body is broken into 10 zones, with 5 on each side of the body. The left foot (and hand) is linked to the left side of the body, while the right foot or hand is linked to the right side. Further, the region from the arch of the foot to the toes represents the body above the waist while the area from the arch to the heel rep-

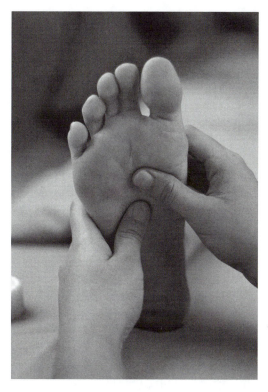

Reflexology is a form of alternative medicine, which applies pressure to feet, hands, or other specific parts of the body using specific techniques. (Photosoup/Dreamstime.com)

resents the body below the waist. The big toe, for instance, corresponds to the head, brain, and the pituitary gland. The ball of the right foot corresponds to the lungs and heart, while the ball of the left foot corresponds to the lungs, and the top of the instep corresponds to the lower back and hips.

The principle behind reflexology is that humans have pressure sensors in the hands and the feet that allow us to detect danger, and that are connected to internal organs that are then put into motion when a danger arises. By pressing the correct zone, stress is released in the corresponding area of the body, unblocking blockages and increasing blood flow.

Reflexology practitioners are trained to use their fingers and thumbs in a particular way when manipulating the hands and feet. Foot rollers can be used too. Unlike acupuncture, reflexology is not regulated and can be practiced by anyone, including laypeople, massage therapists, or nurses and other medical practitioners. Most reflexologists do get some training, however, at locations like the International Institute of Reflexology. A standard course lasts six months and offers 200 hours of training.

The American Reflexology Certification Board (ARCB) has, since 1991, offered certification to reflexologists in the United States, who have concluded at least

110 hours of training and can pass the organization's written and practical tests. According to the ARCB, which provides demographic information on practitioners, the average reflexologist in the United States is white, female, in her 40s, and practices reflexology part-time.

Reflexology is said to reduce stress, and some practitioners claim that reflexology can cure illness. It has been claimed that reflexology can reduce wrinkles, help in weight loss, improve circulation, reduce toxins, balance energy, and bring the body into equilibrium, not to mention treat virtually every illness and disorder. For many practitioners, however, it is primarily used to treat stress and is promoted as an adjunct to Western or Eastern medicine and not as a substitute for it. Sessions last for 30 to 60 minutes and are not focused on particular body parts, as in acupuncture; instead, the whole foot is worked.

Reflexology is also used to assess stress levels, as the presence of calluses, bunions, or hammer toes, for example, is said to indicate stress in other parts of the body.

A number of studies have been conducted in the last 10 years on the benefits of reflexology, and none appear to demonstrate a relationship between receiving reflexology treatments and improvements in health, or in the accurate reflexology diagnoses of medical problems. On the other hand, reflexology, like massage, has been shown to relax patients, leading to a temporary reduction in stress.

The benefits of reflexology can also be attained through wearing reflexology sandals or walking on special reflexology paths. Reflexology sandals are slides with rubber or plastic nubs molded into the sole, which stimulate the feet when walking. Reflexology sandals are only intended to be worn for about 20 minutes per day. A reflexology path is a path laid with stones placed in a particular pattern; walking on the stones will stimulate the reflexology points and thus improve health and relieve stress. Reflexology paths are common in many Asian countries and can also be found in the United States.

*Margo DeMello*

*See also* Acupuncture; Stress.

**References**

Kunz, K., and B. Kunz. *The Complete Guide to Foot Reflexology.* Albuquerque: Reflexology Research, 1993.
Sachs, J., and J. Berger. *Reflexology: The A–Z Guide to Healing with Pressure Points.* New York: Dell, 1997.
Soble, Michelle. *Podiatry for the Reflexologist.* Yellville, AR: Whitehall, 2002.

## REGISTERED DIETITIAN

*Registered dietitian* is the most recognized career in the nutrition field. A registered dietitian is someone who has earned a bachelor's degree in nutrition, finished a period of supervised practice, and passed a registration examination. Registered dietitians work in a variety of basic settings including clinical, community, management, and consultant dietetics. In a clinical setting, registered dietitians will collaborate with doctors and other health care professionals and provide services for patients in hospitals or senior care facilities. They develop nutrition programs, evaluate the results, and continually assess patients' needs.

Those who work in nutrition management often oversee large-scale food service systems in company cafeterias, prisons, health care facilities, or schools. A registered dietitian in this setting would handle the budget and the purchase of food, and enforce sanitary and safety regulations. People with advanced degrees in nutrition and food science also conduct research projects for business, industry, health care institutions, and the government. These experts may investigate the effect of diet on health, or help develop food products.

A number of registered dietitians offer personal nutrition counseling directly to the public. For those not interested in private practice, there are growing opportunities in new areas working with supermarkets, professional sports teams, and other businesses, as well as in traditional settings in home health agencies, public health clinics, and hospitals.

Another emerging area of work for registered dietitians is with specialized diets to deal with chronic disease. Julie Barto, a registered dietitian publicly teamed up with a Food Network celebrity chef to create a program especially for people with multiple sclerosis (MS). The materials are packaged as the MS Active Wellness nutrition program. Barto worked with a team to highlight information aimed at helping those with MS make small cooking adjustments and food choices that will eventually create improvements in their energy and health. The information is available in a series of videos designed to demonstrate cooking techniques as well as featured recipes and a discussion of how certain foods can alleviate some MS symptoms.

Registered dietitians must meet a number of educational criteria to earn the RD credential, including completing a bachelor's degree at an accredited university or college. That course work must be approved by the Commission on Accreditation for Dietetics Education (CADE) of the American Dietetic Association (ADA). Next they need to complete a CADE-accredited supervised practice program lasting from six months to a year in length at some facility, agency, or food service business.

Following completion of all educational coursework and programs each individual must pass a national examination given by the Commission on Dietetic Registration (CDR). Registered dietitians have to meet continuing professional educational requirements throughout their careers to maintain an active certification.

According to the U.S. Bureau of Labor Statistics the job outlook for registered dietitians is expected to increase at least through the year 2014. Reasons for that growth include an increased emphasis on wellness and preventative health, more public interest in nutrition, an expanding senior population, and the continued growth of physician clinics and residential care facilities. The only area where those job numbers are expected to show little growth is in hospital employment of registered dietitians because of anticipated reduced lengths of hospital stays (American Dietetic Association, "Registered Dietitian [RD]").

*Sharon Zoumbaris*

*See also* Nutrition.

## References

"Amanda Freitag of Chopped and Iron Chef America Teams up with Multiple Sclerosis Nutritionist to Create Nutrition Resource for People with MS." December 17, 2010. http:www.benzinga.com.

American Dietetic Association. "Registered Dietitian (RD)." www.eatright.org.

Brown, Amy Christine. *Understanding Food: Principles and Preparation.* Florence, KY: Wadsworth, 2007.

Herbold, Nancie. *Dietitian's Pocket Guide to Nutrition.* Sudbury, MA: Jones and Bartlett, 2008.

Payne-Palacio, June R., and Deborah D. Canter. *The Profession of Dietetics: A Team Approach.* Sudbury, MA: Jones and Bartlett, 2010.

## REIKI

Reiki is a healing practice that originated in Japan. It is derived from two Japanese words, *rei,* or "universal," and *ki,* or "life energy." Reiki seeks to treat the whole person including body, mind, spirit, and emotions. Current Reiki practice can be traced to the spiritual teachings of Dr. Mikao Usui in Japan during the early 20th century. Usui's teachings included meditative techniques and healing practices. Chujiro Hayashi, a student of Usui, placed less emphasis on the meditative techniques. That version of Reiki was then taught to American Hawayo Takata who introduced it to Western cultures in the late 1930s. In the United States today the type of Reiki practiced and taught by Hayashi and Takata is considered traditional Reiki as numerous other variations have been developed and are now widely practiced.

An increasing number of U.S. medical institutions such as hospitals and pain centers are integrating more mind-body and alternative practices into patient care. The National Institutes of Health (NIH) includes Reiki in the complementary and alternative medicine category and is funding studies on its usefulness in treating pain and other symptoms of everything from cancer to AIDS. Through its Center for Complementary and Alternative Medicine, the NIH released statistics that show in the United States some 4 in every 10 adults use some form of complementary and alternative medicine including Reiki, acupuncture, Pilates, and therapeutic touch. The growing interest in alternative therapies may be based on positive anecdotal reports of effectiveness and on studies that indicate Reiki can be effective at reducing pain, anxiety, and stress and increasing a sense of well-being (Hayes, 2008).

According to a 2007 National Health Interview Survey, conducted by the U.S. Department of Health and Human Services, National Institutes of Health, National Center for Complementary and Alternative Medicine (NCCAM), more than 1.2 million adults in the United States had used an energy healing therapy, such as Reiki, in the previous year and more than 161,000 children had used energy healing therapy in that same year.

Reiki practitioners place their hands lightly on or just above the person receiving treatment to facilitate that person's own healing response. Reiki is based on the idea that there is a source of energy that supports the human body's innate healing abilities. According to Reiki's principles, each individual has the innate ability to channel Reiki energy. However, that ability may be difficult to get to without the instruction of a Reiki teacher. Practitioners channel that energy into the body and facilitate healing. While Reiki can be practiced as a form of self-care, it is often received from someone else and is available in a growing variety of health care settings, including medical offices, hospitals, and clinics.

In a Reiki session, the fully clothed client lies down or sits comfortably. The practitioner places her hands lightly on or just above the client's body, palms down, using a series of 12 to 15 different hand positions. Each position is held for anywhere from two to five minutes or until the practitioner can feel the flow

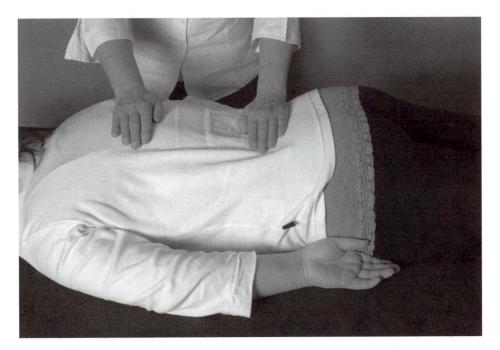

A practitioner performs Reiki on a client. During a Reiki session, the client lies down or sits comfortably while the practitioner places his or her hands lightly on or just above the client's body, palms down, using different hand positions to facilitate healing energy. (Erik De Graaf/Dreamstime.com)

of energy. That energy is often described as heat or tingling in the hands. When it slows or stops the session ends.

The number and duration of sessions depends on the needs of the client. People turn to Reiki for relaxation, stress reduction, and it has been used by people with anxiety, chronic pain, HIV, and other health conditions as well as by people recovering from surgery or experiencing side effects from cancer treatments. Scientific research is underway to learn more about how Reiki may work and its possible effects on health and diseases. In the United States Reiki is considered alternative medicine and is not recommended as a replacement for proven conventional care or as an alterative to seeing a doctor about a medical problem.

Currently, training and certification for Reiki practitioners are not formally regulated. While many of the people who seek training in Reiki have increasingly been licensed health care professionals, there are no licensing or professional standards for the practice of Reiki. Those interested in learning the practice are taught by experienced practitioners, known as Masters. Training has three degrees or levels, each one focused on a different aspect of Reiki. Each degree includes one or more initiations, also known as attunements or empowerments. Reiki energy is activated through these initiations provided by the Reiki Master teacher. Reiki cannot be self-taught. In first-degree training, students learn to perform Reiki on themselves and others. Second-degree training provides training on how to perform Reiki on others from a distance. Master-level training or third-degree is for those students who seek to become a Reiki Master. This process can take years. Although Reiki is spiritual in nature, it is not a religion and has no dogma or belief system. Reiki founder Usui recommended that practitioners of Reiki follow certain ethical ideals to promote peace and harmony.

The NCCAM has supported studies to investigate various aspects of Reiki and its potential uses for treating the symptoms of fibromyalgia as well as if it can reduce nerve pain and cardiovascular risk in people with Type 2 diabetes.

*Sharon Zoumbaris*

*See also* Fibromyalgia; Stress; Therapeutic Touch; Yoga.

## References

Archer, Shirley. "Leading U.S. Trauma Center Using Body-Mind Methods." *IDEA Fitness Journal* 5, no. 1 (January 2008): 90.

Archer, Shirley. "More Than 50 U.S. Hospitals Use Energy Healing." *IDEA Fitness Journal* 3, no. 2 (February 2006): 84.

Buch, Linda J., and Kristen Browning-Blas. "Relief for Your Back Is at Hand: Alternative Remedies from Rolfing to Reiki Hold the Magic Touch Many Sufferers Seek." *Denver Post,* February 12, 2010, C1.

Hayes, Susan. "Calming Vibe: Reiki, a Japanese Healing Treatment, Quiets the Body and Spirit by Tapping into a 'Life Force.'" *Natural Health* 38, no. 3 (March 2008): 96–99.

Narrin, Janeanne. *One Degree Beyond: A Reiki Journey into Energy Medicine.* Seattle: Little White Buffalo, 1998.

Rowland, Amy Zaffarano. *Traditional Reiki for Our Times: Practical Methods for Personal and Planetary Healing.* Rochester, VT: Healing Arts Press, 1998.

Stein, Diane. *Essential Reiki: A Complete Guide to an Ancient Healing Art.* Berkeley, CA: Crossing Press, 1995.

"Yoga Connection: Are Yoga and Reiki Compatible?" *Jakarta Post,* January 20, 2010, 27.

## RELIGION AND SPIRITUALITY

Individuals have held religious and spiritual beliefs since the beginning of recorded history. For some, these religious and spiritual beliefs provide a core sense of identity, purpose, and values that direct life choices. Because religion and spirituality are such strong motivators of human behavior, issues regarding religion and spirituality often bring up strong feelings, both positive and negative. Recently there has been a growing interest and body of research that examines how religious and spiritual beliefs affect one's physical and mental health and wellness. This interest and research has spanned several fields, including psychology, health behavior, medicine, gerontology, epidemiology, and sociology. In this section, we (1) define religion and spirituality and note its prevalence, (2) briefly review the existing research linking religion and spirituality to health and wellness, and (3) discuss possible mechanisms by which religion and spirituality may affect health and wellness.

**What Is Religion?** The majority of Americans report having religious and spiritual beliefs, and many indicate that their religious and spiritual beliefs are important to their lives. For example, surveys indicate that 96 percent of people believe in God or a universal spirit (Gallup, 1995), 92 percent identify with an organized religion (Kosmin & Lachman, 1993), 90 percent pray, 71 percent belong to a church or synagogue, and 42 percent attend worship services weekly (Hoge, 1996). Thus, the impact of religious and spiritual beliefs is widespread. Polls also indicate that the level of interest in religious topics and the number of people who believe that religion is influential has been increasing in recent years (Princeton Religion Research Center, "Dramatic Rise," 1999).

Religion and spirituality are two constructs that have historically been synonymous. Although most individuals still view religion and spirituality as closely linked, researchers have recently clarified the definitions of these constructs. Religion has been defined as the adherence to a belief system and practices associated with a tradition and community in which there is agreement about what is believed and practiced regarding the sacred (Hill et al., 2000). Spirituality, on the other hand, has been defined as a more general feeling of closeness and connectedness with the sacred (Hill et al., 2000). Thus, a person might be (1) both spiritual and religious, (2) spiritual but not religious, (3) religious but not spiritual, or (4) neither spiritual nor religious. Most people, however, experience spirituality in the context of religion. Other types of spirituality include humanistic spirituality (i.e., connection to humankind), nature spirituality (i.e., connection to the environment), and cosmos spirituality (i.e., connection to the whole of creation). Most of the existing research on the connection between religion, spirituality, and wellness has focused on religious involvement rather than personal spirituality. Thus, religion will be the focus of our brief review of research.

**Early Doubts** In the past, scientists have been somewhat antagonistic toward religion and spirituality, and skeptical about research purporting any possible benefits of religion and spirituality on wellness. We present two reasons for this stance. First, in the United States there has been a precedence valuing the separation of church and state. Because many universities are entities of the state, some have considered religion and spirituality to be a topic that should not, or even cannot, be studied scientifically. Second, scientists have often been less religious than the general population. For example, in a national survey, clinical psychologists were less likely to believe in God or report regular involvement with a religious organization than was the general population (Shafranske & Malony, 1990). Furthermore, clinical psychologists also tended to identify more strongly with spirituality than religion (Shafranske & Malony, 1990). A person's values affect what is viewed as an important or valuable topic to study, as well as how research findings are interpreted.

This negativity permeated early writing on the relationship between religion, spirituality, and health. Research on the connection between religion and physical health reminded scientists and readers of charlatans and witch doctors, or of the dangerous "religious" healings of the past. In the area of mental health, Freud (1927) viewed religion as an unhealthy defense mechanism, a strategy that people use to fulfill their wish for an omnipotent father figure. Freud's negative attitudes toward religion seemed to arise from his work with clients; many had unhealthy experiences with religion and were also suffering from mental health problems. Other prominent psychologists also expressed negative views toward religion and spirituality, including B. F. Skinner (1953) and Albert Ellis (1980).

Early research on the relationships between religion, spirituality, and health generally reported a positive relationship, but the early studies lacked scientific rigor (e.g., cross-sectional rather than longitudinal designs; failing to control for other variables that might obscure the relationship between religion, spirituality, and health; Powell, Shahabi, and Thoresen, 2003). Namely, suppose a researcher conducted a study on religion and physical health and found that, on average, the religious participants in the sample were healthier than the nonreligious participants. There are several interpretations of this finding. It could be that (1) religion causes better health, (2) healthier people choose to be more religious, or (3) there is some other variable that is causing people to both be religious and have better health.

Although these concerns have cast some doubt on the veracity of claims that religion and spirituality truly affect health and wellness (see Sloan, Bagiella, & Powell, 1999 for a persuasive argument), there has recently been a marked increase in studies that examine the religion-health connection using high-quality designs that are longitudinal and/or control for possible confounding variables (Miller & Thoresen, 2003). The overall conclusion of these research studies has remained the same. On the whole, there appears to be a positive association between religion and spirituality and both physical health (Powell et al., 2003) and mental health (Koenig & Larson, 2001).

**Physical Health**    In the area of physical health, the most consistent evidence occurs in the area of religious involvement and mortality. Namely, religious individuals have a lower risk of death, even when controlling for possible confounding variables such as demographic and socioeconomic factors, social support, and depression (Powell et al., 2003). For example, in a large nationwide survey of 3,617 individuals, participants who attended religious services at least once a month were 30–35 percent less likely to die over a 7.5-year follow-up period than were participants who attended religious services less than once a month, even after adjusting for possible confounding variables (Musick, House, & Williams, 2004). Evidence for a religion–physical health link has also accrued in the areas of heart disease, hypertension, stroke, cancer, gastrointestinal disease, self-rated health, physical disability, and self-reported physical health symptoms (Ellison & Levin, 1998). For example, in a study of 6,545 individuals, participants who attended religious services weekly were 17 percent less likely to die from cardiovascular disease over a 31-year follow-up period than were those who attended religious services less frequently, even after adjusting for possible confounding variables (Oman, Kurata, Strawbridge, & Cohen, 2002).

**Mental Health**    In the area of mental health, the majority of research again supports a positive relationship between religion, spirituality, and positive mental health. Religious individuals generally report greater well-being, hope, and optimism, as well as less depression, anxiety, and risk of suicide (Koenig & Larson, 2001). For example, in a study of 1,125 individuals, religious attendance was positively related to satisfaction with life, even when controlling for several demographic variables (Levin, Markides, & Ray, 1996). In a study of 111 depressed hospital patients, patients who were more religious reported that their depressive symptoms resolved more quickly than those who were less religious (Koenig, George, & Peterson, 1998). Religious individuals tend to be less likely to abuse alcohol or take illicit drugs (Koenig & Larson, 2001). For example, in a national survey of 7,370 individuals, participants who were religious were more likely to abstain from alcohol than drink, and were also more likely to be moderate drinkers than heavy drinkers (Michalak, Trocki, & Bond, 2007). This relationship held even when controlling for several demographic variables.

Several mechanisms have been proposed to explain the link between religion, spirituality, and physical and mental health (Ellison & Levin, 1998). First, religious involvement may involve the regulation of individual lifestyles and health behaviors. For example, many religious groups advocate a specific set of behaviors (e.g., abstaining from drug use, moderate alcohol intake, and sexual monogamy), as well as resources to promote self-control (e.g., social norms). Second, religious involvement provides a unique source of social integration and support. Religious individuals often have well-developed social networks that they are able to rely on for both instrumental aid (e.g., food, financial assistance) and emotional support. Third, religious involvement provides individuals with meaning. Many religions provide the individual with a worldview that specifies a purpose for religious followers. This may help religious individuals to be more hopeful and optimistic. Fourth, religion provides followers with a useful way to cope with stress. Pargament (1997) has noted that religious individuals often engage the Sacred in order to cope with difficult life events. Religious coping mechanisms such as prayer may help individuals interpret stressful events in ways that reduce stress, such as viewing the event as an opportunity for spiritual growth. In addition, religious or spiritual individuals may see themselves as working alongside God to deal with a difficult situation, giving them greater confidence that they can effectively navigate their circumstances, no matter how difficult.

**Negative Aspects**  Although religion and spirituality are generally linked with positive health and mental health, this does not mean that there are no harmful effects of religion and spirituality on health, or that religious involvement is helpful for all individuals. For example, Pargament (1997) has noted that some styles of religious coping may be maladaptive and actually lead to poorer health outcomes. Examples of maladaptive religious coping styles are passively leaving the responsibility to resolve a problem to divine intervention, praying for God's vengeance on another person, or ruminating about unresolved anger toward God. Also, religious involvement may induce shame and fear, especially for individuals that do not live up to their religious values. Religion has also been associated with certain negative personality traits (e.g., authoritarianism, rigidity, dogmatism, suggestibility, and dependence; Gartner, 1996) that may lead to poorer physical health or mental health. Finally, some traumatic events may cause a person to deeply struggle with or even fall away from his faith. This sort of spiritual struggle is especially stressful and has been found to be associated with poor health outcomes, including increased risk of mortality (Ai, Seymour, Tice, Kronfol, & Bolling, 2009).

In sum, research evidence has accumulated that supports a positive overall relationship between religion, spirituality, and wellness, including both physical and mental health. As scientific rigor of studies has increased, studies have bolstered the conclusion that, overall, religion and spirituality encourage health and wellness through reducing a person's exposure to stress, enhancing social support and meaning, and helping people deal more effectively with stress.

*Joshua Hook and Don E. Davis*

*See also* Depression; Heart Health; Hypertension.

## References

Ai, A. L., E. M. Seymour, T. N. Tice, Z. Kronfol, and S. F. Bolling. "Spiritual Struggle Related to Plasma Interleukin-6 Prior to Cardiac Surgery." *Psychology of Religion and Spirituality* 1 (2009): 112–28.

Ellis, A. "Psychotherapy and Atheistic Values: A Response to A. E. Bergin's 'Psychotherapy and Religious Values.'" *Journal of Consulting and Clinical Psychology* 48 (1980): 635–39.

Ellison, C.G., and J.S. Levin. "The Religion–Health Connection: Evidence, Theory, and Future Directions." *Health Education and Behavior* 25 (1998): 700–20.

Freud, S. "The Future of an Illusion." In *The Standard Edition of the Complete Psychological Works of Sigmund Freud,* edited and translated by J. Strachey. Vol. 21, 1–56. London: Hogarth Press and the Institute of Psycho-Analysis, 1961. Original work published 1927.

Gallup, G., Jr. *The Gallup Poll: Public Opinion 1995.* Wilmington, DE: Scholarly Resources, 1995.

Gartner, J. "Religious Commitment, Mental Health, and Prosocial Behavior: A Review of the Empirical Literature." In *Religion and the Clinical Practice of Psychology,* edited by E.P. Shafranske, 187–214. Washington, DC: American Psychological Association, 1996.

Hill, P.C., K.I. Pargament, R.W. Hood, Jr., M.E. McCullough, J.P. Swyers, D.B. Larson, and B.J. Zinnbauer. "Conceptualizing Religion and Spirituality: Points of Commonality, Points of Departure." *Journal for the Theory of Social Behavior* 30 (2000): 51–77.

Hoge, D.R. "Religion in America: The Demographics of Belief and Affiliation." In *Religion and the Clinical Practice of Psychology,* edited by E.P. Shafranske, 21–41. Washington, DC: American Psychological Association, 1996.

Koenig, H.G., L.K. George, and B.L. Peterson. "Religiosity and Remission of Depression in Medically Ill Older Patients." *American Journal of Psychiatry* 155 (1998): 536–42.

Koenig, H.G., and D.B. Larson. "Religion and Mental Health: Evidence for an Association." *International Review of Psychiatry* 13 (2001): 67–78.

Kosmin, B.A., and S.P. Lachman. *One Nation under God: Religion in Contemporary American Society.* New York: Harmony, 1993.

Levin, J.S., K.S. Markides, and L.A. Ray. "Religious Attendance and Psychological Well-Being in Mexican Americans: A Panel Analysis of Three-Generation Data." *The Gerontologist* 36 (1996): 454–63.

Michalak, L., K. Trocki, and J. Bond. "Religion and Alcohol in the U.S. National Alcohol Survey: How Important Is Religion for Abstention and Drinking?" *Drug and Alcohol Dependence* 87 (2007): 268–80.

Miller, W.R., and C.E. Thoresen (2003). "Spirituality, Religion, and Health: An Emerging Research Field." *American Psychologist* 58 (2003): 24–35.

Musick, M.A., J.S. House, and D.R. Williams. "Attendance at Religious Services and Mortality in a National Sample." *Journal of Health and Social Behavior* 45 (2004): 198–213.

Oman, D., J.H. Kurata, W.J. Strawbridge, and R.D. Cohen. "Religious Attendance and Cause of Death over 31 Years." *International Journal of Psychiatry in Medicine* 32 (2002): 69–89.

Pargament, K.I. *The Psychology of Religion and Coping.* New York: Guilford Press, 1997.

Powell, L.H., L. Shahabi, and C.E. Thoresen. "Religion and Spirituality: Linkages to Physical Health." *American Psychologist* 58 (2003): 36–52.

Princeton Religion Research Center. "Dramatic Rise Seen in Those Who Say Religion Increasing in Influence." *Emerging Trends* 20, nos. 4–5 (1999): 1. Princeton, NJ: The Gallup Poll.

Princeton Religion Research Center. "Index of Leading Religious Indicators at Highest Point in 13 Years." *Emerging Trends* 21, no. 2 (1999): 1. Princeton, NJ: The Gallup Poll.

Shafranske, E.P., and H.N. Malony. "Clinical Psychologists' Religious and Spiritual Orientations and Their Practice of Psychotherapy." *Psychotherapy: Theory, Research, Practice, Training* 27 (1990): 72–78.

Skinner, B.F. *Science and Human Behavior.* New York: Macmillan, 1953.

Sloan, R.P., E. Bagiella, and T. Powell. "Religion, Spirituality, and Medicine." *Lancet* 353 (1999): 664–67.

## RESTING METABOLIC RATE

Resting metabolic rate is the rate at which your body consumes calories during rest. Your body burns up calories simply to support its basic functions. *Total daily energy expenditure* (TDEE) is the term used to describe how much energy is used or how many calories are burned by one person during a 24-hour period. TDEE has three main components, which include resting metabolic rate, the thermic effect of physical activity or exercise, and the thermic effect of food. To create a baseline for the appropriate overall calorie intake, it might be helpful to know your resting metabolic rate. Once you determine it, you can multiply it by another factor, depending on your activity level, to calculate an approximate daily calorie need.

Men and women use different formulas to calculate their resting metabolic rate. For women, start with 655, then add your weight × 4.3, add your height in inches × 4.3, and subtract your age in years × 4.7.

Here's an example for a 20-year-old female, 5'4" or 64 inches tall, weighing 130 pounds.

655 + (130 × 4.3 = 559)
+ (64 × 4.3 = 275) – (20 × 4.7 = 94)

or

655 + 559 + 275 – 94 = 1,395.

That means this young woman's resting metabolic rate is about 1,395 calories per day.

For men, the formula is this:

66 + (weight × 6.2) + (height in inches × 12.7) – (age in years × 6.8)

Our example here is a 22-year-old male, 5'10" (or 70 inches) weighing 190 pounds.

66 + (190 × 6.2 = 1,178)
+ (70 × 12.7 = 889) – (22 × 4.7 = 120)

or

66 + 1,178 + 889 – 150 = 1,983.

Knowing your resting metabolic rate is just a starting point in determining the amount of calories to consume. Your active metabolic rate, or the amount of calories you burn while moving around and doing other physical activities, will obviously be higher. About 65 to 80 percent of the calories your body burns up are consumed while your body is at rest. One rule of thumb is that sedentary people should multiply their resting metabolic rate by 1.2; moderately active people can multiply it by 1.4; and serious athletes can multiply it by 1.8.

The single most important factor is determining resting metabolic rate is lean muscle tissue. Muscle tissue uses up to 22 percent of an individual's daily calories just to exist. For Americans anxious to lose weight, increasing the metabolic rate by developing more muscle tissue is a key weight loss strategy. In fact, resting muscle uses five times as many calories a day as fat does.

One reason women have more trouble losing weight than men is that women have less muscle than men and burn fewer calories. Researchers have also found that yo-yo dieting, which causes a repeated weight loss followed by weight gain, can permanently lower an individual's metabolism, as can certain medications. Aging adds another hurdle for women who, once they reach around age 40, start to lose muscle and gain equivalent amounts of body fat as their metabolism slows. These changes can accelerate in the years after menopause. Still, while some weight gain is inevitable, as Americans get older they can work against this problem with exercise and weight training.

Nutritionists also recommend basic lifestyle changes such as eating a more healthful diet and lowering the amount of food consumed at each meal. Meal content should include a serving of good quality protein at every meal since 25 to 30 percent of the calories from protein are used up in its metabolism.

This is where the thermic effect of food comes into play because a percentage of calories consumed each day are used in digesting what has been eaten. The thermic effect of food accounts for approximately 10 percent of the daily energy expenditure for the average person. For carbohydrates, just 6 to 8 of every 100 calories are used and just 2 to 3 of every 100 fat calories are burned during digestion. For individuals looking to manage their weight or lose weight, the choice of a healthy diet with good protein along with exercise can be a winning combination.

*Marjolijn Bijlefeld and Sharon Zoumbaris*

*See also* Calories; Exercise; Weight Training; Yo-Yo Dieting.

## References

"Avoid Weight Gain in Later Life: Taking Steps to Minimize Excess Fat after Menopause Can Lower Your Risk of Heart Disease and Diabetes." *Women's Health Advisor* 11, no. 4 (April 2007): 4.

Benardot, D., and W.P. Thompson. "Energy from Food for Physical Activity: Enough and on Time." *ACSM's Health and Fitness Journal* 3 (1999): 14–18.

Bowden, Jonny. "Why You Can't Lose Weight: Ditching Pounds Can Be a Challenge, but Some Practical Strategies Can Help You Succeed." *Better Nutrition* (July 2009): 38.

Kinucan, Paige, and Len Kravitz. "Controversies in Metabolism: How Do Resistance Training, Diet and Age Affect Resting Metabolic Rate?" *IDEA Fitness Journal* 3, no. 1 (2006): 20.

Murphy, Sam. "Weekend Wellbeing: Seven Ways to Boost Your Metabolism." *The Guardian,* January 28, 2006, 66.

Sparti, A., J.P. DeLany, J.A. dela Bretonne, G.E. Sander, and G.A. Bray. "Relationship between Resting Metabolic Rate and the Composition of the Fat Free Mass." *Metabolism* 46 (1997): 1225–30.

## RETAIL CLINIC

Health care is a business. In the 19th and early 20th centuries, doctors bartered their services, often accepting farm products or crafts from patients in exchange for treatment. The transaction between the patient and provider was arm's length. But all of that changed with the introduction of health insurance in the mid-20th century. Increasingly, third-party payers (i.e., government, insurers, and employers) assumed control of the pricing and purchasing of health care (Starr, 1982). Providing health care services became more of a *wholesale* business with doctors and hospitals selling their services to third-party payers instead of directly to patients (Honaman, 2006).

However, the emergence of the retail clinic offers consumers an alternative to wholesale health care. Retail involves selling small quantities of goods and services directly to the consumer. Consequently, there is no middleman (third-party payer) so the costs are reduced.

Retail clinics, also known as retail-based health clinics or convenient care clinics, have become one of the fastest-growing segments of the health care sector (Costello, 2008). Even though thousands of freestanding primary care clinics have been operating across the United States, including many in shopping mall locations, they have been staffed primarily by physicians. The retail health clinics represent a new model for primary care services for the consumer. They offer a limited number of services at lower prices and almost always are staffed by a nurse practitioner (Turner, 2007).

Despite rapid growth and increasing national attention to retail clinics, these clinics are still a fairly new phenomenon, and little is known about them. There are few sources of reliable information and studies that detail and describe these clinics. However, what has been suggested by consumers and researchers alike is that retail clinics represent an affordable alternative for primary care. They offer increased access to groups that typically have difficulty accessing health care services, especially the uninsured and minorities. Yet, as of 2007, only 2.3 percent of families in the United States reported ever having visited a retail clinic (Tu & Cohen, 2008).

At the beginning of 2006, there were only 60 retail clinics in the United States (Consumer Reports, 2009). By the end of 2008, industry expert Merchant Medicine reported a year of record growth for retail clinics. There were approximately 1,175 retail clinics located in 37 different states, with Florida reporting the highest number of retail clinics in operation (122) than any other state. This represents a net increase of 274 clinics from 2007. In addition, a total of 55 retail clinic operators were identified, and 43 different retailers were reported as "hosting" these clinics in their stores. In the host capacity, the retailer functions as a landlord and leases space to the clinic operator (Merchant Medicine, *Retail Clinics and the Changing Primary Care Landscape*).

In the face of such positive growth, however, there was a more significant development: clinic closures. Approximately 150 retail clinics were closed during 2008, and about 80 of the closures were the result of some privately backed clinic operators going out of business while others exited because they were not willing to wait up to two years for profits (Merchant Medicine, *Retail Clinics and the Changing Primary Care Landscape*).

In addition, the retailers associated with retail clinics began to change their strategies. Some retail pharmacy chains began pursuing acquisition strategies and buying clinic operators. Meanwhile, the world's largest discount retailer, Wal-Mart, has rejected buying clinic operators and prefers to function as a landlord. However, Wal-Mart continues to experiment and test different clinic models, including a telemedicine model, as well as partnering with hospital system–owned clinics in an effort to cobrand the retail clinic.

**What Do We Know about Retail Clinics?**   Retail clinics are in many ways an experiment that links retailers and health care. Clinics are typically located in retail stores such as Wal-Mart, Target, Walgreens, and CVS, and grocery chains such as Publix or Kroger. Therefore, instead of the consumer entering the health care system in the routine manner by visiting a physician in his office or the emergency room, patients may now access health care when they go shopping. This means that there is a new portal of entry to the health care system for the consumer, one that lies outside of *mainstream* health care (Tu & Cohen, 2008).

By offering patients a new portal for medical care, retailers are separating basic health care services from traditional providers and offering patients a means of escaping what has previously been a captive system. This captive system has contained few alternatives for patients, especially within the restrictions of tightly managed medical care. Retailers are also revising the relationship with the patient's physician, who is not involved in the decision to seek services at a retail health care clinic. Such changes will require a new logic about marketing as customers toggle between retail and traditional health care system boundaries.

**New Portal of Care**   Retail clinics function as a *portal* to the primary care system, especially for those who do not have a regular source of care. In the Rand Corporation Study (2008), which analyzed data for 1.3 million clinic visits from 2000 through 2007, fully 60 percent of those surveyed did not have a primary care physician (PCP). Young adults (ages 18–44) in particular did not have a regular source of care, and they accounted for 43 percent of all clinic visits (Mehrotra et al., 2008).

Most of the users of retail clinics appear to understand that retail clinic visits are for basic medical needs, including minor injuries and illnesses. Only 2.3 percent of clinic patients end up being referred to the emergency department. Listed below are the 10 simple conditions and preventive care that were identified in the Rand Corporation Study as reasons for visiting a retail clinic. They represented approximately 90 percent of retail clinic visits:

Upper respiratory infections
Sinusitis
Bronchitis
Sore throat
Immunizations

Inner ear infections
Swimmer's ear
Conjunctivitis
Urinary tract infections
And either a screening test or a blood test (Mehrotra et al., 2008).

Meanwhile, another major study looked at family use of retail clinics. The researchers analyzed data from the 2007 Health Tracking Household Survey that was conducted by the Center for Studying Health System Change. The analysis revealed that users tended to be younger families and people who had difficulty gaining access to the health care system, including the uninsured and minorities. Uninsured families accounted for 27 percent of retail clinic visits. The finding that such families used clinics at a much higher rate than their share of the population is consistent with previous research about uninsured consumers (Tu & Cohen, 2008).

Most clinics offer extended hours, including evening hours and weekends. Typically no appointments are needed, and there is little waiting time. Clinic visits tend to be brief or about 15 minutes. Patients usually can use waiting time productively by shopping elsewhere in the store (Andrews, 2004; Rice, 2005; Spencer, 2005). The charges for services at a retail clinic tend to be much lower than what would be expected in an emergency department or physician practice.

Health care innovations precipitated the development of retail clinics. Retail clinics are possible because of cost-reducing innovations in health care such as the development of inexpensive yet reliable tests for strep throat and other infections. They are also possible because of the development of rules-based treatment protocols that expand diagnostic and treatment capabilities of nonphysician providers such as nurse practitioners (Robinson & Smith, 2008).

**What Does the Future Predict for Retail Clinics?** The impact of the retail clinic is potentially very substantial. It includes lower costs for services, increased access to primary care especially for the uninsured and underinsured, increased convenience for the customer, and perhaps a solution for the shortage of primary care physicians. Even though these clinics may appeal to consumers, they directly challenge existing models of physician-directed care that have prevailed in the United States for more than a century (Winkenwerder, 2008).

However, the larger question remains regarding the future of retail clinics: Will they be profitable? If the clinics are not profitable, retailers will look for other means of entering health care markets. Because retail clinics are capital-intensive, they take time to return a profit. Many private investors that initially backed retail clinic operators thought that they could make a quick return off of their investment. They were not prepared for a long-term commitment. Smart Care, one of the privately backed retail clinic operators that closed, saw investors exit before clinics were launched (Merchant Medicine, *Primary Care Meets Private Investor*). But retailers and large investors and entrepreneurs appear to still be in the game and willing to continue to revise their business models to achieve success.

Retail clinics have a short history in health care. Yet because of the "fast" nature of the retail industry, they have undergone an accelerated evolution of growth and development in search of profitability. The early "host" model in which retailers leased store space to privately backed clinic operators still exists, but there have been some revisions to the model. Larger pharmacy retailers have transitioned to owners of clinic companies through acquisition and have shifted from opening new clinics to also developing new markets, products, and services such as pharmacy benefits management programs with self-insured employers (Merchant Medicine, *Retail Clinics: 2008 Year-End Review and 2009 Outlook,* 2009). Furthermore, the growth of hospital-linked retail clinics bears watching as hospitals have discovered that these clinics perform as feeder systems for them (Freudenheim, 2009).

**Putting Consumers First**  In *Money Driven Medicine* (2006), author Maggie Mahar suggests that the purchase of health care is different from other purchases because the transaction is based on trust and the belief that the physician will put the patients' interests first. This is contrary to what occurs among corporate retailers who may put their shareholders' interests ahead of their customers.

Corporate retailers such as Wal-Mart and McDonald's are expected to be honest, but they are not expected to be selfless; they are not expected to put their customers' interests ahead of their shareholders'. But physicians are not retailers, and health care is not a retail industry or even a service industry in the ordinary sense of the term (Mahar, 2006, pp. 343–44).

Given the trend toward retail clinics, especially hospital-linked retail clinics, the nature of the health care industry may be changing.

*Myron D. Fottler and Donna M. Malvey*

*See also* Health Insurance; Medicaid; Medicare; Primary Care Physicians.

## References

Andrews, M. "Next to the Express Checkout, Express Medical Care." *New York Times,* July 18, 2004. www.nytimes.com.

Bohmer, R. "The Rise of In-Store Clinics—Threats or Opportunity?" *New England Journal of Medicine* 356, no. 8 (2007): 765–68.

Consumer Reports. "When You Need Care Fast." *Consumer Reports on Health* (April 2009): 6.

Costello, D. "Report from the Field—A Checkup for Retail Medicine." *Health Affairs* 27, no. 5 (2008): 1299–1303.

Fenn, S. "Integrating CCCs into the Hospital System." *Frontiers of Health Services Management* 24, no. 3 (2008): 33–36.

Freudenheim, M. "Hospitals Begin to Move into Supermarkets." *New York Times,* May 12, 2009. www.nytimes.com/2009/05/12/business/12clinic.html.

Goldstein, J. "Wal-Mart Clinics Close in 23 Stores." *Wall Street Journal,* January 29, 2008. http://blogs.wsj.com/health/2008/01/29/wal-mart-clinics-close-in-23-stores/?mod=homeblogmod_healthb.

Honaman, C.J. "Going Retail—New Leadership Skills to Keep up with Healthcare's Market Shift." *Healthcare Executive* (November/December 2006): 49–50.

Litch, B. "Retail Clinics: Making the Decision to Join the Game." *Healthcare Executive* 23, no. 5 (September/October 2008): 27–33.

Mahar, M. *Money Driven Medicine.* New York: HarperCollins, 2006.

Mehrotra, A., M.C. Wang, J.R. Lave, J.L. Adams, and E.A. McGlynn. "Retail Clinics, Primary Care Physicians, and Emergency Departments: A Comparison of Patients' Visits." *Health Affairs* 27, no. 5 (September/October 2008): 1272–82.

Merchant Medicine. *Feature: Retail Clinics and Primary Care, Will the Scope of Care Always Be Simple Episodic Illnesses?* 2008. www.merchantmedicine.com/Home.cfm.

Merchant Medicine. *Primary Care Meets Private Investor: Former Retail Clinic Operators Share Lessons Learned.* April 2, 2009. www.merchantmedicine.com/news.cfm?view=29.

Merchant Medicine. *Retail Clinics and the Changing Primary Care Landscape.* April 2, 2009. www.merchantmedicine.com/news.cfm?view=25.

Merchant Medicine. *Retail Clinics by Metro Area: A Geographic Look at Clinic Saturation and Demand.* Vol. 2, no. 4. March 1, 2009. www.merchantmedicine.com/news.cfm?view=40.

Merchant Medicine. *Retail Clinics: 2008 Year-End Review and 2009 Outlook: Many Closures in 2008 but the Market Continues to Expand.* April 2, 2009. www.merchantmedicine.com/news.cfm?view=21.

Merchant Medicine. *A Travel Industry Giant Drops in on Healthcare: A Profile of Hal Rosenbluth.* April 2, 2009. www.merchantmedicine.com/news.cfm?view=36.

Rice, B. (2005). *In-Store Clinics: Should You Worry?* 2005. http://medicaleconomics.modernmedicine.com/memag/article/articleDetail.jsp?id=179078.

Robinson, J.C., and M.D. Smith. "Perspective—Cost-Reducing Innovation in Health Care." *Health Affairs* 27, no. 5 (September/October 2008): 1353–56.

Scott, M. "Health Care in the Express Lane: The Emergence of Retail Clinics." Report prepared for the California Healthcare Foundation, 2006.

Scott, M.K. *Health Care in the Express Lane: Retail Clinics Go Mainstream.* California Health-Care Foundation. 2007. www.chcf.org/topics/view.cfm?itemid=133464.

Spencer, J. "Getting Your Healthcare at Wal-Mart." *Wall Street Journal,* 266(70), October 5, 2005, D1–D5.

Starr, P. *The Social Transformation of American Medicine.* New York: Basic Books, 1982.

Tu, H.T., and G.R. Cohen. "Checking up on Retail-Based Health Clinics: Is the Boom Ending?" *The Commonwealth Fund* 48 (2008): 1–12.

Turner, G. "Customer Health Care." *Wall Street Journal,* May 14, 2007, A17.

Winkenwerder, W. (2008). *Retail Medical Clinics: Here to Stay?* 2008. www.deloitte.com/dtt/article/0,1002,sid%253d127087%2526cid%253d192739,00.html.

# RITALIN

Ritalin is the trade name for a drug developed and distributed by Novartis. Its chemical composition is methylphenidate hydrochloride. It is packaged in 5-, 10-, and 20-milligram tablets to be taken orally, and is freely soluble in water. Ritalin contains such inactive ingredients as lactose, magnesium stearate, polyethylene glycol, starch, sucrose, talc, and tragacanth. It is available in slow release (SR) form as well as the standard form.

Ritalin is a central nervous system stimulant. The primary approved medical use of Ritalin is in treatment of narcolepsy, hyperactivity, attention deficit disorder

(ADD), and attention deficit hyperactivity disorder (ADHD) in children, though it also is prescribed for adult use in specifically indicated conditions. While little is understood about the way in which Ritalin affects the central nervous system, it is presumed that it activates the medulla of the brain and the cortex to produce the stimulation. It increases the production of dopamine and norepinephrine in the brain. The affects Ritalin has in children are something of a mystery, in that it reduces hyperactivity. The mechanism by which this is accomplished may be an overstimulation that produces an increased compensatory reaction in the child's chemistry or neurology that causes an actual decrease in stimulation or activity.

In children, the affects of Ritalin peak between two (standard) and four (SR) hours after ingestion and 33 percent of the dosage is effectively absorbed into the child's system. In adults the effective absorption is 14 percent. Effective rates of absorption are generally greater in females than in males, which may suggest lower effective doses for females in individual cases. ADD and ADHD specify a general syndrome that may be identified as hyperkinetic child syndrome, minimal brain damage, minimal cerebral dysfunction, and minor cerebral dysfunction. All of these respond effectively to the application of Ritalin.

Typically the prescription of Ritalin for such conditions is effective when combined with other types of therapy such as psychotherapy, educational support, and guided or structured socialization. Symptoms of the syndrome suggesting this combined approach to treatment tend to be a cluster of developmentally inappropriate behaviors including moderate or severe distractibility, short attention span, hyperactivity, emotional instability, and impulsivity. In some cases an abnormal EEG, learning disability, and other neurological indications may be present.

Ritalin should not be prescribed for patients with significant anxiety, tension, agitation, hypertension, cardiac abnormalities, instability or anomalies in pulse rate, hypersensitivity to medications, glaucoma, underlying medical conditions, motor tics or Tourette's syndrome, and tendencies toward psychosis. These conditions are likely to be aggravated by the application of Ritalin, and instances of blurred vision, seizures, strokes, and sudden death have been reported. This medication should be avoided in patients who are treated with monoamine oxidase inhibitors and for two weeks following the termination of such treatment. It should not be prescribed for children less than six years of age. Pregnant and nursing mothers should avoid Ritalin if possible.

A large, long-term study of the drug's effects on preschoolers underscored the importance of careful monitoring of preschoolers with ADHD who take Ritalin according to Thomas R. Insel, director of the National Institute of Mental Health in Bethesda, Maryland. The findings, reported in the fall of 2006, showed that some preschoolers developed more stimulant-related side effects, including irritability, insomnia, and weight loss than older children with ADHD have in prior studies. The U.S. Department of Health and Human Services list of medications approved for use with ADHD patients suggests Adderal as the top choice for children age 3 and older, and Ritalin for children age 6 and older.

Methylphenidate was first synthesized in 1944 and beginning in the 1960s was used to treat children with ADHD or ADD. Production and prescription rose

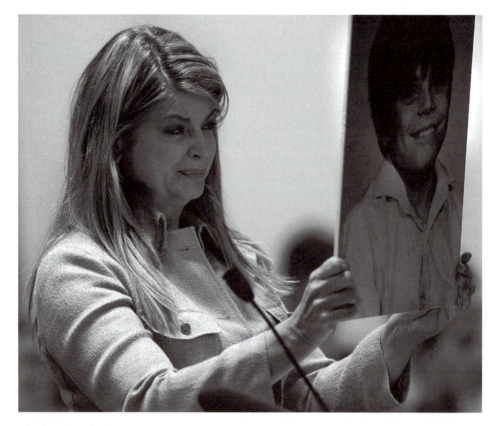

Kirstie Alley displays a picture of Raymond Perone, a 10-year-old suicide victim, while testifying in front of the Florida House Education Council for a bill to limit the prescribing of psychotropic drugs like Ritalin in Tallahassee, Florida, on April 19, 2005. According to Marla Filidei of the Citizens Commission on Human Rights, Raymond committed suicide while withdrawing from the use of Ritalin. (AP/Wide World Photos)

significantly in the United States in the 1990s as the diagnosis was more widely accepted. The medication comes in short-acting, long-acting, or slow-release varieties. In each variety, the active ingredient is the same but it is released differently in the body. Long-acting or slow-release (SR) forms are often preferred for school-aged children because the medicine only needs to be administered once a day before school. This means less disruption for the child as she no longer needs to make a daily trip to the school nurse for another dose. Dosage amounts are determined by many factors, including if the child needs medication only for the school hours or for evening and weekends, too.

In the company's advertisement brochure, Novartis has issued a specific warning regarding drug addicts. "Ritalin should be given cautiously to patients with a history of drug dependence or alcoholism. Chronic abusive use can lead to marked tolerance and psychological dependence with varying degrees of abnormal behavior. Frank psychotic episodes can occur, especially with parenteral or injected abuse. Careful supervision is required during withdrawal from abusive use, since severe depression may occur. Withdrawal following chronic therapeutic use may unmask symptoms of the underlying disorder that may require follow-up."

A recent form of abuse of the drug is now occurring among high school and college students who are using the drug in increasing numbers to help them learn and complete mentally challenging work. While it is still unproven whether Ritalin or Adderal provide any significant boost, students believe they do. Figures from the U.S. poison control centers showed a 76 percent increase in calls concerning teens and ADHD medications from 1998 to 2005. The pills are sometimes provided by students who already have a prescription for treatment of their hyperactivity or attention disorders, but Ritalin and other prescription medications are increasingly available through Internet sales.

*J. Harold Ellens*

*See also* Attention Deficit Hyperactivity Disorder (ADHD).

## References

"Attention Deficit Hyperactivity Disorder (ADHD)." U.S. Department of Health and Human Services National Institutes of Health. NIH Publication No. 08–3572, revised 2008. www.nimh.nih.gov/health/publications/attention-deficit-hyperacitivty-disorder/complete-index.shtml.

Aue, Pamela Willwerth. *Teen Drug Abuse.* Detroit: Thompson Gale, 2006.

Bower, B. "Med-Start Kids: Pros, Cons of Ritalin for Preschool ADHD." *Science News* (October 28, 2006): 275–77.

Coghill, D., and S. Seth. "Osmotic, Controlled-Release Methylphenidate for the Treatment of Attention-Deficit/Hyperactivity Disorder." *Expert Opinions in Pharmacotherapy* 7, no. 15 (October 2006): 2119–38.

Diller, Lawrence H. *Running on Ritalin: A Physician Reflects on Children, Society and Performance in a Pill.* New York: Bantam Books, 1998.

DSM–IV–TR Workgroup. *Diagnostic and Statistical Manual of Mental Disorders.* 4th ed., text rev. Washington, DC: American Psychiatric Association, 2000.

Hahn, Laura. "Rx Drug Alert." *Good Housekeeping* 250, no. 4 (April 2010): 109.

Mucha, Peter. "Smart Pills a Smart Idea, Penn Prof Tells '60 Minutes.'" *Philadelphia Inquirer,* April 26, 2010. www.philly.com/philly/health_and_science/9208779.html.

## RODALE, JEROME

Long before organic food was considered fashionable Jerome I. Rodale bought a farm in a small Pennsylvania town and set out to learn how to grow food without chemicals. In the decades that followed Rodale become one of the first and best-known advocate for sustainable agriculture and organic farming in the United States. Over the decades and long after his death, his publishing company continues to introduce the concepts of organic food and its health benefits to millions of Americans through its magazines and books.

Rodale learned about organic theories for food and for living through Sir Arthur Howard, a British agronomist whose own views were shaped by Eastern spiritual concepts and a belief in a connected circle of life. Howard's organic philosophy started when he was sent by the British government to India in 1905 to establish an agricultural research base.

In India, Howard saw how local farmers fertilized with composted animal and vegetable wastes, and he concluded that their soil fertility, abundant crops, and livestock that appeared to be immune to pests and diseases were the result of these methods. Howard used his research and his firsthand experiences to develop a philosophy that recognized what he saw as a dangerous connection between increased animal diseases and the use of chemical fertilizers. Rodale discovered Howard's writings in the early 1940s, which coincided with American agriculture's embrace of chemical fertilizers. In fact, from 1940 to 1941 U.S. fertilizer use increased sevenfold (Green, 1971). Fertilizer usage has continued to grow; USDA figures for 2009 showed conventional U.S. agriculture spent more than $20 million on chemical fertilizer that year, almost double that of 2005 ("Chemical, Fertilizer").

After Rodale read Howard's work he bought a 60-acre Pennsylvania farm and continued to correspond with Howard about farming ideas and methods. His publishing company, which he started with his brother with the profits from his business, launched *Organic Farming* magazine. Unfortunately, subscriptions were slow. Rodale then widened the scope of the publication to include home gardeners and rereleased the magazine in 1942 as *Organic Farming and Gardening,* with Howard working as a long-distance associate editor. The magazine remains a successful publication with readership of up to 70 million subscribers according to its website.

Rodale's interest in health may have come from his early childhood. He was born in 1898 in New York City and was frequently ill as a youngster. He worked as an accountant before going into the electrical equipment business with his brother. In 1930 they moved the company to Pennsylvania where he eventually bought his farm. In 1947 Rodale formed the Soil and Health Foundation to promote scientific research, education, teaching, and training on organic farming. He continued to promote organic farming and gardening techniques on his farm through the 1960s.

In 1971 the Rodales bought a 333-acre farm, also in Kutztown, Pennsylvania, to use for scientific experiments, which they hoped could educate others about the environmental sustainability and economic viability of larger-scale organic farm production methods. Named the Rodale Research Center, today it is called the Rodale Institute. Research continues in organic agriculture according to the Rodale Institute website, where researchers compare conventional agriculture with organic methods. According to the institute, new research continues on issues including carbon sequestration in chemical versus organic plots and new techniques for weed suppression.

Less than a decade after he launched his first magazine, Rodale introduced another publication in 1950 devoted entirely to health and named it *Prevention*. The magazine was designed to promote preventing disease rather than trying to cure it and in later editions it also focused on alternative health methods including the benefits of eating organic foods.

In 1971 the *New York Times Magazine* named Rodale "Guru of the Organic Food Cult." His farming theory was based on three key elements. First, the long-range health of the soil is paramount to healthy food and is enhanced by a high level of organic matter. Second, organic matter offers a more balanced delivery of nutrients to plants than do chemical fertilizers. Finally, the third point was that a delicate balance in the soil keeps pathogenic organisms in check but chemical fertilizers and pesticides upset that balance (Green, 1971).

At that time Rodale's beliefs contradicted the official USDA position on organic plants, which stated that there was no evidence that organic plants were any better than their conventionally grown counterparts. Tragically, Rodale died in 1971 just after the *New York Times* magazine article was published, leaving his son Robert in charge of Rodale Press and of the company's educational efforts on organic farming. Robert took the organic point of view and expanded it into other social and environmental issues. He called for an America that would promote more responsible use of the land and its resources through recycling and other methods.

Rodale also initiated a comparison of organic and conventional farming methods in 1981 called the Farming Systems Trial. The project started as research on the economic viability of larger-scale organic agriculture with the goal of documenting the steps necessary to convert from conventional farming to organic. However, at the same time it illustrated that comparable crop yields could be obtained without the use of chemical pesticides or fertilizers. Results showed that organic crop yields were comparable to conventional yields.

By 1985 the USDA was interested in the research being done by the Rodale Institute and together the two sponsored the first workshops on regenerative agriculture that year. Encouraged by this success, Robert Rodale and the institute were able to win the first federal funding for what was called the Low Input Sustainable Agriculture Program. This has since grown into the more-than-$9-million Sustainable Agriculture Research and Education Program, which supports joint public and private studies and efforts between conventional agriculture and organic agriculture. During the 1980s Rodale introduced the Cornucopia Project, which documented the cost of energy and chemicals used in conventional food production and distribution. They also advocated the use of local and regional food production systems to lower food costs.

Robert Rodale planned to expand his father's vision throughout the world and in 1983 sent a delegation of Rodale experts to Tanzania, East Africa, to teach resource-efficient farming workshops. This trip and others resulted in the development of the institute's Regenerative Agriculture Resource Center (RARC) program, which focuses on farm research, farmer-to-farmer training, and exchange of information to support sustainable agriculture. Unfortunately, Robert Rodale was killed in an automobile accident on a trip to the Soviet Union in September 1990. He was there for discussions on a joint venture to publish materials on regenerative agriculture in the Soviet Union.

His widow, Ardath Rodale, took over following her husband's death, and in 2008, J. I. Rodale's granddaughter, Maria Rodale, was named Chairperson of Rodale Inc. Eighty years after the company's inception, the commitment to J. I. Rodale's principles continues to grow. In 2010 Maria Rodale published *Organic Manifesto: How Organic Farming Can Heal Our Planet, Feed the World and Keep Us Safe.* Other accomplishments over the years by the Rodale Institute include a partnership with Pennsylvania State University to establish the Penn State/Rodale Center for Sustaining Agriculture and Natural Resources in Urbanizing Environments. Its mission is to sponsor research and educational programs that highlight rural/urban community practices that are profitable, environmentally sound, and socially acceptable.

The institute also expanded its research into composting and established the Compost Utilization trial to study a variety of issues involving the impact of using organic waste for soil enrichment in urban and rural areas. The institute partnered with the Pennsylvania Department of Environmental Protection to produce a series of educational materials on backyard composting and developed best management practices guidelines for composting for the Chesapeake Bay Program. It has partnered with the USDA and the W.K. Kellogg Foundation to advance the study of soil nutrients and pest management projects. The early vision of J. I. Rodale has had a lasting effect on efforts in this country to support sustainable agriculture and farming practices and has linked the Rodale name with health and nutrition for millions of Americans.

*Sharon Zoumbaris*

*See also* Organic Food; U.S. Department of Agriculture (USDA).

## References

Alexander, Anna B. "Welcome to *Prevention* Magazine's 50th Anniversary." *Prevention* 52, no. 9 (September 2000): 145.

"Chemical, Fertilizer, Labor and Feed Expenses by Year—United States: 2005–2009." National Agriculture Statistics Service (NASS), U.S. Department of Agriculture (USDA). www.naas.usda.gov.

Green, Ward. "Guru of the Organic Food Cult." *New York Times Magazine,* June 6, 1971, 57.

Holden, Patrick. "Howard's Way," *The Ecologist* 31, no. 5 (June 2001): 30.

"Jerome Irving Rodale." *Contemporary Authors Online.* Detroit: Gale, 1998. Gale Biography in Context. September 14, 2010.

Rodale, Maria. "The Organic Solution." *Women's Health* 7, no. 3 (April 2010): 86.

"Rodale Publishes 'Our Roots Grow Deep, the Story of Rodale.'" *Agriculture Business Week,* May 14, 2009, 10.

Vaccariello, Liz. "Growing up Organic: Maria Rodale." *Prevention* 62, no. 4 (April 2010): 118.

# S

## SALMONELLA

*Salmonella* Enteritidis (SE) bacterial infections associated with eggs are never very far from the news. In fact, eggs have become the most common food source of salmonella outbreaks. For example, from May to November in 2010, almost 2,000 illnesses were reported to be linked to a salmonella infection from eggs, according to the Centers for Disease Control and Prevention (CDC, 2010). In the spring of 2010, public health investigators from 11 states worked to determine that shell eggs were the cause of this latest salmonella outbreak, and they pinpointed two farms in Iowa as possible sources of contamination. By August of 2010, both Wright County Egg of Galt, Iowa, and the Hillandale Farms, Inc. of Iowa conducted nationwide voluntary recalls of shell eggs in an effort to stop the nationwide outbreak that filled the nightly news.

The connection between salmonella and poultry has intensified in recent decades. Beginning in the 1980s, scientists detected salmonella bacteria inside the chickens, which meant the hens were passing it internally into their eggs. Back in the 1960s and 1970s this was extremely rare. However, by the 1990s, the number of cases of salmonella infection from transovarian transfer had increased dramatically.

Scientists acknowledge that the contaminated eggs are linked to U.S. industrial farming practices and to the crowded conditions of laying hens. With so many birds in such close quarters, the bacteria are easily passed from one hen to another. Many chickens have infected ovaries, even though they show no signs of sickness, and they shed the bacteria into the egg white. Once the shell has secreted around the egg, the bacteria is invisibly sealed inside.

In 1994, more than 200,000 Americans got salmonella from a contaminated ice-cream truck that was eventually linked to eggs containing salmonella. After a great deal of investigative work, government officials pinpointed a specific brand of ice cream as the cause of the outbreak. Researchers discovered that the ice cream had been transported by tanker trucks that previously carried unpasteurized eggs.

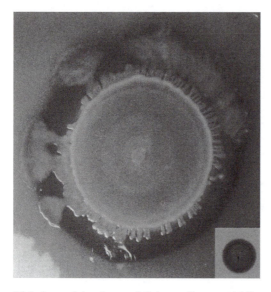

This bacterial colony of Salmonella enteritidis, when injected into a chicken egg, grew rapidly. (U.S. Department of Agriculture)

Those eggs had been infected with salmonella bacteria, which then became part of the ice cream.

The United States Department of Agriculture (USDA) estimates that more than 70 billion eggs are sold each year in the United States, and that approximately 19 percent contain salmonella bacteria (Callaway et al., 2008). This means American consumers are buying millions of salmonella-infected eggs each year. In 2006, the USDA Food Safety and Inspection Service (FSIS) launched a "salmonella attack plan" to lower the rate of infection in U.S. eggs, and, at this point, their figures show some success. According to statistics released by the CDC Foodborne Diseases Active Surveillance Network, or FoodNet, the incidence of illnesses from salmonella decreased by 10 percent in 2009 (FSIS 2011).

Salmonella is just one of more than 250 foodborne diseases the CDC tracks each year. The CDC estimates that 48 million people get sick, 128,000 are hospitalized, and 3,000 die each year from foodborne diseases (FSIS, 2011). Other diseases include *Echerichia coli* (*E. coli*), *Campylobacter jejuni*, *Shigella*, *Listeria* and *Clostridium botulinum* along with the *Norovirus*. A salmonella bacteria infection mimics the flu with symptoms that include fever, cramps, muscle aches, vomiting and diarrhea. Foods suspected of carrying salmonella most frequently include eggs, poultry, cheese, raw vegetables and fruit, and unpasteurized milk and juices.

How does salmonella spread? It lives in the intestine of infected people or animals, and the germs are released during bowel movements. It can then be found in soil, food, water, or on surfaces that the bacteria touch. It is sometimes spread due to lack of hand washing after a bowel movement or after changing a baby's diaper. Once on other surfaces, the bacteria are easily spread by touch or by eating something that touched the infected surface.

The symptoms of the infection appear two or three days after ingestion and can last for up to a week. While most people recover without treatment, some individuals do require hospitalization, especially in cases of severe diarrhea and the dehydration that accompanies it. In some cases, severe illness develops and the infection spreads from the intestines to the bloodstream. Individuals with weak immune systems, the elderly, or the very young face a more serious illness, and if the infection spreads, it may require immediate treatment with antibiotics to prevent organ failure and death.

Other problems that can result from a salmonella infection include infection of the gall bladder and bile ducts, known as cholangitis; meningitis, or swelling of the brain covering and spinal cord; a bone tissue infection known as osteomyelitis; and pneumonia. These may develop if a salmonella infection worsens and is untreated.

While eggs have become a very common food source for causing salmonella infections, there have been other, equally serious infections from other foods. The summer of 2008 will be remembered for an outbreak of salmonella that sickened at least 1,440 people across the United States and at the time was considered the worst foodborne outbreak in at least a decade. Although the early evidence suggested that the bacteria traced to fresh tomatoes from Florida, the CDC and Food and Drug Administration (FDA) eventually placed the blame on peppers grown in Mexico and imported to the United States.

The outbreak began in April, and the majority of the cases appeared during May and June. A salmonella outbreak of this size is not cheap. The Economic Research Service (ERS) of the USDA estimated the economic cost of salmonellosis alone in 2010 as more than $2 billion (ERS 2010). The ERS measured medical expenses, lost work, and premature death to calculate those figures. Whatever the cost, salmonella now has a major effect on people and the economy.

With the increase in salmonella showing up in raw fruits and vegetables, scientists have initiated new research to focus on preventing contamination before and during the harvesting of produce. A study from Purdue University, released in June 2011, examined the effectiveness of three technologies that did not use heat to prevent or inactivate salmonella and E. coli on tomatoes, lettuce, and cantaloupe seeds. Those technologies included chlorine dioxide gas, ozone gas, and e-beam irradiation. Researchers concluded that these methods could potentially control and reduce bacteria contamination of the seeds (Trinetta et al., 2011).

The growing number of food-safety incidents has also heightened government scrutiny of the industry and increased congressional legislation aimed at improving the laws and regulations governing food handling and production. Several food-safety bills have called for new food-tracing systems and for increasing access to records so that food can be followed from farm to table. While food-safety experts agree that an improved system should look at potential hazards at the farm level, there are differing opinions on the need for government safety standards that could also restrict how farms and agribusiness raises food. In July of 2010, the FDA released details about its egg-safety rule that called for flock-based salmonella programs that include mandatory testing for poultry producers with more than 50,000 hens. The testing will look for microbiologic problems in the chickens.

Salmonella also occurs when people eat raw eggs, undercooked eggs, or chicken or sauces, salad dressings, or desserts such as cookie dough made with raw eggs. It is also important to be careful about cross contamination when handling raw chicken. It is important to use different cutting boards and to wash hands so that bacteria cannot be spread from the uncooked chicken to other foods.

Children face a bigger threat to infection because their hand-washing skills may be less thorough. Besides careful hand washing, other ways to avoid salmonella include keeping eggs refrigerated at all times or buying and using pasteurized eggs. Avoid eating raw eggs in such items as eggnog, cookie dough, homemade ice cream, or sauces such as hollandaise or Caesar salad dressing. Leftover foods made with eggs should be refrigerated immediately, and it is important to discard any cracked or dirty eggs. Pets that can carry salmonella include turtles, iguanas, chicks, or ducklings.

The best way to avoid salmonella is to thoroughly cook all foods that could possibly contain the bacteria. Heat is the only way to kill the bacteria, freezing and drying are not enough. Cooking chicken to 165 degrees Fahrenheit kills salmonella and prevents illness.

*Sharon Zoumbaris*

*See also* Antibiotics; Bacteria; Centers for Disease Control and Prevention (CDC); Food and Drug Administration (FDA); Food-borne Illness.

### References

Callaway T.R., T.S. Edrington, R. C. Anderson, J. A. Byrd, and J. D. Nisbet. "Gastrointestinal Microbial Ecology and the Safety of Our Food Supply as Related to Salmonella," *Journal of Animal Science* 86, no. 14 (April 2008): E163–E172.

Centers for Disease Control and Prevention. "Investigation Update: Multistate Outbreak of Human Salmonella Enteritidis Infections Associated with Shell Eggs." December 2, 2010. www.cdc.gov.

Johnson, Renee. "Food Safety on the Farm: Federal Programs and Legislative Action." *Congressional Research Service (CRS) Reports and Issue Briefs. CRS Report 34612*. October 2010. www.nationalaglawcenter.org/assets/CRS/RL34612.pdf.

Trinetta, V., N. Vaidya, R. Linton, and M. Morgan. "A Comparative Study on the Effectiveness of Chlorine Dioxide Gas, Ozone Gas and E-Beam Irradiation Treatments for Inactivation of Pathogens Inoculated onto Tomato, Cantaloupe and Lettuce Seeds." *International Journal of Food Microbiology* 146, no. 2 (March 30, 2011): 203–206.

United States Department of Agriculture Economic Research Service. "Foodborne Illness Cost Calculator: Salmonella." December 28, 2010. www.ers.usda.gov/Data/Food borneillness.

United States Department of Agriculture Food Safety and Inspection Service. "Statement of Dr. Elisabeth Hagen: Fiscal Year 2012 Budget Request for Food Safety." March 15, 2011. www.fsis.usda.gov/News__Events/Testimony_Hagen_031511/index.asp.

## SCHOOL MEALS INITIATIVE

The Child Nutrition Act, signed into law by President Barack Obama at the end of 2010, will mandate new standards for school lunches. This is the first time since the 1995 School Meals Initiative (SMI) for Healthy Children that concern over the nutritional content of school food has prompted government action.

The SMI was designed to put guidelines in place that would answer critics who saw the school meals as being unhealthy and too high in fat.

Before the changes proposed by the SMI, it had been almost 50 years since the United States Department of Agriculture (USDA) had changed the school lunch nutritional standards. The SMI was the USDA's attempt to bring school meals in line with the 1990 Dietary Guidelines for Americans and to ensure that children were eating breakfast and lunch foods that provided solid nutrition while reducing the percentage of calories from fat and saturated fat.

Fast forward to 2010. As the Child Nutrition Act made its way through the legislative process, the concern among lawmakers was not about the staggering obesity rates among U.S. school children or how school districts could afford the hefty prices of healthy food, but how the federal government would find the money to pay billions of dollars for this increase in federal funding. This increased funding for school lunches will cost the federal government an additional $4.5 billion a year.

However, supporters of the bill say lawmakers should be worried, since statistics from the Centers for Disease Control and Prevention (CDC) show that over the past three decades childhood obesity rates in America have tripled, with nearly one in three children today considered overweight or obese (CDC, 2010).

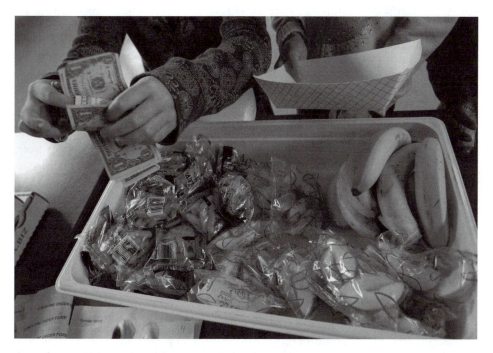

A student at Fairmeadow Elementary School pays for fruits and vegetables as part of a school lunch program in Palo Alto, California, on December 2, 2010. President Obama signed the Child Nutrition Act into law in 2010 with the goal of improving the nutritional value of school lunches. (AP/Wide World Photos)

While there are many culprits to blame for the current obesity rates among the nation's children, supporters of the SMI and the newest Child Nutrition Act say local school districts need the increase in funding to pay the cost of buying healthy, low-fat food. According to school nutrition officials, the USDA-proposed increase or subsidy to school meals translates into an additional 6 cents per meal. The changing rules will require significant increases in the amount of fruits and vegetables schools must serve. Local school districts spend on average less than $150 to feed a child for the entire 180-day school year. That amounts to less than $1 per day to feed the nation's children. According to 2011 figures from the USDA, over 32 million U.S. school children buy their lunch as part of the National School Lunch Program (NSLP), and over 11 million children participate in the school breakfast program.

School food managers have faced an increasingly difficult budgetary balancing act since the late 1960s and early 1970s, when President Richard Nixon dramatically increased funding for the NSLP. The problem arose when Congress increased federal dollars for food costs but not for operating expenses, equipment, or labor, making it necessary for school food-service programs to choose between cost and nutrition. School lunch programs are nonprofit, and, given the tight budgets faced by many school districts, they have had to rely on sales of a la carte lunch items to stay within their budget.

Still in place are the 1995 SMI-specific minimum standards for calories and key nutrients. Also designated in the 1995 SMI are four options for menu planning. Different options are allowed in different schools, and different options are even allowed for breakfast and lunch in the same school. Those tools for planning school menus include Enhanced Food Based Menu Planning, Traditional Meal Pattern, Nutrient Standard Menu Planning, or Assisted Nutrient Standard Menu Planning.

Still, no matter what form of menu planning each school food manager selects, they all must meet the same goals: School breakfasts and lunches must have less than 30 percent of calories from fat and less than 10 percent of calories from saturated fat over the course of a week. The SMI requires that meals meet one-third of the Recommended Dietary Allowances (RDA) for protein, calcium, iron, vitamin A, vitamin C, and specific levels of calories for specified age groups. And, lastly, menus must meet the Dietary Guidelines for Americans of 1990 for children over the age of two years.

Based on USDA statistics released at that time, the nutritional quality of the meals was in need of change. In school year 1991 to 1992, for example, only 1 percent of all school lunches met the standard for keeping total fat under 30 percent and none met the standard for serving meals with less than 10 percent of calories from saturated fat ("School Meal Study," 2001). Saturated fats are found in whole milk, red meats and other animal products as well as in palm oil and processed foods such as margarine and pastries. Saturated fats encourage the body to make more LDL cholesterol. LDL cholesterol, considered to be the harmful type of cholesterol, eventually damages artery linings and forms deposits on artery walls. Nutritional studies have linked saturated fats and cholesterol to a variety of health problems in adults, including greater risk of heart attack, heart disease, and stroke.

School meals may again be asked to meet changing nutritional standards. The USDA announced in early 2011 plans for an update to the nutrition standards for the school lunch and breakfast programs. Agriculture Secretary Tom Vilsack said in a prepared statement that, "With many children consuming as many as half their daily calories at school, strengthening nutritional standards is an important step in the Obama administration's effort to combat childhood obesity and improve the health and well-being of all our kids" (Gauthier, 2011).

*Sharon Zoumbaris*

*See also* Dietary Guidelines for Americans; National School Lunch Program (NSLP); Obesity.

### References

Centers for Disease Control and Prevention. "Vital Signs: State Specific Obesity Prevalence among Adults–United States, 2009." *Morbidity and Mortality Weekly Report.* August 3, 2010. Accessed January 19, 2011. www.cdc.gov.

Gauthier, Kelli. "School Lunch Revamp Would Cause Challenges." *Chattanooga Times/Free Press,* January 25, 2011. Accessed January 26, 2011. www.timesfreepress.com.

Havala, Suzanne. "USDA School Meals Initiative for Healthy Children." *Vegetarian Journal,* November/December 1994. Accessed January 25, 2011. www.vrg.org/journal/school lunch.htm.

Ogden, C. L., M. D. Carroll, L. R. Curtin, M. A. McDowell, C. J. Tabak, and K. M. Flegal. "Prevalence of Obesity among Children and Adolescents: United States, Trends 1963–1965 through 2007–2008." *Centers for Disease Control and Prevention (CDC).* www.cdc.gov/nchs/data/hestat/obesity_child_07_08/obesity_child_07_08.htm.

"President Obama Has Signed into Law the Child Nutrition Act, which Mandates New Standards for School Lunches." *National Review,* 62 no. 24 (December 31, 2010): 10.

"School Meal Study Shows Higher Nutritional Activity." *Food Service Director* 14, no. 2 (February 15, 2001): 12.

United States Department of Agriculture. "Annual Summary of Food and Nutrition Service Programs." January 5, 2011. www.fns.usda.gov/pd/annual.htm.

## SCOLIOSIS. *See* BONE HEALTH

## SEASONAL AFFECTIVE DISORDER (SAD)

Seasonal Affective Disorder (SAD) is a type of significant depression that consistently relates to, or appears in, a specific time of year, namely the fall and winter. Spontaneous remission takes place consistently in the spring. This disorder is related to the relative amount of light, thus the relative length of days and nights, in the patient's geographical region. SAD is consistent with the darker periods of the year and goes into remission with the increase of sunlight. The *Diagnostic and Statistical Manual of Mental Disorders* (APA, 2000) indicates that this disorder seems to fall within the general category of Major Depressive Disorder, or Bipolar I and II Disorders. The regular pattern for onset of SAD is not related to special stressors that are present at various times of year such as holiday seasons.

Mayo Clinic research distinguishes SAD from "cabin fever" and the "blahs." While these latter terms are not scientifically technical, most people readily understand their references to common experiences. This research also indicates that a frequency of low energy, headaches, feelings of stress unrelated to any situation or stimulus, free-floating anxiety, and crying spells that have no identifiable provocation are associated with or components of this disorder. Statistics show that SAD affects nearly 6 percent of the U.S. population, and 80 percent of those affected are women.

SAD usually manifests in late adolescence and is most frequently seen in young adult or mid-life women. Most children who are affected have a close relative who also has SAD or another psychiatric condition. The condition manifests in irritability, excessive sleep need, increased consumption of carbohydrates, consequent weight gain, and discernibly flattened affect. National Institute of Mental Health research indicates that 92 percent of humans experience a subclinical pattern of seasonal mood changes, 43 percent of humans have some degree of clinical-level SAD, and 27 percent have problems that cause distortions of normal relationality and other life-changing dysfunctions.

Melatonin levels are indicated as the biochemical mediator of SAD. Light that is taken in through the eyes affects the pineal gland and thence regulates melatonin secretion. Darkness increases the melatonin and is the factor that mediates sexual cycles and hibernation functions in some mammals. As spring returns, activity levels spontaneously increase, sexual activity increases, even to the point of a kind of manic overactivity, as melatonin levels fade in the face of the longer days and brighter sunlight. This is undoubtedly the source or reason for the poet's line, "In the spring a young man's fancy, lightly turns to thoughts of love." Some humans have a greater capacity to adjust their function to situation-appropriateness, while others do not. This variance between persons is likely to be related to a genetic predisposition to differences in the volume of melatonin secreted by each individual.

Diagnosis of SAD requires at least two major depressive episodes occurring consistently at the season(s) of decreased sunlight in the region in which the patient lives, together with the absence of any nonseasonal depressive episodes during the same period. The patient may have suffered from other types of major depressive episodes over his or her lifetime, but the pattern of seasonal episodes, with the absence of the nonseasonal episodes, must substantially outnumber any general seasonal episodes to arrive at a diagnosis of SAD.

Management and treatment of SAD is limited in scope and effectiveness. Fluorescent light therapy is helpful for many patients with severe SAD, as is moving to a consistently sunnier climate, such as the U.S. desert southwest. One of the antidepressant medications can be of great help to patients if taken consistently year round and of less effective help when taken only during the season of the disorder. Living in the darker regions of the planet, such as Alaska, northern Siberia, northern Scandinavia, and the like, tend to exacerbate the symptoms and suffering of patients with SAD. Psychotherapy by itself does not help much with the management of SAD, though it can be very useful in curing the psychological side effects or bad habits the patient has developed over the years as a result of or in trying to cope with SAD. The disorder is not curable, but a combination of light therapy, medication, and supportive psychotherapy is very helpful in managing SAD.

Dr. Norman E. Rosenthal (2005), a psychiatrist at Georgetown University Medical Center who was among the first to describe SAD, suggests the root cause lies in insensitivity to light. Investigations are underway to see if timing the exposure to light to match changes in individual melatonin levels may show improvement in treatment levels. Studies are also underway to test the effectiveness of "dawn simulation," a way to gradually increase exposure to light before a patient awakens.

*J. Harold Ellens*

*See also* Bipolar Disorder; Depression.

### References

American Psychiatric Association (APA). *Diagnostic and Statistical Manual of Mental Disorders.* 4th ed. text rev. Arlington, VA: American Psychiatric Association, 2000.

Larson, David E., ed. *Mayo Clinic Family Health Book.* New York: William Morrow and Company, 1990.

Moran, Sarah. "Shedding Light on SAD: It's Not Uncommon for Winter Blues to Become Something More Serious-A Recurring Depression Known as Seasonal Affective Disorder." *Minneapolis Star Tribune,* January 25, 2010, 1E.

"Renewed Research for Seasonal Affective Disorder." *Health News* 15, no. 1 (January 2009): 2.

Rosenthal, Norman E. *Winter Blues: Everything You Need to Know to Beat Seasonal Affective Disorder.* New York: Guilford Press, 2005.

"A SAD Story: Seasonal Affective Disorder." *Harvard Health Letter* (January 1, 2008).

"Seasonal Affective Disorder." *The Columbia Encyclopedia.* 6th ed. New York: Columbia University Press, 2000: 34685.

## SECONDHAND SMOKE

Secondhand smoke, or environmental tobacco smoke (ETS), is the smoke inhaled by individuals who themselves are not actively smoking, and for this reason it is also sometimes referred to as passive smoking. Though secondhand smoke has existed since smoking began, it was not until the 1970s, when scientific research began to discover the health hazards it poses, that it became a serious matter of public policy. With a growing recognition of the dangers of ETS, numerous smoking restrictions, such as the Clean Indoor Air Act, have been passed in order to protect the nonsmoking public from inhaling secondhand smoke.

According to the American Cancer Society, secondhand smoke is responsible for an estimated 46,000 deaths each year in the United States alone from heart disease in nonsmokers who live with smokers. It also estimates there are 3,400 lung cancer deaths in nonsmoking adults, along with breathing problems that include coughing, chest discomfort, and reduced lung function. The American Cancer Society also estimates that secondhand smoke increases the number and severity of asthma attacks for the 200,000 to 1 million children who have asthma. The Centers for Disease Control and Prevention (CDC) detailed other health effects for children exposed to secondhand smoke, including increased ear infections and respiratory infections and a greater risk for sudden infant death syndrome (SIDS).

Until the 1950s, few Americans viewed smoking cigarettes as a major health threat, and consequently, even fewer considered secondhand smoke a hazard. In the early 1950s, however, a wave of scientific reports, including *Reader's Digest's* 1952 blockbuster, "Cancer by the Carton," which linked smoking to lung cancer, reached a popular audience and created a major shift in American attitudes toward tobacco. In the wake of these reports, some 40 percent of Americans believed that smoking caused lung cancer. Public fears were temporarily allayed by the public relations efforts of the Tobacco Industry Research Committee (TIRC), a tobacco industry-financed entity that worked to create uncertainty and doubt as to whether cigarettes were carcinogenic by distorting, discrediting, or suppressing findings that concluded that smoking represented a serious health threat. But with the Surgeon General's 1964 report, which concluded that smoking causes serious disease, the true dangers of lighting up were quite evident.

With the Surgeon General's report irreversibly establishing the act of smoking a cigarette as a major health risk, a few science reporters in the late 1960s took the next logical step and reasoned that if tobacco smoke was so dangerous to a smokers' health, it might also represent a considerable health threat to individuals breathing in the vicinity of smokers. Testing this hypothesis proved to be a difficult and time-consuming endeavor, though, and the studies that would confirm the serious health effects of inhaling secondhand smoke were not published until after a grassroots movement to curb smoking in public places had emerged in the early 1970s.

The first groups to argue for smoke-free air as a nonsmokers' right drew upon the civil rights, antiwar, and environmental movements as inspirations. They enlisted volunteer activists and formed organizations like Americans for Non-Smokers' Rights, which was based in Berkeley, California, and Group Against Smoking and Pollution (GASP), which was founded by Clara Gouin in 1971 and had fifty-six local chapters spread across several states by 1974. GASP's newsletter, *Ventilator,* advanced the notion that nonsmokers had a right to breathe smoke-free air. Each chapter of the organization aggressively pushed for the passage of local and state ordinances that would regulate smoking in places of public accommodation, such as restaurants and office buildings. Beyond their legislative efforts, GASP members went directly to restaurant owners, and numbers of them agreed to create nonsmoking sections in their businesses well before the passage of any laws mandating such areas. In some cases, restaurant owners even expanded these sections upon discovering how popular they were with nonsmoking customers.

These local-level developments led to more far-reaching restrictions on secondhand smoke, particularly after the 1972 Surgeon General's report on smoking identified ETS as a potential health hazard to nonsmokers. Though the Surgeon General did not yet define the precise nature of the threat that secondhand smoke posed to nonsmokers, there was enough momentum for the Civil Aeronautics Boards to require, in 1973, the creation of a nonsmoking section on all U.S. airlines. That year also marked the passage of the first state law restricting smoking in public places. Following two years of grassroots organizing and campaigning from Arizonans Concerned About Smoking, Arizona banned smoking in buses, theaters, elevators, museums, and libraries. The state further legislated the creation of designated smoking areas in public spaces such as government buildings and hospitals. Minnesota soon followed Arizona's lead by becoming, in 1975, the first state to pass a comprehensive Clean Indoor Air Act. In large part the result of work by the Twin Cities' local chapter of the Association for Non-Smokers' Rights, Minnesota's act forbade smoking in all public places, unless specifically allowed, and it stipulated that at least 30 percent of restaurant seating needed to be reserved for nonsmokers. By 1981, thirty-six states had smoking restrictions of some form, and by the mid-1980s, almost all states had some restrictions on public smoking. As such, around 80 percent of the nation's population lived in areas that were covered by these laws, and by 1988, all domestic flights had become nonsmoking.

The tobacco industry did not passively accept these tremendous changes to the place of smoking in public life, and their fight against nonsmokers' rights took place on two fronts. On one level, the tobacco industry attempted to cast secondhand smoke as an issue of manners rather than one of health. Though their efforts were, for the most part, unable to prevent the passage of most smoking restrictions, the tobacco industry argued that legislative regulation on behalf of nonsmokers' rights amounted to an un-American violation of smokers' rights. To counter what they argued was an undue governmental intrusion into an individual smoker's personal life, Philip Morris even went so far as to offer a Bill of Rights for smoking. It also helped fund the National Smokers' Alliance as a counter organization to grassroots groups like GASP. On a second level, the tobacco industry put its considerable resources behind a push to discredit the scientific link between secondhand smoke and cancer or other serious illnesses. After the Tobacco Institute's 1978 survey confirmed a fairly widespread public support for bans on smoking in public places, the tobacco companies decided to create an institution along the lines of the TIRC (which by then had been renamed the Council for Tobacco Research) that would fund scientific research into indoor air quality so as to suggest that other elements in the air supply were responsible for the diseases and illnesses being linked to secondhand smoke. The Center for Indoor Air Research (CIAR) was thus founded in March 1988 to create uncertainty about the risk ETS posed to nonsmokers, and the reports it produced consistently trumpeted the line that there was insufficient evidence to conclude that secondhand smoke posed any health risk.

Despite the CIAR's undertakings, the tobacco industry was unable to convince many people of ETS's harmlessness, especially after two major studies on secondhand smoke appeared in 1986. One came from the National Academy of Sciences (NAS), which reported that children of smokers were twice as likely to suffer from respiratory illnesses as children with nonsmoking parents. The Surgeon General's report from the same year was even more damaging to the CIAR's efforts, as it concluded that the best way to protect nonsmokers from the dangers of ETS would be to establish entirely smoke-free work sites, and not just nonsmoking areas. The two reports even put a number on the amount of lung cancer deaths in the United States attributable to the secondhand smoke, with the Surgeon General claiming it be around 3,000, while the NAS estimated the figure to somewhere between 2,500 and 8,400. These arresting estimations were further buttressed by a 1992 report by the Environmental Protection Agency, which found tobacco smoke to be a Class A human lung carcinogen—putting it in the same category as asbestos and benzene. The report also suggested that 20 percent of lung cancer cases among nonsmokers resulted from secondhand smoke. Subsequent studies have concluded that secondhand smoke is even more dangerous than previously thought, with some research indicating that as many as 50,000 Americans die each year as a result of ETS-related illnesses.

Reports about ETS such as these were central to the legal difficulties the tobacco industry experienced in the 1990s. The most salient example is *Broin v. Philip Morris,* a class-action lawsuit filed on behalf of Norma Broin, an American Airlines flight attendant who had never smoked but still contracted lung cancer at an early age, and approximately 60,000 other nonsmoking flight attendants who sought roughly $5 billion in redress from big tobacco as a result of illnesses and injuries suffered as a result of their exposure to secondhand smoke. Facing a difficult case, the tobacco companies avoided admitting to secondhand smoke's health risks to nonsmokers by agreeing, out of court, to a $349 million settlement. ETS's health hazards were thus, by the late 20th century, firmly established, even if the tobacco industry was reluctant to publicly admit it.

In recent years, secondhand smoke regulation has been extended, in many places, to traditional bastions of public smoking such as bars. Many cities have also banned smoking at sports stadiums, beaches, and parks as a result of ETS health effects. California has been one of the most vigorous states in its restriction of smoking on behalf of nonsmokers, with recently passed legislation banning the act of smoking in a vehicle that contains minors. Some communities within the state have even recently taken the controversial step of restricting smoking within private residences, such as apartment buildings, in order to shield neighboring nonsmokers from the hazards of secondhand smoke.

Secondhand smoke is also being blamed for technology problems. Consumer blogs have posted accounts of computer users who were smokers and experienced problems with their computer hardware. Several bloggers suggested smoking around a laptop or desktop does have a negative impact on the machine and creates a sticky, heavy dust that can create problems.

*Howard Padwa and Jacob Cunningham*

*See also* Asthma; Cancer; Smoking.

## References

American Cancer Society. *Cancer Facts & Figures 2009.* Atlanta, GA: American Cancer Society, 2009.

American Lung Association. *Secondhand Smoke Fact Sheet.* August 6, 2010. www.lungusa.org/site/pp.asp?c=dvLUK9O0E&=35422.

"Apple Refuses to Fix Smokers Computers Suggest Customers." *eWeek,* November 23, 2009. www.eweek.com.

Brandt, Allan M. *The Cigarette Century: The Rise, Fall, and Deadly Persistence of the Product that Defined America.* New York: Basic Books, 2007.

Cordry, Harold V. *Tobacco: A Reference Handbook.* Santa Barbara, CA: ABC-CLIO, 2001.

Environmental Protection Agency. *Respiratory Health Effects of Passive Smoking: Lung Cancer and Other Disorders.* Washington, DC: Environmental Protection Agency, 1992 (report # EPA/600/6-90/006F). www.epa.gov.

Goodman, Jordan, ed. *Tobacco in History and Culture: An Encyclopedia.* Detroit: Thomson Gale, 2005.

Lynette, Rachel. *Tobacco.* Chicago, IL: Heinemann Library, 2008.

Parker-Pope, Tara. *Cigarettes: Anatomy of an Industry from Seed to Smoke.* New York: The New Press, 2001.

National Cancer Institute. *Cancer Progress Report 2003.* Washington, DC: Public Health Service, National Institutes of Health, U.S. Department of Health and Human Services, 2004.

National Toxicology Program. *Report on Carcinogens.* 11th ed. Washington, DC: U.S. Department of Health and Human Services, Public Health Service, National Toxicology Program, 2005.

U.S. Department of Health and Human Services. *Healthy People 2010: Understanding and Improving Health.* 2nd. ed. Washington DC: U.S. Government Printing Office, 2000.

## SEXUALLY TRANSMITTED DISEASES (STDs)

A group of diseases known collectively as sexually transmitted infections (STIs) were at one time (and still among many individuals) known as sexually transmitted diseases (STDs) or venereal diseases (VDs). Diseases that fall into this category include amebiasis, bacterial vaginosis, campylobacter fetus, candidiasis, chancroid, chlamydia, condyloma acuminata, cytomegalovirus, enteric infections, genital mycoplasmas, genital warts, giardiasis, gonorrhea, granuloma inguinale, hepatitis, herpes, HIV disease, lymphogranuloma venereum, molluscum contagiosum, pediculosis pubis, scabies, shingellosis, syphilis, trichomoniasis, yeast infections, and vaginitis.

Some of these diseases are rare and unfamiliar to most people; others are common and affect many people. Some diseases are mild and pose little threat to a person who develops the condition; others are life-threatening. In any case, all STIs are medical problems; that is, they are caused by specific microorganisms, such as bacteria or viruses; they can be recognized by certain characteristic signs and symptoms; they may have both short- and long-term consequences for one's overall health; and they usually can be treated and, in many cases, cured.

But, like many medical issues, sexually transmitted infections have nonmedical consequences (i.e., social, moral, ethical, legal, and emotional) in one's life. For example, the possibility of an individual having syphilis means more than simply going to the hospital, being tested, and being treated. It also means having the possibility of assessing his or her own sexual practices, talking with close friends and family, and reconsidering what he or she knows and believes about him- or herself as a person. These issues come wrapped not only in the experience of dealing with STIs, but in dealing with any issue related to one's sexual health, including pregnancy and contraception, and one's sexual identity and sexual orientation. Medical issues that almost anyone can deal with in a relatively emotion-free state become especially troubling when they have to do with one's reproductive system.

**An Ancient Issue** Venereal diseases have been a major medical problem in the world for at least five centuries. Unraveling the history of these diseases is problematic because ancient records do not offer unambiguous clinical symptoms that allow a modern reader to determine precisely what disease a person had. For example, some scholars find that passages in the Bible appear to indicate that Abraham's wife, Sarah, might have had syphilis (Cohen, 1991). Considerable debate among experts has developed over attempts to decide the sexually transmitted diseases to which ancient writers from China and Egypt may have alluded (see Goldman 1971; Heymann 2006; Rothschild 2005; Willcox 1949).

The first mention of sexually transmitted infections in Western Europe dates to about 1495, when a disease called the great pox (to distinguish it from smallpox) broke out among French troops besieging Naples (McAllister, 2000). As was to become a common pattern, the French blamed the disease on their enemies and called it the Italian disease. Later, the Italians themselves called the disease the French disease; the Dutch called it the Spanish disease; the Russians called it the Polish disease; the Turks called it the Christian disease; and much later, the Tahitians called it the British disease. These names reflected the fact that the disease commonly showed up in port cities, where it was presumably introduced by sailors arriving from another country.

In any case, the epidemiology and symptomology of syphilis were poorly known until at least the end of the 18th century. It was not until 1767 that syphilis and gonorrhea were even recognized as separate diseases. In that year, Scottish physician John Hunter infected himself with pus from a patient with gonorrhea, only to discover that he later developed symptoms not only of that disease, but also of syphilis. He was able to track the development of the latter disease, describing in careful detail for the first time the stages through which the disease developed until, in 1793, it caused an aneurysm that was responsible for his death (Androutsos, Magiorkinis, & Diamantis, 2008).

**Types of Infections**   Sexually transmitted infections can range from harmless but annoying diseases to serious and potentially fatal conditions. An example of the former is the condition known as pediculosis pubis. The term "pediculosis" refers to a group of infections caused by a group of insects that belong to the order Phthiraptera. These are tiny insects that live off blood and typically attach themselves to the base of a hair, from which they feed off their host. Perhaps the best-known example of the pest is *Pediculosis capitis,* the common head louse. Its close cousin, *Pediculosis pubis,* occurs most commonly in the pubic region, although it may also be found in other hairy areas, such as the eyelashes or in underarm hair. The most common symptom of an infection by this insect is itchiness, which becomes more severe over time. The only long-term problem is that scratching of infected areas may produce sores, which themselves may lead to more serious infections. The disease is readily treated with a variety of over-the-counter medications which, although not necessarily 100 percent effective, will eventually cure the problem.

Most STIs are of considerably more concern than *Pediculosis pubis.* The American Social Health Association has assembled a number of important statistics about these diseases. First, more than half of all Americans will contract a sexually transmitted infection at some point during their lifetime. Second, about 65 million Americans are currently living with some type of STI, and about 19 million new cases are reported every year. Third, about half of all new cases of STI occur among men and women age 15 to 24. Fourth, each year in the United States, about one in four teenagers contract one type of STI. Fifth, less than a third of all U.S. physicians routinely screen for STIs. Sixth, about one half of all sexually active men and women will contract at least one STI before the age of 25 (American Social Health Association, 2009).

The most common sexually transmitted infection in the United States is chlamydia. In 2007, 1,108,374 cases of chlamydia were reported to the U.S. Centers for Disease Control and Prevention (CDC) in the 50 states and the District of Columbia. Experts believe that the true number of cases is probably much larger, perhaps as many as 2,291,000, because many women do not realize that they have the infection. Such is the case with other STIs, which always raises questions about the accuracy of STI statistics. Not only are people sometimes unaware or unwilling to report an STI, but also figures for various diseases are difficult to compare because some public health departments may be required by law to report the number of cases for some diseases but not for others.

**Symptoms and Treatment**   For each specific sexually transmitted infection, a set of basic information is useful. The first is the signs and symptoms of the disease and the physical conditions associated with the disease, such as fever, nausea, blurred vision, and achy muscles. The second set of information concerns prognosis, the likely course of the disease. The third set of information relates to available treatments for prevention of the disease, for relief of symptoms, and for a possible cure. This outline serves as the basis for the discussion of the following sexually transmitted infections.

*Chlamydia*  Chlamydia is the most common sexually transmitted infection in the United States. It is caused by the bacterium *Chlamydia trachomatis,* which is transmitted most commonly by any type of sexual activity in which body parts come into contact with each other. The disease can also be transmitted from a woman to a newborn baby during childbirth. The disease occurs most commonly among women, causing abnormal vaginal discharge, discomfort during urination, and some itchiness.

Men who have chlamydia may experience an unusual discharge from the penis and some pain and burning during urination. Perhaps the most important point about chlamydia, however, is that no symptoms may appear, and a person may be unaware that he or she has the infection. This fact is troublesome because in women the infection may spread from its initial site in the vagina into the urethra and cervix, where it can cause long-term reproductive problems, such as sterility. The most serious consequence of untreated chlamydial infection is pelvic inflammatory disease (PID), which can cause permanent damage to the fallopian tubes and other parts of the reproductive system. Experts estimate that 40 percent of all untreated chlamydial infections eventually result in a PID infection. The most serious health consequence of PID is an ectopic pregnancy (a pregnancy that occurs outside the uterus), which can result in death.

As with many STIs, the more serious consequences of chlamydia can be avoided by early detection and treatment. The *Chlamydia trachomatis* bacterium is easily killed with antibiotics, azithromycin or doxycycline being the drugs of choice. The best way to avoid a chlamydial infection is abstinence, not having sexual contact with another person, but that option is difficult or impossible for most people. Alternatively, one should be open with a sexual partner about her or his health status in order to avoid contact with someone who is or may be infected. The CDC also recommends annual tests for chlamydia for all sexually active women under the age of 25 and for older women who have risk factors for the disease, such as a number of sexual partners or many new partners.

*Syphilis*  Historically, the most feared of all STIs, syphilis, has gradually come under control in the United States and most other parts of the world. In the United States, the number of syphilis cases has fallen from more than 485,000 in 1941 to less than 32,000 in 2000. It has since increased moderately to just over 40,000 in 2007 (Division of STD Prevention, 2008).

Syphilis is caused by the microorganism *Treponema pallidum,* belonging to the Spirochaetaceae family, which gets its name from the spiral-shaped appearance of its members. The microorganism survives reasonably well in the warm, moist environment of the mucous membranes that line the mouth, vagina, rectum, and other parts of the human body, but it dies quickly in almost any other environment.

It is transmitted from one person to another during any act in which two individuals come into close contact, such as during oral, anal, or vaginal sexual contact. Because the organism is fragile, however, contact between an infected and uninfected person does not guarantee that the second individual will develop the disease.

If transmission does occur, symptoms do not appear until the organism has become established and has started to multiply. This period of incubation may range anywhere from 9 to 90 days, with an average of about three weeks, during which time a person is asymptomatic (does not shown signs of infection). At this point, an ugly sore, or chancre, may appear at the site of contact. The chancre is a symptom of the primary stage of syphilis. The chancre may develop on the penis, vagina, rectum, or mouth and, in some cases, may appear to be no more than a simple pimple that is easy to ignore. In other cases, it is larger and may break open, forming an ugly, hard-to-ignore open sore. In any case, if left untreated, the chancre or sore heals within two to four weeks. An individual may easily conclude that the disease has disappeared and requires no further attention.

Such is not the case, however, as the spirochetes that caused the disease remain in the body, growing and multiplying within the bloodstream. At some point— at any time between one and six months, with an average of six to eight weeks— a new set of symptoms will appear. These symptoms include a skin rash that covers all or part of the body, most characteristically on the palms of the hands or soles of the feet, where rashes normally do not occur. In about a quarter of all cases, an individual will also experience flu-like symptoms, including headache, sore throat, runny nose, nausea, and constipation. Other symptoms include fever and weight loss and, in some cases, loss of hair. A person is most contagious during this stage of the disease.

If untreated, these symptoms may also disappear, again prompting a person to conclude that the disease has disappeared. Again, this conclusion is erroneous because the spirochete remains in the body, although it has now stopped growing and multiplying. No further symptoms may appear for a very long time— known as the latent period—before reappearing months or years after the initial infection. At that point, the most serious stage of syphilis—known as late or tertiary syphilis—develops. This stage of the disease is characterized by a number of very serious disorders affecting the muscular, cardiovascular, and nervous systems that disable and damage a person's body. The disease may eventually end in death.

Shortly after the first cases of syphilis had been reported on the Italian peninsula in about 1495, a method for treating the disease had been developed—the use of mercury salts, which had previously been used to treat leprosy and other diseases of the skin. In fact, for more than 500 years, mercury compounds remained the drugs of choice for dealing with the disease, in spite of the fact that such compounds are themselves poisonous. Thus, in many cases, the cure was worse than the disease, prompting the famous saying, "Spend one night with Venus [the goddess of love]; spend the rest of your life with Mercury" (Candida Martinelli's Italophile Site, 2009). That situation finally changed in 1910, when

German bacteriologist Paul Ehrlich (1854–1915) discovered a chemical called arsphenamine that was effective in killing the syphilis spirochete. Arsphenamine was marketed under the name of Salvarsan, or 606, the latter name reflecting the fact that it was the 606th drug that Ehrlich had tried in his effort to find a treatment for syphilis. Today, syphilis is easily treated in its early stages. A single dose of penicillin given during the primary stage will kill the spirochetes that cause the disease. For individuals who are in more advanced stages of the disease, a series of inoculations are necessary, and for anyone allergic to penicillin, alternative antibiotics are available. Thus, the disease that once was the scourge of most of the world can be cured more easily than the common cold.

*Gonorrhea*   Gonorrhea is caused by the bacterium *Neisseria gonorrhoeae,* which like the causative agent of all STIs, grows in any moist, warm region of the body, ranging from the reproductive tract to the anus to the mouth and eyes. Women are often asymptomatic for gonorrhea, or symptoms may be so mild as to be mistaken for a simple bladder or vaginal infection. Men may also be asymptomatic, although they more commonly experience a burning sensation or pain during urination and/or a discharge from the penis. These symptoms appear anywhere from 1 to 30 days after exposure, with an average of 3 to 5 days. As with syphilis, untreated cases of gonorrhea eventually go into remission and symptoms disappear. But also as with syphilis, disease organisms have not disappeared from the body and may cause more serious problems at a later date. For men, these problems may include urethritis, prostatitis, and epididymitis, which can result in sterility. For women, the most serious complication from untreated gonorrheal infection is pelvic inflammatory disease (PID), which can range from mild to severe. About a million American women develop PID each year, with gonorrheal infections being an important cause. In the most serious cases, PID can be very painful, causing damage to the fallopian tubes and increasing the chance of an ectopic pregnancy.

Although the *Neisseria gonorrhoeae* bacterium is killed by a number of antibiotics, treatment of the disease has become more difficult in recent years because of the evolution of drug-resistant strains of the microorganism. In 2007, the CDC issued new recommendations for the treatment of these drug-resistant forms of the disease which make use of the antibiotics ceftriaxone, cefixime, or spectinomycin (Centers for Disease Control and Prevention, 2008b).

*Hepatitis*   Hepatitis is an inflammation of tissues in the liver. The disease can be caused by a number of factors, including alcohol abuse. Hepatitis can be either acute, in which case the disease lasts less than six months, or chronic, in which case it continues for an extended period of time. Most cases of acute hepatitis are caused by a group of viruses designated as hepatitis virus A, hepatitis virus B, hepatitis virus C, hepatitis virus D, and hepatitis virus E. Other possible hepatitis viruses have been hypothesized but not yet confirmed. The diseases caused by these viruses have the same names as the viruses themselves: hepatitis A, hepatitis B, hepatitis C (originally called non-A, non-B), hepatitis D, and hepatitis E. The first two of these forms are the most common sexually transmitted forms of hepatitis.

Hepatitis A was formerly called infectious hepatitis. It is transmitted through contaminated food or water and by means of oral–anal sex. Symptoms of the disease normally appear about two to six weeks after exposure and mimic flu symptoms: fever, nausea, diarrhea, abdominal pain, fatigue, and loss of appetite. One of the clearest symptoms, as it is for all forms of hepatitis, is jaundice, a yellowing of the skin and the whites of the eyes. The disease usually runs its course in about two to six months, after which most people recover completely.

The disease does not recur because the immune system develops antibodies to the virus, and long-term serious effects are rare and generally due to other infections that may be present at the same time. No treatment is available for a hepatitis A infection, although a vaccine is available.

Hepatitis B was formerly called serum hepatitis because it can be transmitted through contaminated blood and blood products. It is one of the most common diseases in the world, with an estimated two billion individuals having been exposed to the hepatitis B virus. The most important means of transmission are blood transfusions that involve contaminated blood, unprotected sexual activities, sharing of contaminated needles, and transmission from a woman to her child during childbirth.

The symptoms associated with hepatitis B are similar to those for hepatitis A but include the appearance of clay-colored bowel movements, a very distinctive symptom of the infection. Symptoms may appear anywhere from six weeks to six months but appear most commonly about 90 days after exposure. In the vast majority of cases, symptoms clear (disappear) after a few weeks or months, and reoccurrence of the disease is unlikely. In a small number of cases, the disease becomes chronic, with the virus remaining in a person's bloodstream for many years.

In the most serious cases, the infection may eventually lead to cirrhosis of the liver (in which normal liver tissue is replaced by scar tissue), liver cancer, and even death. A vaccine for hepatitis B is available and is recommended for travelers who plan to visit areas in which the risk for infection is high and for other individuals at risk for infection in their daily lives, including those who are sexually active with a number of different partners.

*Herpes*   The term "herpes" refers to a large number of diseases in humans and other animals caused by one of more than a dozen different viruses. Eight of those diseases affecting humans are caused by viruses classified as human herpesvirus 1 through 8, which are responsible for diseases such as chicken pox and shingles (human herpesvirus 4), infectious mononucleosis (human herpesvirus 5), and Kaposi's sarcoma (human herpesvirus 8). The two sexually transmitted forms of the disease are caused by human herpesvirus 1 and 2, better known as herpes simplex virus type 1 and type 2 (HSV-1 and HSV-2). HSV-1 and HSV-2 are very similar to each other, sharing about 50 percent of their DNA.

The most important difference between the two types is their preferred sites in the body. HSV-1 most commonly resides in nerve cells near the ear, while HSV-2 tends to become established in nerve tissue at the base of the spine. When HSV-1 becomes active, it most commonly causes the painful but relatively harmless condition known as cold sores or fever blisters. When HSV-2 becomes active, it is responsible for the development of the condition known as genital herpes, a painful infection of the genital area. Either form of the virus can cause an infection in either part of the body, although the distribution described here tends to be most common.

As with all STIs, herpes infections are spread by intimate contact between an infected person and an uninfected person. The first signs of the disease include blister-like sores that may be very painful and may be accompanied by fever and flu-like symptoms. In many cases, symptoms do not appear, and a person may not be aware that she or he has been infected with the virus. According to some estimates, more than one in five American adults have been infected with HSV-2 at some time in their lives, and most of them are not aware of it (Herpes.com, 2009).

The incubation period for the disease is about two weeks, and any sores that appear tend to disappear two to four weeks later. As with other STIs, the disappearance of symptoms is not an indication that the disease has been cured, however. Instead, the viruses responsible for the disease remain embedded in nerve tissue and may become activated again at a future date.

The number and severity of additional outbreaks vary significantly from person to person and appear to be dependent on three major factors: (1) the severity of the first outbreak (that is, the ability of a person's immune system to combat the first appearance of the virus); (2) the length of time a person has been infected (the number and severity of infections tend to decrease over time); and (3) the variety of virus causing the infection (HSV-1-caused genital herpes tends to be less severe than HSV-2-caused genital herpes).

Genital herpes tends to receive bad press from the general public, largely because people are embarrassed to have sexual partners or others find out about their condition. From a medical standpoint, however, the disease is usually no more serious (although just as uncomfortable and inconvenient) as a cold sore (Herpes.com, 2009). Somewhat uncommonly, genital herpes may progress to more serious conditions and, perhaps, may be associated with increased risk for other viral infections, especially HIV/AIDS.

The most serious consequence of genital herpes is potential infection of a newborn child during birth to a woman with the infection, a condition that is potentially fatal for the child. There is currently no cure for genital herpes, although medications are available to relieve its symptoms. Three commonly recommended drugs are the antivirals famciclovir, acyclovir, and valacyclovir.

***HIV/AIDS*** The acronym HIV stands for human immunodeficiency virus, the agent responsible for acquired immune deficiency syndrome (AIDS). The first cases of HIV/AIDS were seen in the United States in the early 1980s. HIV spread rapidly through the gay community, among intravenous drug users and Haitians, among hemophiliacs, and finally to the heterosexual community, both in the United States and throughout the world. Today the disease is regarded as a worldwide pandemic, meaning an epidemic that has spread over a wide geographical area.

In 2008, the CDC estimated that there were 1,056,400–1,156,400 people in the United States living with AIDS, of whom 21 percent were undiagnosed. An additional 56,300 new cases of the disease were reported in 2006, the last year for which data are available. The CDC also estimated that 583,298 people had died of AIDS since it was first reported in the 1980s, with 14,561 of those deaths having occurred in 2006 (CDC, August 2008; Department of Health and Human Services, 2008).

The term "HIV/AIDS" is often used to describe an infection that has a very long incubation period. A person who has become infected may not show symptoms of the disease for many months or years. The average time between infection and so-called full-blown AIDS has been estimated at about 10 years. During this period, an individual is usually not aware that he or she has been infected. Only a blood test can detect the presence of the AIDS virus, and that test may not show results for at least six months after infection.

During the incubation period, the AIDS virus slowly attacks and disables the immune system, exposing an infected individual to ever greater risk from a number of diseases against which the body is usually able to protect itself. HIV/AIDS is, thus, a progressive disease in which a person's health gradually worsens. The CDC now defines the transition of an HIV infection to full-blown AIDS as the point at which a person has a CD4 T-cell count of less than 200 or has had one or more opportunistic infections. CD4 cells are a critical component of the immune system. When they decrease sufficiently in number, the body is no longer able to combat diseases effectively.

The term "opportunistic infection" refers to a number of conditions that are usually relatively harmless because the immune system is able to combat them effectively. Some typical opportunistic infections are a form of pneumonia called *Pneumocystis jirovecii* (formerly *Pneumocystis carinii*); a rare type of cancer, Kaposi's sarcoma; a type of streptococcus caused by the bacterium *Streptococcus pyogenes*; and a yeast infection caused by the fungus *Candida albicans*.

For the first decade of the HIV/AIDS epidemic, no treatment was available for the disease and death rates were very high, generally over 95 percent. However, a number of medications have been developed for treating the infection. The most effective therapy involves the use of a combination of at least three drugs to destroy or deactivate the virus. The availability of this cocktail has dramatically reduced the death rate from HIV/AIDS. Efforts have been made to develop a vaccine against the virus, but without success thus far. One problem is that the virus tends to evolve rapidly so that a vaccine developed against one strain of the virus may not be effective for very long. By far the most important approach to dealing with the HIV/AIDS epidemic is education. The more individuals know about the disease and the better they understand the value of and methods for practicing safer sex, the better their chances of avoiding becoming infected with HIV. The term "safe sex" refers to all those practices that one can employ during sexual acts that are likely to reduce the risk of contracting HIV/AIDS or, for that matter, any other sexual infection.

*David E. Newton*

*See also* Acquired Immune Deficiency Syndrome (AIDS); Hepatitis; Human Immunodeficiency Virus (HIV); Human Papillomavirus (HPV).

### References

American Social Health Association. "STD/STI Statistics > Fast Facts." 2009. www.ashastd. org/learn/learn_STDSTIstatistics.cfm.

Androutsos G., E. Magiorkinis, and A. Diamantis. "John Hunter (1728–1793): Father of Modern Urology." *Balkan Military Medical Review* 11 (2008): 52–55.

Candida Martinelli's Italophile Site. 2009. http://italophiles.com/carnevale.htm.

Centers for Disease Control and Prevention. *MMWR Weekly.* October 3, 2008. www.cdc. gov/mmwr/preview/mmwrhtml/mm5739a2.htm.

Centers for Disease Control and Prevention. "Updated Recommended Treatment Regimens for Gonococcal Infections and Associated Conditions—United States, April 2007." August 21, 2008. www.cdc.gov/std/treatment/2006/updated-regimens.htm.

Cohen, Mark Nathan. *Health and the Rise of Civilization.* New Haven, CT: Yale University Press, 1991.

Department of Health and Human Services, Public Health Service, Centers for Disease Control and Prevention. *HIV/AIDS Surveillance Report.* Atlanta, GA: Centers for Disease Control and Prevention, December 2008.

Division of STD Prevention. *Sexually Transmitted Disease Surveillance 2007.* Washington, DC: Department of Health and Human Services; Centers for Disease Control and Prevention; National Center for HIV/AIDS, Viral Hepatitis, STD, and TB Prevention; Division of STD Prevention, December 2008.

Goldman, Leon. 1971. "Syphilis in the Bible." *Archives of Dermatology* 103, no. 5 (May): 535–36.

Herpes.com. "The Truth about HSV-1 and HSV-2." 2009. www.herpes.com/hsv1-2.html.

Heymann, Warren R. "The History of Syphilis." *Journal of the American Academy of Dermatology* 54, no. 2 (February 2006): 322–23.

McAllister, Marie E. "Stories of the Origin of Syphilis in Eighteenth-Century England: Science, Myth, and Prejudice." *Eighteenth-Century Life* 24, no. 1 (Winter, 2000): 22–44.

Rothschild, Bruce M. "History of Syphilis." *Clinical Infectious Diseases* 40, no. 10 (May 2005): 1454–63.

Willcox, R.R. "Venereal Disease in the Bible." *British Journal of Venereal Diseases* 25 (1949): 28–33.

## SKIN CANCER. *See* CANCER

## SLEEP

A good night's sleep is not a luxury, it's a necessity for good health. When we sleep our bodies are busy doing a myriad of activities, including committing new information to memory and repairing cell damage. While more research is needed to explore the links between sleep loss and health, scientists are certain that sleep is too important to shortchange. In fact, chronic sleep problems are considered a public health problem in the United States according to the Centers for Disease Control and Prevention (CDC), whose latest statistics show 50 to 70 million Americans have chronic sleep and wakefulness disorders (CDC, 2009).

Sleep is defined as a series of complex, natural, physiological rhythms. The National Sleep Foundation (NSF) estimates that we spend one-third of our lives sleeping (NSF, 2004). We achieve sleep based on our need for sleep and the time of night when we get sleepy. Is sleep determined only by physiological events? No, behaviors also influence sleep patterns. Depending on what these behaviors are, they can actually interfere with or promote sleep.

We have allowed a flurry of responsibilities and obligations to impede our sleep. From a physiological perspective, it does not take much to induce sleep, yet we thwart our sleep by our voluntary activities and behaviors (e.g., *venti*-sized coffees that are consumed at varying times during the day and evening, Internet surfing, socializing); these behaviors accentuate the extended wakefulness (Sexton-Radek, 2004). Additionally, our student population tends to condense class schedules to accommodate full-time work schedules in conjunction with a busy social calendar. Teens and children have also extended the wake day to include homework, athletics, and Internet use. Taken together, record numbers of children, teens, young adults, adults, and the elderly are living each day in a sleep-deprived state.

Why is sleep deprivation such a big concern? Results of a Gallup poll reported that 56 percent of the adult population reported daytime drowsiness as a problem. In that grouping, 31 percent stated that they had fallen asleep at the wheel at least once in their lifetime. Sleep deprivation is a very serious threat to safety and overall emotional and physical well-being. This accumulation of sleep loss does not dissipate; it does, however, reduce our capacity to function (Coren, 1996; Engle-Friedman et al., 2003).

What effects does shortened sleep have on health or wellness? The most likely outcome is excessive daytime sleepiness resulting in personality changes (e.g., irritability), memory and concentration difficulties, safety concerns (employment and automobile accidents), and an overall decrement in quality of life.

Other potential health problems linked to lack of sleep include weight gain and obesity, as chronic sleep deprivation may affect how our bodies process and store carbohydrates. Serious sleep disorders have been linked to hypertension, increased stress hormone levels, and irregular heartbeat. Research has shown that sleep deprivation also alters immune function, and lack of sleep may decrease an individual's ability to learn or memorize new information.

The first step in solving sleep problems is to identify and determine signs of poor sleep. In addition to sleepiness, the quality and quantity of sleep must also be addressed. Ratings of *poor, good,* or *excellent* or *light, fair,* or *deep* are some ways to describe how quality and quantity of sleep may be classified.

If your sleep is disturbed, you are more likely to rate the quality of your sleep as poor. If you are sleeping less than your ideal number of hours, you are most likely going to rate your quantity of sleep as poor. If you do not know the number of hours your body requires for restorative sleep, there is an easy way to figure it out. Think back to the last time you took a vacation. Ignore the first few nights of sleep (it is generally catch-up sleep). What was the length of your sleep? Generally, this question is a good heuristic to follow to determine your personal sleep need. If you experience less than good or fair sleep on a consistent basis, you most likely will experience excessive daytime sleepiness.

**Understanding Sleep** Approximately 55 years ago, sleep was thought of as a "dormant state of passive activity or no consequence" (Sexton-Radek, 2004). This period of "no consequence" was hypothesized to serve as a much-needed downshifting in physiological activity from the day's events. We know much more today, however, especially with the burgeoning field of sleep medicine focusing on the diagnosis, assessment, and treatment of sleep disorders. Sleep is considered now to be an active state of being; the mind is a 24-hour mind, and it does stop working—a surprising fact of which we often are not aware. We spend roughly one-third of our lives sleeping in this active state. Although the specific function of sleep still eludes researchers, many substantiated theories now point to the necessity of good-quality sleep to our existence and overall well-being.

Different brain-cell chemicals and neurotransmitters regulate our sleep–wake states by acting on a variety of cells in the brain. Sleep–wake functioning is analogous to a light switch with on and off features. A type of switch setting systematically turns on sleep, including turning on different types of sleep (e.g., Stages 1–4 and dream sleep), and systematically turns off each sleep stage correspondingly.

This switch setting easily explains how our sleep progresses from light sleep to deep sleep and then transcends to dream, or rapid eye movement (REM), sleep. The neurochemical signaling begins when we fall asleep. An exact sleep chemical is still considered to be controversial, yet a number of studies suggest adenosine (a nucleoside) binds to cells and causes a cascade of events that promotes drowsiness (Chokroverty, 1999).

Adenosine levels in the blood increase during waking hours and have a cumulative effect throughout the day, causing drowsiness. During sleep, adenosine levels decline (unbind to cells), promoting wakefulness toward the end of the nocturnal period (Johns, 1991). The cycle begins again once we are awake. It is not surprising that stimulants such as caffeine cause wakefulness, because caffeine competes for the same receptors to which adenosine binds. If more receptors have caffeine bound to them, sleepiness is less likely to happen.

**Sleep Stages** Sleep architecture refers to the various stages in the sleep–wake cycle, typically defined by a brainwave recording. In healthy individuals without sleep problems, these stages occur in a regular pattern throughout a 24-hour period. There are two types of sleep: dream or rapid eye movement (REM) sleep, which occurs every 1.5 hours throughout the sleep interval, or 18 percent to 25 percent of the sleep period (Graci, 2005; Graci & Sexton-Radek, 2005). REM periods vary from a number of minutes to an hour or more. REM sleep has a characteristic physiological pattern distinguished by the lateral saccadic (left to right) rhythm of the eyes, absence of muscle movement (atonia), and heightened cardiovascular arousal. Studies of the REM period by self-report have revealed that the changing themes from everyday events to surreal wish fantasies occur toward the end of the sleep period.

In contrast, non-REM (NREM) sleep occupies a greater portion of the sleep period. NREM is further subdivided into Stages 1, 2, 3, and 4, with corresponding physiological activity to each. Stage 1 is considered light sleep and is estimated to be approximately 5 percent of the sleep period. Stage 2 sleep is about 60 percent of the sleep interval and is formally considered to be sleep. Stages 3 and 4 sleep are often collapsed together and are classified as deep sleep, a physiological event characterized by slow brain wave patterns and increased immune system activity. Non-REM makes up approximately 10 percent to 15 percent of the sleep period.

A night of sleep is characterized as a predicted pattern beginning with the initiation of sleep onset (Stage 1) and progression to Stages 2, 3, and 4. Within 90 minutes after sleep onset, the first REM episode (generally four to five REM episodes per night) occurs. Following this sleep period, the cycle repeats itself, with at least four cycles of sleep per night. An excess or deficit in the amount of a type of sleep (e.g., no REM), a misordering of the timing of sleep (e.g., sleep begins with REM), or an intrusion into sleep represent conditions for further study to determine if a sleep disorder exists.

**Function of Sleep**  Sleep is needed for survival (Coren, 1996). In animal studies, sleep-deprived rats subjected to extended periods of sleep loss developed disease and illness, with some resulting in death (Chokroverty, 1999). What does sleep loss do to our bodies? Our immune system becomes less efficient and productive with reduced sleep (Chokroverty, 1999; Horne, 1988). Our ability to fight off infection under increased stress levels can become compromised.

For instance, increased reports of cold- and flu-like symptoms are reported at college health clinics in response to surveys about high stress-response levels (commonly presented as sleep loss) (Engle-Friedman et al., 2003). It is during deep (Stage 4) sleep when our immune system regenerates. Stage 4 sleep is also the time when growth hormone (the hormone responsible for growth and metabolism) is released, thus implicating the importance of a good night's sleep for children.

The biological systems of our body follow a natural rhythm of activity and rest (Monk, 1991). Many of these rhythms (cycles) are activated during the stages of sleep, usually deep sleep (Stages 3 and 4) or dream (REM) sleep. Overall, all cycles follow an approximate 24-hour schedule; hence the term "circadian" (i.e., "about a day") is used. When an individual's 24-hour schedule becomes skewed or altered due to work, travel, or personal habits, the timing of the sleep in terms of bedtime and wake time is offset. For instance, when traveling across time zones, we will experience a change in our sleep schedule (Notti, 1990).

This change may present as either a delay (sleep occurs at a later time) or advancement (sleep occurs at an earlier time) in our sleep time. Last, our natural drive for sleep is strongest during the day (A.M.) and nighttime (P.M.) between the hours of 1:00 and 4:00. This feeling of sleepiness that occurs during the hours between 1:00 P.M. and 4:00 P.M. is often misinterpreted as sleepiness resulting from having lunch.

Taken together, problem sleepiness occurs if we alter our schedule of activity and sleep at a time when the drive for sleepiness is the strongest. Treatment efforts address this change or desynchronization of our normal wake–sleep rhythms by scheduling naps, implementing light physical activity to the schedule and utilizing light therapy at varying times during the day to promote either sleepiness or wakefulness.

We are generally aware of our level and ratings of sleepiness. We are all familiar with stories of businesspeople traveling and staying up late to prepare for a big presentation. Or there is the scenario of young adults and teens altering their sleep schedules with in-house socializing (e.g., instant messaging) by staying up into the late hours of the night. Additional examples include patients who are recovering from medical procedures who may easily awaken from experiencing pain or restlessly shifting positions while dipping in and out of sleep during the night. In each of these scenarios, poor sleep is experienced, and if these sleep patterns remain unabated, the individual is at risk for mood alterations and performance and health consequences.

A mounting sleep debt—regardless of the process that triggered it—has the same result: decreased performance efficiency, mood instability, and poor health and disease and disorder formation (Monk, 1991). Our defensive response to the challenges we face with poor sleep is weakened and remains that way. Poor sleep, especially when continuously experienced, lowers the immune system response. Couple poor sleep with exposure to environmental toxins, disease and infection exposure, and/or mental or physical stress and we may see how the immune system can significantly be lowered.

**Treatments for Sleep Disturbances**   The treatments for sleep disturbances have been the focus of outstanding research investigations. Complex and rigorous scientific studies have yielded robust treatment outcomes. The rationale for utilizing various treatment interventions is based on the level of distress and behavioral discomfort experienced by patients (Nelson, 2006).

Sources of sleep disturbance in individuals are many, varied, and complex (Sexton-Radek, 1998). It is helpful to think of these sources in terms of predisposing, precipitating, and perpetuating factors (Dement & Vaughn, 1999; Nelson, 2006; Sexton-Radek, 1998). The condition of chronic insomnia is conceptualized as starting from what are termed "predisposing" factors (Nelson, 2006; Sexton-Radek, 1998). These factors are events or actions that significantly disturb one's sleep, such as anxious or tense feelings, and are sufficient factors leading to sleep disturbance (i.e., not being able to fall asleep and/or stay asleep).

Precipitating factors are viewed as disturbing events that interrupt and worsen sleep. Examples of precipitating factors include experiencing a medical illness that causes extended wakefulness or being subjected to continued environmental disturbance such as loud music from a neighbor's apartment. Individuals then engage in behaviors to "fix" their sleep. These behaviors actually perpetuate the sleep disturbance instead of fixing sleep. For instance, individuals may decide to stay up really late by watching television to increase sleepiness. In this example, staying up late does not enhance sleep initiation, it succeeds only in making the individual more aroused instead of achieving a state of relaxation.

Two empirically validated sleep treatments are stimulus control and sleep restriction therapies. These approaches are quite effective with insomnia diagnoses and may even be applied to complaints of poor sleep that do not meet insomnia criteria. Occasional insomnia is common, and many factors may precipitate the sleep disturbance. Researchers have hypothesized an interrelationship between anxiety, depression, and insomnia (Sexton-Radek, 1998).

**Sleep Restriction Therapy**   Individuals undergoing sleep restriction therapy will be asked to go on a so-called sleep diet. This type of intervention is formally called sleep restriction and represents one of the most effective means to regulate sleep. By keeping track of sleep with a sleep log, individuals will be able to convey to a sleep specialist the times during the day that they are sleeping.

The logic behind the use of sleep restriction has been demonstrated in many research studies of sleep quality. Consolidating sleep to the actual time when one is sleeping (on a regular basis) provides the necessary cues to the brain that it is time to sleep (Dement & Vaughn, 1999; Johnson et al., 1992).

A person may be able to fall asleep but then wake up and be unable to return to sleep until the body is ready for sleep. It is common for individuals to lie awake in bed and focus on not sleeping, worrying about how this lack of sleep is going to affect them during the day.

Sleep restriction generally involves creating a mild state of sleep deprivation with the goal of increasing sleep pressure so that patients are able to consolidate their sleep. The overarching goal is to have the patient sleep continuously throughout the night. A general heuristic is that if you complain of difficulty falling asleep and report lying awake in bed for more than 30 minutes, your sleep specialist may restrict your bedtime to the actual time (on a consistent basis) that you report falling asleep. For instance, if a patient reports going to bed at 10:00 P.M. but does not fall asleep until midnight, it is appropriate to suggest going to bed at midnight.

**Stimulus Control Therapy**   Wakefulness after sleep onset arising from an environmental trigger or behavioral factors has been studied extensively (Johnson et al., 1992). It seems that the longer an individual lies in bed ruminating or worrying about not sleeping can be the stimulus that produces the arousal or anxiety that is associated with either walking into your bedroom or getting into bed at night. Once the bedroom is associated with anxious feelings or sensation, the bed is no longer considered a safe haven. The wakefulness associated with worrying about not sleeping is sufficiently potent to cause not sleeping to be habit forming.

Stimulus control therapy is the treatment that involves breaking up these false bedroom associations or the conditioned arousal that we have taught ourselves to experience when we get into bed. If we learn to dread sleep, we can unlearn it through stimulus control treatment. The primary objective of stimulus control therapy is to train the patient, through a learning paradigm, to associate the bed with sleeping and sleeping with the bed. In addition, the patient learns to set their sleep–wake cycle. To achieve these goals, the following behaviors are suggested:

- Go to bed only when sleepy.
- Pursue only sleep in bed. No other activity except sexual activity is permitted; in other words, reading, eating, watching television, or completing homework is to be done not in bed but in another area of the home.
- Get out of bed if sleep does not come within 15 or 20 minutes of retiring at night, and engage in relaxing behavior, returning to bed only when sleepy (this may be repeated as often as needed throughout the night).
- Wake at the same time every day, regardless of the amount of sleep achieved during the night.
- Avoid daytime naps.

Essentially, the intervention entails having an individual get out of bed and go into another room if he is unable to sleep within 15 minutes and engaging in a boring, nonmentally stimulating activity. The key is that the activity has to be boring and nonmentally stimulating. The selection of a boring task is designed to neutralize one's dreadful thinking and, in effect, to promote relaxation that can elicit sleep. The boring task activity is done outside of the bedroom so as to break the link of the bedroom and sleeplessness. In numerous studies of this intervention, it has been consistently found to be one of the most effective (Johnson et al., 1992). Some individuals may have to repeat the procedure more than once a night in order to reduce or eliminate bodily tension and replace it with one of relaxation experienced from performing a boring task in the middle of the night.

*Kathy Sexton-Radek and Gina Graci*

*See also* Basal Metabolism; Immune System; Insomnia.

## References

APA (American Psychiatric Association). *Diagnostic and Statistical Manual of Mental Disorders,* 4th ed. Washington, DC: APA, 1994.

Centers for Disease Control and Prevention. "Insufficient Rest or Sleep in Adults, United States, 2008." December 7, 2009. www.cdc.gov/features/ds/sleep.

Chokroverty, S. *Sleep Disorders Medicine: Basic Science, Technical Considerations, and Clinical Aspects.* Boston: Butterworth Heinemann, 1999.

Coren, S. *Sleep Thieves: An Eye-opening Exploration into the Science and Mysteries of Sleep.* New York: Free Press, 1996.

Dement, W.C. and C. Vaughn. *The Promise of Sleep.* New York: Random House, 1999.

Engle-Friedman, M., S. Riela, R. Golan, A. M. Ventenac, C. Davis, A. Jefferson, et al. "The Effect of Sleep Loss on Next Day Effect," *Journal of Sleep Research* 12 (2003):113–24.

Graci, G. M. "Pathogenesis and Management of Cancer-Related Insomnia," *The Journal of Supportive Oncology* 3 no. 5 (September–October, 2005): 349–59.

Graci, G. and K. Sexton-Radek. "Treating Sleep Disorders Using Cognitive Behavioral Therapy and Hypnosis." In *The Clinical Use of Hypnosis in Cognitive Behavior Therapy: A Practitioner's Casebook,* edited by R.A. Chapman, 348. New York: Springer, 2005.

Horne, J. *Why We Sleep.* Oxford: Oxford University Press, 1988.

Johns, M.W. "A New Method of Measuring Daytime Sleepiness: The Epworth Sleepiness Scale." *Sleep* 14 (1991): 540.

Johnson, M.P., J.F. Duffy, D. J. Dijk, J. M. Ronda, C. M. Dyal, and C. A. Czeisler. "Short-term Memory, Alertness and Performance: A Reappraisal of Their Relationship to Body Temperature," *Journal of Sleep Research* 1 (1992): 642–56.

Monk, T.H. *Sleep, Sleepiness and Performance.* Chichester, UK: Wiley, 1991.

National Sleep Foundation. *Sleep and America Poll.* Washington, DC: National Sleep Foundation, 2004.

Nelson, G. "Conquering Sleep: Move Over Nature, We're Taking Control," *The New Scientist* 2539 (February 2006): 43–9.

Notti, L. *Losing Sleep: How Your Sleeping Habits Affect Your Life.* New York: Morrow, 1990.

Sexton-Radek, K. "Pre-sleep Autonomic Arousal as a Distinguishing Factor of Sleep Pattern Type," *Perceptual and Motor Skills* 87 (1998): 261–2.

Sexton-Radek, K. *Sleep Quality in Young Adults.* New York: Mellon Press, 2004.

# SMOKING

In the United States, an estimated 24 million men and 21 million women are smokers (American Heart Association, 2011). Today, almost everyone knows that smoking causes cancer, emphysema, and heart disease. The habit costs smokers thousands of dollars year. So why are people still lighting up? The answer can be found in the substances people are smoking and in one word: addiction. This article will examine smoking in regard to tobacco, cannabis, and crack cocaine.

**Smoking Tobacco**   Tobacco is a plant that belongs to the same family that includes tomatoes, belladonna, and petunias, and most of the tobacco available on the commercial market today comes from a mild, broad-leafed variety of the plant called *Nicotiana tabacum*. While the leaves of tobacco can be crushed and snorted, sucked, or chewed, most of the tobacco used in the United States is smoked and inhaled into the lungs, either through cigars or cigarettes.

Though smoking is the most prevalent form of tobacco use, smokeless tobacco remains popular as well, particularly in the form of moist snuff, powder snuff, and loose-leaf tobacco, which can be consumed in a variety of ways. Though one of the most addictive substances known to man (it is harder to quit smoking than it is to stop using opiates or alcohol), the physical and mental effects of nicotine are less intense than the sensations caused by other drugs. When chewed or sucked, it takes about five to eight minutes for the effects of nicotine to reach the brain, while smoking and inhaling the drug gets it to the brain much faster, usually between five and eight seconds.

The average cigarette contains about 10 milligrams of nicotine, though only one to three milligrams of that nicotine are delivered to the lungs when smoked; chewing tobacco delivers more nicotine to the body (4.5 milligrams per chew), while a pinch of snuff delivers 3.6 milligrams. This makes the effects of smokeless tobacco slightly more intense than those of cigarettes. Nicotine acts as a stimulant by disrupting the natural balance between several neurotransmitters—endorphins, epinephrine, acetylcholine, and dopamine. By affecting acetylcholine, it increases the heart rate, blood pressure, memory, learning, mental activity, and aggression.

The epinephrine that nicotine causes to be released creates a surge of energy, leading to a rise in glucose levels in the blood as well as a higher heart rate, increased blood pressure, and more rapid respiration. In addition to these physiological effects, the drug also suppresses appetite and increases the body's metabolism, and the average regular smoker weighs between six and nine pounds less than nonsmokers. The drug also enhances the body's release of dopamine, a neurotransmitter that makes users feel satisfied and calm. Thus, while it creates a feeling of calm and satisfaction on the one hand, nicotine is also a very strong stimulant on the other. The stimulant effects of nicotine, particularly the release of dopamine, are usually short-lived, lasting only a few minutes. To maintain the sense of satisfaction triggered by dopamine, people who use tobacco naturally want to take additional doses of the drug. This is a major reason that the drug is highly addictive.

On average, a heavy tobacco smoker will consume between 30 and 40 cigarettes a day, which translates to over 10,000 cigarettes per year. Even knowledge of the potentially harmful effects of smoking is not enough to get many smokers to quit, as 80 percent of them know their habit can cause cancer but nonetheless continue to smoke.

Appearing on an almost annual basis after the inaugural report in 1964, the Surgeon General's reports on tobacco have scientifically established the many health hazards of smoking. The first Surgeon General's report on tobacco, which appeared when almost half of American adults smoked, was a groundbreaking document that culled years of research and concluded, among other things, that smoking was a cause of lung and laryngeal cancer. Similarly repercussive was the 1988 report

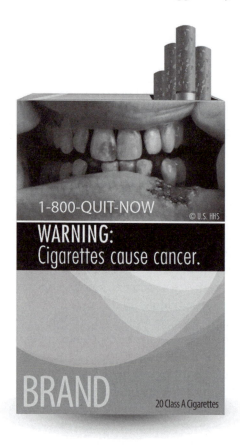

New government warning labels on cigarette packages are designed to send a stark health message. (Food and Drug Administration)

on nicotine addiction, which concluded that cigarettes were addicting, nicotine was the drug that causes addiction, and the pharmacologic and behavioral processes at work in nicotine addiction were similar to those determining addiction to drugs like heroin or cocaine.

The first Surgeon General's report on smoking was born out of a committee that started to come together in 1962. In that year, President Kennedy's Surgeon General, Luther Terry, announced that he would be forming a committee to investigate the impact of smoking upon health, and the group he judiciously convened consisted of five smokers and five nonsmokers. The committee was not opposed by the tobacco industry's pseudoscientific institution, the Tobacco Industry Research Committee (TIRC), thereby making it all the more difficult for the conclusions the committee eventually reached to be called into question by big tobacco.

The committee's groundbreaking findings, which were based upon a review of more than 7,000 articles about smoking, health, and disease, were published on January 11, 1964, under the title *Smoking and Health.* Cognizant of the potential impact of the committee's findings, Terry scheduled the news conference surrounding the report's release on a Saturday so as to avert any panic that might arise on Wall Street. Similarly, Terry made sure that information as potent as that contained in the report made its way into the hands of as few people as possible before the news conference. As such, the White House received a copy of *Smoking and Health* only two hours before its official release.

The historic report constituted both the most authoritative and direst assessment of the health effects of tobacco use up that point. It concluded that cigarette smoking was a cause of both lung and laryngeal cancer in men; in the case of women, cigarette smoking was described as a probable cause. Chronic bronchitis and emphysema were found to be far more common in smokers than nonsmokers, and the report also determined that the rates of coronary artery disease were 70 percent higher among smokers. Additionally alarming to a nation of some 70 million regular smokers was the report's conclusion that the fatality rate from lung cancer was 1,000 percent higher among smoking men than nonsmoking men. In response to these findings, the committee stated that smoking represented a health hazard of such a degree as to warrant appropriate remedial action, though they left such an action undefined.

These conclusions represented a tremendous blow to the tobacco industry, which had successfully weathered the first wave of reports linking cigarette smoking to cancer and other diseases in the early 1950s by hiring the public relations firm, Hill & Knowlton, which helped form the TIRC and which was behind the publication, in hundreds of newspapers across the country in 1954, of "A Frank Statement to Cigarette Smokers." That letter-form advertisement had alleviated growing concern over the health effects of smoking by claiming that there was no proof that cigarette smoke was a cause of lung cancer, but *Smoking and Health* made such a stance no longer scientifically tenable. The TIRC tried to regain some of the legitimacy it lost in the wake of the report by changing its name to the Council for Tobacco Research, but the superficiality of this move highlighted that the tobacco industry could have no significant answer to *Smoking and Health*.

American smokers, too, were hit hard by the committee's conclusions, and in January and February of 1964 many smokers tried to quit in what was called "The Great Forswearing." In March, however, even the knowledge of smoking's dangers was not enough to prevent what soon came to be known as "The Great Relapse." The continued smoking of cigarettes surprised Terry, who believed that *Smoking and Health* would be enough to convince Americans to quit an extremely hazardous practice, and he suggested that the addictiveness of cigarettes was stronger than had been indicated the conclusions of the first Surgeon General's report on smoking.

The Surgeon General in the 1980s, C. Everett Koop, had no such reservations, and the report he released in May 1988 was based upon a significant amount of new research. *The Health Consequences of Smoking—Nicotine Addiction: A Report of the Surgeon General* concluded that cigarettes were addicting and that nicotine was the drug causing addiction. It additionally determined that the pharmacologic and behavioral processes at work in nicotine addiction were similar to those determining addiction to drugs like heroin or cocaine. Koop even explicitly explained that his document overturned the 1964 report's conclusion that cigarette smoking was habituating instead of addicting.

Koop's report was yet another blow to the tobacco industry, which by then had been denying the addictiveness of cigarettes in important lawsuits such as *Cipollone v. Liggett Group Inc. et al.* Internal industry documents, however, revealed big tobacco's longstanding knowledge of nicotine's addictiveness, and whistleblower Jeffrey Wigand provided further confirmation of this. Food and Drug Administration (FDA) head David Kessler would later utilize the conclusions reached by Surgeon General's reports like those from 1964 and 1988 when he declared, in 1996, that cigarettes were essentially nicotine-delivery devices and should thus be brought under the regulatory authority of the FDA.

**Smoking Cannabis** Human beings have been using the leaves of the hemp plant (also known as cannabis or marijuana), which probably originated in China or Central Asia, for a variety of purposes for at least 10,000 years. There are many uses for the plant, as its fibers can be used to produce rope and cloth, its seeds are edible, it contains an oil that can be used as a fuel, and it also contains active ingredients that have been used as medicines throughout history. Even today, some recommend using marijuana to alleviate pain, and as a medicine for the treatment of certain forms of glaucoma and muscular sclerosis.

The drug is usually smoked, though it can be eaten if added to food. Most users, however, prefer to smoke cannabis since it takes longer to feel the psychoactive effects of the drug if it is eaten, and consuming the drug orally increases the likelihood that the drug will have unpleasant effects.

Of the 420 chemicals in the cannabis plant, over 60 of them, called cannabinoids, are believed to have some psychoactive properties. The main psychoactive ingredient in cannabis is the chemical delta-9-tetrahydrocannabinol (THC), which makes up somewhere between 1 percent and 3 percent of the cannabis leaf as it grows in nature. Illegal growers, however, have adopted new techniques for growing the plant to enhance its psychoactive effects, and much of the marijuana available on the black market today has THC concentrations as high as 15 percent.

The main sensations produced by marijuana include euphoria, a slightly altered sense of sight and sound, and a distortion of the sense of time. The main reason marijuana users use the drug is to gain the overall sense of pleasure, calm, and relaxation that it produces, especially in small doses. When used in social settings, the initial feelings brought on by marijuana—euphoria, talkativeness, and sometimes uncontrollable laughter—are similar to the initial effects of alcohol. In doses of about 2.5 milligrams, the changes in perception become more intense, with users experiencing decreases in feelings of tension and depression, a disrupted short-term memory, increased drowsiness, hallucinations, flashbacks, and a sense of being mentally separated from the outside world.

For individuals unaccustomed to these effects, this can lead to anxiety and paranoia, though regular users grow to find the experience a pleasant one. These mental effects are accompanied by physical feelings of relaxation and sedation, the attenuation of physical pain, bloodshot eyes, diminished muscular coordination, increased feelings of hunger and thirst, and nausea. Within an hour of use, the effects of marijuana begin to diminish, and generally dissipate within four to six hours. The high induced by the drug lasts longer when it is eaten than when it is smoked, though it also takes much longer to take effect.

Users develop a tolerance to marijuana relatively quickly, and the drug can remain in the bodies of chronic users for up to three months after they last smoked it. The withdrawal symptoms experienced by marijuana users, however, are relatively mild when compared to most other addictive drugs. Part of the reason withdrawal symptoms from marijuana are minimal is that the THC chemical remains in the brain for a long period after the drug was last used, and it sometimes takes weeks for chronic users to start feeling any unpleasant side effects when they stop taking the drug.

Some people report never feeling any withdrawal symptoms when they stop using it, though studies show that in the long-run, most regular users can experience a variety of symptoms, including anger, irritability, depression, an inability to concentrate, trouble sleeping, and a craving to start using marijuana again. Nonetheless, the side effects of marijuana withdrawal are not nearly as severe as those caused by withdrawal from nicotine, alcohol, opiates, or other commonly abused drugs. Many individuals who first try the drug casually do wind up becoming habitual users, even if they do not suffer from extreme and immediate withdrawal symptoms when they stop.

Most of the negative consequences of chronic cannabis use are physical, with regular users developing respiratory problems largely because the drug is smoked, and some studies have shown that prolonged use can have negative effects on the immune system and cognitive functioning, while impairing short-term memory, attention span, and motivation. Other studies have also found a correlation between cannabis use and the development of psychotic disorders, though scientists have not found any causal link between marijuana and mental illness.

In the United States, cannabis was a common plant (even George Washington grew it on his plantation), though it was cultivated more for use as a fiber than anything else. The practice of using cannabis recreationally probably came over to the United States with slaves, who brought it with them from Africa, and then with migrant laborers who came to the United States from Latin America during World War I.

The association of the drug with minorities who, according to some of the racist beliefs of the time, were amoral and dangerous, spawned opposition to the drug, as did some early 20th-century research that argued it was potentially just as harmful as alcohol and opium. With the passage of the Pure Food and Drug Act of 1906, cannabis became less prevalent in common medical preparations, though it was not subject to the same tight controls as other drugs, such as opiates, under the 1914 Harrison Narcotics Act.

Political pressure to institute federal controls, however, grew in the 1930s, and in 1937 the federal government took action with the passage of the Marihuana Tax Act, which gave the Treasury Department the power to regulate cannabis. But despite these controls, marijuana use exploded in the 1960s when the drug became a favorite of hippies and others in the counterculture. Largely in response to the spread of cannabis use, the federal government passed the Comprehensive Drug Abuse Prevention and Control Act of 1970, which raised the penalties for growing, importing, exporting, and dealing the drug to up to 10 years in prison, while making possession of the drug punishable by up to two years in jail.

In 1972, the National Organization for the Reform of Marijuana Laws (NORML) petitioned the government to reclassify the drug and lighten the restrictions on it. After years of legal wrangling, NORML finally got the DEA to hear its case in 1987, and the judge in the case agreed that the drug should be reclassified so it could be used as a medicine. In spite of the recommendation, the DEA refused to reclassify the drug, and in federal law, it remains a Schedule I drug—the most highly controlled class of drug—to this day.

Beginning in the 1970s, many states took action to either decriminalize possession of marijuana or to allow for it to be used as a medicine, though the legal status of these statutes remains in limbo. While states can pass whatever laws they want concerning marijuana, federal law, which still classifies it as a highly controlled substance, technically trumps state laws when there is a conflict between the two. As a result, the fate of medical marijuana laws and state efforts to decriminalize the drug remains up in the air.

Meanwhile, recreational use remains prevalent in the United States today, with some 14.8 million people in the United States reporting using the drug in the last month in a National Survey on Drug Use and Health that was conducted in 2006. Marijuana use continues to remain common among the young, as over 63.3 percent of the people who tried the drug for the first time were under

18 years. In 2007, 14.2 percent of eighth graders reported trying marijuana at least once, while over 40 percent of high school seniors have used the drug at some point in their lives.

**Smoking Crack Cocaine**   The most typical form of cocaine use in the 1970s and early 1980s was the snorting of cocaine powder, but the mid-1980s saw the emergence of a new form of cocaine use—crack smoking. Far cheaper than cocaine in its powder form, crack found a sizeable market in impoverished, inner-city neighborhoods in the 1980s. Some scholars, however, believe that the "crack epidemic" of the period was more media exaggeration than social reality, resulting from misinformation about crack's addictiveness combined with crack's greater visibility amongst the lowest classes in urban ghettos.

Though controlled by federal drug laws since the early 20th century, cocaine reemerged as a popular drug the 1970s, when its use by celebrities and musicians transformed it into a glamorous substance in many circles. The rise of Latin American drug trafficking organizations also played a significant role in the reemergence of cocaine in American life, as they smuggled it into the United States and distributed it on American streets on a large scale. Nonetheless, cocaine remained relatively expensive, costing between $80 and $100 per gram in the 1970s.

Crack emerged in the mid-1980s as a more potent, low-cost alternative to powder cocaine. Underground chemists in Los Angeles first devised crack in the early 1980s by mixing cocaine with baking soda and boiling down the mixture into a smokable rock form. The new form of cocaine was on the black market by late 1984, and it soon spread throughout lower-class neighborhoods of Los Angeles, Miami, and New York City.

Originally dubbed "cocaine-rock," the substance soon came to be known as "crack," getting its name from the cracking or crackling sound that is made when the substance is heated and smoked in glass pipes. Crack was more powerful than powdered cocaine, faster acting (it got users high within seconds), and also significantly cheaper, costing just $5 to $10 per rock. Crack's potency and relative cheapness, authorities feared, could make the drug spread like wildfire. Street dealers stood to benefit from crack since its effects wore off quicker than cocaine, meaning that users would need to come back to buy more of the drug more regularly. Users, drug policymakers feared, would turn to crack instead of cocaine since it was relatively inexpensive and created a high that was more powerful.

The emergence of crack generated calls of alarm, as many claimed that the country was in the midst of a crack epidemic from the mid-1980s through the early 1990s. Members of the media, politicians, and public health officials alike contributed to a seeming consensus that crack represented the most dangerous drug ever created or known. Characterized as extremely destructive and almost instantaneously addictive, crack came to be seen as a kind of narcotic juggernaut that jeopardized the well-being of Americans of all stripes.

Newspaper, magazine, and television reports spoke of crack's rapid spread beyond the ghettos of the big cities in which it originally appeared thus and alarmed suburban and rural readers and viewers, who feared a crack epidemic that could cut across social, racial, and geographic lines. In particular, the media seized on the problem of "crack babies"—children who were born to crack-addicted mothers with serious health problems. Fear that crack use had reached epidemic proportions and had tremendous social costs became a driving force behind national drug policies in the 1980s, and Congress passed tough antidrug legislation—the Anti-Drug Abuse Acts—largely in response to the dangers the drug seemingly posed to the American public.

Despite (or perhaps because of) this intense focus on the crack epidemic, the true place of crack in American life was obscured in the 1980s. Lost amidst the hubbub over crack was the fact that the drug was never widely used by Americans, and in further contradiction of media reports about the instantaneous addictiveness of the drug, few people who tried crack continued using it. One reason that only a small percentage of people who smoked crack a first time opted to do it again is that the drug has a strong, almost overwhelming, impact.

The repeated use of a drug of this strength and impact is generally limited to the small segment of the population that uses heroin heavily. As such, even amongst cocaine users, only a small percentage of them smoked crack heavily. National Institute on Drug Abuse (NIDA) surveys from the 1980s and 1990s confirm the relative rarity of crack use during the so-called crack epidemic. The NIDA-led National Household Survey on Drug Abuse of 1990 revealed that in the first years after crack's emergence, overall drug use, including that of cocaine and its derivatives, declined.

The survey from the following year showed that the percentage of Americans between the ages of 12 and 25 who had ever tried cocaine and related drugs peaked in 1982—well before the appearance of crack—and continued to decline thereafter. NIDA's 1986 study measuring crack use among high school seniors found that 4.1 percent had tried crack at least once in the previous year, but as the crack scare continued, yearly surveys showed this figure dropped each subsequent year. Through the early 1990s, this number hovered around just 1.5 percent, clearly indicating that Americans were not using crack in epidemic proportions. An explanation for the disconnect between Americans' sense in the late 1980s and early 1990s that they were living in the midst of a crack epidemic and the reality that crack never truly threatened wide swaths of the population may lie in the fact that those most affected by crack were the impoverished, blacks, and Latinos. Because they had little financial means of combating their addiction and a greater visibility in the nation's ghettos and barrios than middle-class cocaine users, crack users and addicts attracted media scrutiny and political attention disproportionate to the true level of crack use in the country. Racial prejudices, too, likely contributed to suburban and rural Americans' fears of a crack epidemic.

By 1990, a number of media reports emerged that called into question the phenomenon of a crack epidemic. These stories revealed that crack was not nearly as addictive as it had been built up to be, nor had it made significant inroads beyond inner-city neighborhoods. By the election year of 1992, fears of a crack epidemic had essentially come to an end. George H. W. Bush said little about illicit drugs during his reelection campaign, and the Clinton administration did not continue to address the drug problem in the same way as its Republican predecessors had done, so the concerns about crack began to fade by the mid-1990s.

*Howard Padwa and Jacob Cunningham*

*See also* Cancer; Cigarettes; Drugs, Recreational; Secondhand Smoke.

### References

American Heart Association. *Cigarette Smoking Statistics.* 2010. www.americanheart.org.

American Psychiatric Association. *Diagnostic Criteria from DSM-IV.* Washington, DC: American Psychiatric Association, 1994.

Belenko, Steven R., ed. *Drugs and Drug Policy in America: A Documentary History.* Westport, CT: Greenwood Press, 2000.

Brandt, Allan M. *The Cigarette Century: The Rise, Fall, and Deadly Persistence of the Product that Defined America.* New York: Basic Books, 2007.

Coombs, Robert Holman, ed. *Handbook of Addictive Disorders: A Practical Guide to Diagnosis and Treatment.* Hoboken, NJ: John Wiley & Sons, Inc., 2004.

Cordry, Harold V. *Tobacco: A Reference Handbook.* Santa Barbara, CA: ABC-CLIO, 2001.

Erickson, Patricia G., Edward M. Adlaf, Reginald G. Smart, and Glenn F. Murray, eds. *The Steel Drug: Cocaine and Crack in Perspective.* New York: Lexington Books, 1994.

Goodman, Aviel. "Neurobiology of Addiction: An Integrative Review." *Biochemical Pharmacology* 75 (2008): 266–322.

Gwinnell, Esther and Christine Adamec. *The Encyclopedia of Addictions and Addictive Behaviors.* New York: Facts on File, 2006.

Hirschfelder, Arlene B. *Encyclopedia of Smoking and Tobacco.* Phoenix, AZ: Oryx Press 1999.

National Institute on Drug Abuse. *InfoFacts: Marijuana.* November 1, 2008. www.nida.nih.gov/Infofacts/marijuana.html.

Reinarman, Craig and Harry G. Levine, eds. *Crack in America: Demon Drugs and Social Justice.* Berkeley: University of California Press, 1997.

U.S. Drug Enforcement Administration. "Cocaine." November 1, 2008. www.usdoj.gov/dea/concern/cocaine.html.

U.S. Public Health Services, Office of the Surgeon General. *The Health Consequences of Smoking—Nicotine Addiction: A Report of the Surgeon General.* 1988. http://profiles.nlm.nih.gov/NN/B/B/Z/D/_/nnbbzd.pdf.

U.S. Surgeon General's Advisory Committee on Smoking and Health. *Smoking and Health: Report of the Advisory Committee to the Surgeon General of the Public Health Service.* 1964. http://profiles.nlm.nih.gov/NN/B/B/M/Q/_/nnbbmq.pdf.

## SODIUM

Sodium, an element identified as "Na" in the periodic table, is present in many different compounds and was first isolated in 1807 by Sir Humphrey Davy. It is the most abundant element among the alkali group of metals. These days, people also associate sodium with salt and recognize it for its role in helping foods taste flavorful. However, salt is actually made of sodium chloride, NaCl, the most common compound containing sodium. NaCl is made up of 40 percent sodium and 60 percent chloride (Larson-Duyff, 2006).

In the human body, sodium is an electrolyte. Electrolytes are minerals that exist in blood and other bodily fluids and that carry an electric charge. The body must have a balance between water and these electrolytes to maintain blood pressure and to ensure nerves and muscles work properly. Sodium, among other electrolytes, moves fluid in and out of cells. This fluid carries in nutrients and eliminates waste (Larson-Duyff, 2006).

Hyponatremia is a metabolic condition in which there is not enough sodium in the body's fluids outside of its cells. When the amount of sodium in fluids outside of cells drops, water moves into the cells. This excess of fluid causes the cells to swell. While the condition is treatable, in some cases it can be life-threatening. Symptoms include abnormal mental status, convulsions, fatigue, headache, irritability, and vomiting, among other signs. A primary care physician or health care provider should be contacted if a person experiences these symptoms (National Center for Biotechnology Information, 2011b).

On the other hand, too much sodium can also cause problems for the human body. According to the American Heart Association, people only need about 1,500 milligrams per day of sodium (American Heart Association, 2007). Unfortunately, many of today's prepared foods contain high amounts of sodium. In fact, 1 teaspoon of salt contains approximately 2,300 milligrams of sodium. Adults who take in more milligrams of sodium than they should on a daily basis could experience high blood pressure, also known as hypertension (Larson-Duyff, 2006).

Blood pressure is the measure of the force against the walls of the body's arteries as the heart pumps blood throughout. A normal blood pressure is considered 120 systolic pressure over 80 diastolic pressure. When these numbers are elevated by 10 or more points most of the time, then a person blood pressure is considered to be high. When these numbers are consistently above the normal range and below the high range, then a person is considered to be pre-hypertensive. Often called the "Silent Killer," symptoms of hypertension are not always easy to recognize making it difficult for individuals to know when the condition develops.

Pre-hypertension and hypertension according to statistics released by the Institute of Medicine (IOM) are seen most frequently among African Americans, who also tend to be salt-sensitive (American Heart Association, 2010). Hyponatremia, when individuals have a lack of sodium, is the most common electrolyte disorder in the United States. It is seen among burn victims, high-endurance athletes who may perspire faster than they can replace their electrolytes, individuals with congestive heart failure, or those with kidney diseases. Balance is the key in maintaining healthy sodium levels.

*Abena Foreman-Trice*

*See also* Blood Pressure; Hypertension; Minerals; Water.

## References

American Heart Association. *Why Should I Limit Sodium?* October 2007. www.heart.org/ldc/groups/heart-public@wcm/@hcm/documents/downloadable/ucm_300625.pdf.

American Heart Association. "Statement by American Heart Association President Clyde Yancy, M.D. on IOM Report on Hypertension." February 22, 2010. www.newsroom.heart.org/index.php?s=43&item=967&printable.

Bentor, Yinon. *Periodic Table: Sodium.* February 21, 2011. www.chemicalelements.com/elements/na.html

Burnier, Michel. *Sodium in Health and Disease.* Informahealthcare.com, 2007.

Kurlansky, Mark. *Salt: A World History.* New York: Walker and Co., 2002.

Larson-Duyff, Roberta. *American Dietetic Association Complete Food Guide.* Hoboken, NJ: John Wiley and Sons, 2006.

National Center for Biotechnology Information. *Pub Med Health-Electrolytes.* February 21, 2011a. www.ncbi.nlm.nih.gov/pubmedhealth/PMH0003004.

National Center for Biotechnology Information. *Pub Med Health-Hyponatremia.* February 21, 2011b. www.ncbi.nlm.nih.gov/pubmedhealth/PMH0001431.

## SOY

Around 3,000 years ago, soybeans originated in China. They were introduced to Japan in the eighth century, and, later, they traveled to other parts of Asia including Thailand, Malaysia, Korea, and Vietnam.

Soybeans first appeared in the United States in the 18th century, planted by Americans who brought them from China. Today, the United States leads the world in the commercial production of soybeans. Soybeans are sold in a wide variety of forms. Fresh soybeans are known as edamame. But, soybeans may be processed into foods such as dried soybean seeds, soymilk, soynuts, and tofu (George Mateljan Foundation, n.d.).

Soybeans contain excellent amounts of molybdenum and tryptophan. They are a very good source of manganese and protein, and a good source of iron, omega-3 fatty acids, phosphorus, dietary fiber, vitamin K, magnesium, copper, vitamin B2, and potassium (George Mateljan Foundation, n.d.). But what have researchers learned?

### Cancer

*Breast Cancer*    In a Korean study that was published in 2008 in *Nutrition and Cancer,* researchers compared the soy protein intake of 362 women who had been diagnosed with breast cancer to the same number of healthy women matched for age and menopausal status. The researchers found that the women with the highest intake of soy protein had a significantly lower risk of breast cancer than the women with the lowest intake of soy. The researchers noted that, "Increased regular soy food intake at a level equivalent to traditional Korean consumption levels may be associated with a reduced risk of breast cancer, and this effect is more pronounced in premenopausal women" (Kim et al., 2008).

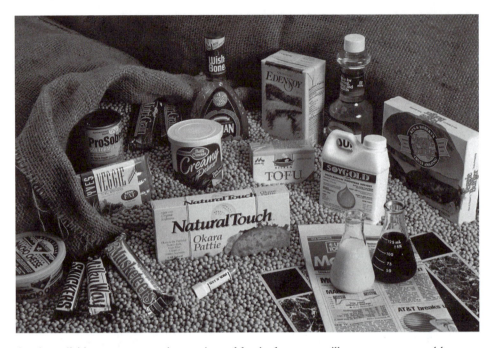

Soy is available to consumers in a variety of foods, from soy milk to soy yogurt and burgers. (U.S. Department of Agriculture)

In a study published in 2009 in *Cancer Epidemiology, Biomarkers & Prevention*, researchers investigated the consumption of soy during childhood in women of Chinese, Japanese, and Filipino descent who lived in San Francisco, Oakland, or Los Angeles, California, or in Hawaii. Of the women, 597 had a history of breast cancer, and 966 were considered healthy. They ranged in age from 20 to 55. The researchers found that a high intake of soy during childhood was associated with a 58 percent reduction in rates of breast cancer. Furthermore, a high level of soy intake during adolescence and adulthood caused a 20 percent to 25 percent reduction (Korde et al., 2009).

***Ovarian Cancer*** In a European study published in 2008 in the *International Journal of Cancer*, researchers compared the flavonoid intake (including the flavonoid known as isoflavone, which is found in soy foods) of 1,031 women who were diagnosed with epithelial ovarian cancer to 2,411 women who were hospitalized for an acute, noncancer medical problem. The researchers found that the women with a high intake of isoflavones reduced their risk of ovarian cancer by about half. "On the basis of our findings and the relevant literature," the researchers wrote, "we infer that isoflavones . . . may have favorable effects with respect to ovarian cancer risk" (Rossi et al., 2008).

***Colorectal Cancer*** In a study published in 2009 in *The American Journal of Clinical Nutrition*, researchers prospectively examined 68,412 women between the ages of 40 and 70 who were initially free of cancer. During the mean follow-up period of 6.4 years, there were 321 cases of colorectal cancer. The researchers determined that the women who ate the highest amount of soy had 30 percent fewer cases of colorectal cancer. These benefits were primarily seen in postmenopausal women (Yang et al., 2009).

**Cardiovascular Support** In a study published in 2008 in the *European Heart Journal,* Chinese researchers reviewed the effects on blood-vessel functioning of the 12-week consumption of 80 mg/day of isoflavone supplementation or a placebo by 102 patients who had previously suffered from a stroke. When compared with the control group, the researchers found that the subjects who took the isoflavone supplementation had significant improvement in blood-vessel functioning. Even more encouraging was the finding that the response was best for those with the more severe cardiovascular disease. Moreover, the isoflavone supplementation reduced levels of C-reactive protein, an indicator of vascular inflammation. The researchers concluded that their findings "may have important implication for the use of isoflavone for secondary prevention in patients with cardiovascular disease, on top of conventional interventions" (Chan et al., 2008).

**Menopausal Women** Soy supplements do not appear to help women in menopause, based on a two-year, $3 million study conducted at the Miller School's Osteoporosis Center at the University of Miami. Funded by the National Institutes of Health to determine if soy could preserve bone mineralization and ease menopausal symptoms in the first few years after menopause, the study found that soy did not. The results show that, "contrary to popular belief, soy isoflavone supplements neither prevent bone loss nor reduce menopausal symptoms" ("U.M. Soy Study," 2011). The SPARE Study findings (standing for "Soy Phytoestrogens As Replacement Estrogen)," were published in the August 8, 2011, issue of the *Archives of Internal Medicine.*

For postmenopausal women, a study published in 2009, in *Menopause,* also reported lack of benefit for soy supplements, with or without isoflavones. Researchers randomly divided 203 healthy postmenopausal women into one of three groups. For two years, one group took 25 grams of soy protein without isoflavones; a second group took 25 grams of soy protein with 90 milligrams of isoflavones; and the third (control) group took 25 grams of milk protein (casein and whey). At the end of two years, the women in all three groups had significant decreases in the bone mineral density of the lumbar spine and femoral neck. In addition, all three groups had decreases in physical performance measurements. The researchers concluded that "twenty-five grams of soy protein with 90 mg of isoflavones has no added benefit in preventing bone loss or improving physical performance" (Vupadhyayula et al., 2009).

**Weight Control** A study published in 2008 in the *European Journal of Nutrition* examined whether soy products may play a role in controlling weight gain. Researchers in Seattle and Honolulu reviewed the association between lifetime intake of soy foods and body mass index (BMI) of 1,418 women who lived in Hawaii. The researchers found that the women with higher soy consumption in adulthood had lower levels of BMI. However, this association was only significant for Caucasian and postmenopausal women. "The women in the highest category also experienced a smaller annual weight change since age 21 (by 0.05 kg/year) than the low soy intake group . . . " (Maskarinec, 2008).

**One Caveat**   Much of the world's soybean crop is genetically modified. People who wish to avoid genetically modified foods should eat organic soy products. Should soy products be part of the diet? For most people, there is no reason to exclude them. And, they may well have some benefits.

*Myrna Chandler Goldstein and Mark A. Goldstein*

*See also* Cancer; Genetically Modified Organisms (GMOs); Heart Health; Proteins.

### References

Chan, Yap-Hang, Kui-Kai Lau, Kai-Hang Yiu, Sheung-Wai Li, Hiu-Ting Chan, Daniel Yee-Tak, Sidney Tam, Chu-Pak Lau, Hung-Fat Tse. "Reduction of C-Reactive Protein with Isoflavone Supplement Reverses Endothelial Dysfunction in Patients with Ischaemic Stroke." *European Heart Journal* 29, no. 22 (2008): 2800–07.

George Mateljan Foundation. www.whfoods.com.

Kim, Mi Kyung, Jin Hee Kim, Seok Jin Nam, Seungho Ryu, Gu Kong. "Dietary Intake of Soy Protein and Tofu in Association with Breast Cancer Risk Based on a Case-Control Study." *Nutrition and Cancer* (September 5, 2008) 60: 568–76.

Korde, Larissa A., Anna H. Wu, Thomas Fears, Abraham Nomura, Dee W. West, Laurence N. Kolonel, Malcolm C. Pike, Robert N. Hoover, Regina G. Ziegler. "Childhood Soy Intake and Breast Cancer Risk in Asian American Women." *Cancer Epidemiology, Biomarkers & Prevention* 18, no. 4 (April 1, 2009): 1050–59.

Maskarinec, Gertraud, Alison G. Aylward, Eva Erber, Yumie Takata, Laurence N. Kolonel. "Soy Intake Is Related to a Lower Body Mass Index in Adult Women." *European Journal of Nutrition* (April 2008) 47(3): 138–144.

Rossi, Marta, Eva Negri, Pagona Lagiou, Renato Talamini, Luigino Dal Maso, Maurizio Montella, Silvia Franceschi, Carlo Va Vecchia. "Flavonoids and Ovarian Cancer Risk: A Case-Control Study in Italy." *International Journal of Cancer* 123, no. 4 (2008): 895–8.

"U.M. Soy Study Shows Soy Does Not Help Women during Menopause." University of Miami Miller School of Medicine." August 8, 2011. www.med.miami.edu/news/um-soy-study-shows-no-benefit-for-menopausal-women.

Vupadhyayula, Phanni M., J.C. Gallagher, Thomas Templin, S.M. Logsdon, L.M. Smith. "Effects of Soy Protein on Bone Mineral Density and Physical Performance Indices in Postmenopausal Women—A 2-Year Randomized, Double-Blind, Placebo-Controlled Trial." *Menopause* (March-April 2009) 16(2): 320–328.

Yang, Gong, Xiao-Ou Shu, Honglan Li, Wong-Ho Chow, Hui Cai, Xianglan Zhang, Yu-Tang Gao, Wei Zheng. "Prospective Cohort Study of Soy Food Intake and Colorectal Cancer Risk in Women." *The American Journal of Clinical Nutrition* 89, no. 2 (February 2009): 577–583.

## SPAS, MEDICAL

In the 1980s and 1990s, globalization, the Internet, and worldwide travel contributed to increased consumer awareness and fueled demand for integrated wellness, spa, alternative medical services, and traditional healing arts from around the world. As visitors to health resorts—such as Canyon Ranch in the United States or Chiva-Som in Thailand, or to hotels with spa and medical services in spa cities such as Baden-Baden, Germany—sampled therapeutic benefits of such time-honored healing therapies ranging from traditional Chinese and Ayurvedic medicine, Kneipp therapies, acupuncture, nutrition, therapeutic massage, and exercise not typically offered at their conventional doctor's offices and hospitals, they began to seek out facilities offering diverse services in spa therapies, medical programs, and traditional healing arts in growing numbers.

Since the 1980s, influenced by pioneering destination spa resorts such as Rancho La Puerta, the Golden Door, Canyon Ranch, and Cal-a-Vie, thousands of day spas were established across the country, and by the 1990s the spa boom was in full swing, giving birth to industry associations, conferences, and trade publications. Growth has been fueled by consumer demand, and as of 2006 U.S. spas were a $15 billion per year industry (Spa Finder, n.d.). As the fourth-largest leisure industry in the United States, it generates more revenue than ski resorts, amusement/theme parks, and box office receipts (Spa Finder, n.d.). That figure is expected to grow with continued industry expansion and diversification, influencing secondary markets such as residential and commercial design and architecture, spa-inspired furnishings, personal care products, lifestyle accessories, travel and leisure industries, and real estate developments.

**Spas as the New Hospitals** As the industry continues to evolve, spas that bridge centuries of healing arts traditions with 21st-century health care have emerged as respected centers for integrative medicine—that is, places where wellness and spa treatments are offered side by side with medical diagnostics and prevention-based health care services. According to the International Spa Association, between 2002 and 2004, the medical spa segment expanded faster than any other segment, growing by 109 percent compared to 26 percent for the U.S. spa industry as a whole (International Spa Association, n.d.).

According to the International Spa Association, a medical spa is a facility that operates under the full-time, on-site supervision of a licensed health care professional whose primary purpose is to provide comprehensive medical and wellness care in an environment that integrates spa services as well as traditional, complementary, and alternative therapies and treatments. A medical spa facility operates within the scope of practice of its staff, which can include both aesthetic/cosmetic and prevention/wellness procedures and services (International Spa Association, 2004).

Healing-oriented spas have become a source of information about and inspiration for new ways to live and live well—where ideas, information, and resources about healing, fitness, nutrition, beauty, and spirituality converge. Spa categories continue to evolve, addressing broad and niche markets from day spas, wellness spas, aesthetic-medicine spas, age-management spas, dental spas, and hospital spas to residential spa lifestyle communities. As the demand for optimizing health and managing stress grows, and the health care industry transitions toward wellness and prevention, the spa industry is uniquely positioned to contribute centuries of spa culture to current and emerging wellness and health care models.

**What Is Fueling the Surge in Spas?**   In an age when modern medicine usually means rushed office visits, a maze of fragmented services, and costly and invasive procedures, many consumers are finding that practitioners and health centers that offer a menu of nonmedical therapies along with medical treatments or diagnostic services that put them in charge of their own health are very appealing. In a growing number of cases, spas fill the bill because many are staffed by a host of practitioners—MDs, naturopaths, acupuncturists, chiropractors, nutritionists, and meditation teachers—who view patients as partners and are skilled in offering an array of therapy options that are customized to the needs of the individual and coordinated by a physician, nurse practitioner, or medical concierge professional.

Again, the overall aim is not so much to treat disease but to provide an opportunity and environment with ongoing support for the body to heal itself. This approach is common in many non-Western medical modalities around the world, and, in 1978, the World Health Organization recognized holistic medical systems as "viewing humans in totality within a wide ecological spectrum, and emphasizing the view that ill health or disease is brought about by imbalance or disequilibrium of humans in the total ecological system and not only the causative agent and pathogenic mechanism" (Marcozzi, 2006, p. 11).

At a time when the long-term sustainability of the current high-cost U.S. health care system is in doubt, it is important to note that primary health care for 80 percent of the world's population utilizes modalities that are called "alternative medicine" in the United States—such as therapeutic approaches associated with health traditions of India, China, and Europe and medical systems such as chiropractic, homeopathy, herbal medicine, naturopathy, and osteopathy. These approaches stem from a philosophy that addresses the whole person in diagnosis, treatment of illness, disease and injury, and prevention of illness.

For managing minor pain conditions, such as back pain, the leading cause of job-related disability in the United States, massage, a mainstay of spa menus, can be an attractive alternative to painkillers and a comforting treatment before and after medical procedures. Massage is the most requested treatment at spas, and, according to the Associated Bodywork and Massage Professionals (a national membership association for massage therapy and esthetic professionals), as of 2005, over 240,000 massage and bodywork professionals are licensed in the United States, providing 120 to 135 million massage sessions representing a $7 billion to $10 billion industry (Associated Bodywork & Massage Professionals, 2010).

The Touch Therapy Institute at the University of Miami School of Medicine, the first center in the world devoted to the study of touch and its application in science and medicine, has identified various attributes and benefits of massage. These include reduced pain from migraines and arthritis; decreased glucose levels in patients with diabetes; greater attentiveness in children who have autism; less pain, nausea, and depression for oncology patients; improved immunity, stress reduction, and better work performance for employees receiving on-site massage treatments (Touch Research Institute, 1997). In the 2003 annual list of the 100 Best Companies for Working Mothers, published by *Working Mother* magazine, 77 of the top 100 companies offered work-site massage (Associated Bodywork & Massage Professionals, 2010).

**Evolution of Spas as Modern-Day Healing Centers**   As spas continue to evolve and partner with hospitals, hotels, resorts, and research centers, more consumers can expect to find everything from high-tech MRI diagnostic scans and cholesterol-lowering strategies on the spa menu, alongside massage, stress-management techniques such as meditation, yoga, and a host of other nondrug therapies and techniques. Whether Americans are seeking methods to cope with cancer, shed unwanted pounds, keep their hearts healthy, or stave off the effects of everyday stress, spas are emerging as a viable resource for services, guidelines, and support for healthy-living practices.

Responding to increasing numbers of people affected by cancer, many spas specialize in programs that address this condition by teaching skills for managing pain and addressing challenging symptoms and side effects associated with radiation and chemotherapy. At the California-based Greet the Day program—partnered with Spa Gregories in Newport Beach, Pacific Water Spa at the Hyatt Regency in Huntington Beach, and nine participating hospitals—cancer patients receive a complimentary day of rejuvenation, relaxation, and empowerment; network with cancer survivors; and learn take-home tools for managing their health. According to Johnnette du Rand, Greet the Day cofounder, the program's goal is "to create a timeout from regular hospital visits and provide a place in which guests can reconnect with themselves as a whole" (du Rand, 2006).

A typical Greet the Day program begins with yoga or meditation, followed with spa treatments such as massage, facials, and relaxation techniques. Social networking activities designed to minimize the feelings of isolation and disempowerment that often accompany radiation, surgery, and chemotherapy help establish a sense of community. Numerous studies confirm the importance of friends in the healing process, demonstrating that patients heal faster when they feel supported (du Rand, 2006).

In addition to providing an extensive selection of therapies, with many customized to specific health problems, spas are also uniquely positioned to address lifestyle solutions for what experts have dubbed America's leading lifestyle diseases: obesity, heart disease, diabetes, and depression. To treat, prevent, and, in some cases, reverse these conditions, spas that help consumers make healthy lifestyle choices—dietary, fitness, and stress management among them—can be a powerful prescription.

Centers that offer a wide range of lifestyle strategies and customized programs especially for preventing and treating problems such as coronary heart disease (the leading cause of death in the United States) are in demand. Since opening its doors in 1970, Cooper Clinic at the Cooper Aerobics Center in Dallas, Texas, says it has helped over 70,000 people reduce their risk of heart disease and stress-related illness through nutrition, exercise, education, and motivation to live a healthy and active lifestyle (Cooper Wellness Program, n.d.).

Prevention appears to be especially important to the burgeoning aging population who wants to live a full life not debilitated by chronic disease. According to the National Institute of Aging, nearly 8,000 people turn 60 each day (National Institute of Aging, n.d.). In addition, life expectancy continues to lengthen. As baby boomers look forward to living longer, they are eager for healthy lifestyle strategies and services to help them continue to function without being disabled by obesity, diabetes, heart disease, mental decline, and other chronic conditions. People want to feel and look fit, stay active, and remain independent well into their advanced senior years.

Looking as good as one feels is another priority for the aging population, and aesthetic services combined with wellness programs are predicted to be the largest growth segment for years to come. Many organizations offer hope and make impressive claims, but the results-oriented leaders of the future will be delivering science-based evaluations to assess biomarkers of aging, genomics testing (risk of developing age-related conditions such as heart disease, diabetes, and osteoporosis), and personalized programs for lifestyle enhancing services such as cosmetic procedures. The Miami Institute for Age Management and Intervention at the Four Seasons Hotel is an example of medical facilities within a hotel, offering personalized medical evaluations, hormone replacement therapy, weight-management strategies, nutrition, exercise, and wellness programs in addition to noninvasive and surgical cosmetic procedures (Miami Institute for Age Management and Intervention, n.d.).

**A Vision for the Future** As the current primary-care system experiences a long overdue reorganization, more spa, health, and wellness-based organizations will appear on the horizon and will change the face of health care. However, the place of greatest potential change is not with the government, medical community, spas, insurers, universities, or service providers but within each individual. Through open access to information and education, consumers have a tremendous opportunity to enjoy good health individually and collectively and to support organizations and policymakers committed to offering the best of science, medicine, and technology, balanced with practical tools and resources for healthy living. The principles of spas and health have a long and rich history. Coming full circle from its ancient roots, the new horizon promises an inspiring vision of opportunity and possibility.

*Janice Gronvold*

*See also* Acupuncture; Homeopathy; Naturopathy; Nutrition; Tai Chi.

## References

Answers.com. *Eclectic Medicine.* n.d. www.answers.com/topic/eclectic-medicine.
Associated Bodywork & Massage Professionals. *Massage Therapy Fast Facts.* October 2010. www.massagetherapy.com/_content/images/Media/Factsheet1.pdf.

Chez, R., K. Pelletier, and W. Jonas. *Toward Optimal Healing Environments in Health Care.* New Rochelle, NY: Mary Ann Liebert.

Cooper Wellness Program *Cooper Wellness Program, Fitness, Weight Loss, Stress Management.* n.d. www.cooperwellness.com/.

du Rand, Johnnette. Interview with the author, Newport Beach, California. November 2006.

International Spa Association. "How Fast is the Spa Industry Growing?" *ISPA 2004 Spa Industry Study.* November 15, 2004. www.experienceispa.com/articles/index.cfm?action=view&articleID=89&menuID-75.

International Spa Association. "Spa." n.d. www.experienceispa.com.

La Ferla, R. "Hospitals Are Discovering Their Inner Spa." *New York Times,* August 13, 2000. www.nytimes.com/library/style/weekend/081300medical-spa.html.

Marcozzi, M. "Culture and Complementary Medicine." *Seminars in Integrative Medicine* 2, no. 3 (2004): 11.

Miami Institute for Age Management and Intervention. n.d. www.miami-institute.com.

National Center for Complementary and Alternative Medicine. *Mission and History.* October 18, 2011. http://nccam.nih.gov/about.

National Institute of Aging. *Health and Aging.* n.d. www.nia.nih.gov.

Pratt Design Studio. *Condell Medical Center.* n.d. www.prattdesign.com/site/epage/13356_417.htm.

Spa Finder. *Rancho La Puerta Highlights and Awards.* n.d. www.spafinder.com/Spas/overview.jsp?spaID=37&pageType=highlights.

Spa Finder. *Spa History.* www.spafinder.com/spalifestyle/spa101/history.jsp.

Szekely, D. *Vegetarian Spa Cuisine from Rancho La Puerta.* San Diego, CA: Rancho La Puerta, 1992.

Tai Sophia Institute. *The Report A3* 4, no. 2 (2006, Summer/Fall): Touch Research Institute, University of Miami School of Medicine. *General Information about TRI Research.* 1997. www6.miami.edu/touch-research.

Warner, Jennifer. *Alternative Medicine Goes Mainstream: 1 in 4 Hospitals Offer Services Such as Acupuncture, Yoga and Homeopathy.* CBS News, July 20, 2006. www.cbsnews.com/stories/2006/07/20/health/webmd/main1823747.shtml.

# STAPHYLOCOCCUS

Staphylococcus is a common bacterium, which, under the microscope, appears as a bunch or cluster of grapes. There are a variety of staphylococci, and they can be found everywhere in the air, on the human body, or on animals. Many types of staphylococci are harmless, but others can cause diseases such as impetigo, skin infections, pneumonia, and blood poisoning. The most common form of food poisoning is caused by staphylococcus contamination in food.

In fact, a report released by the Translational Genomics Research Institute in Arizona raised concerns about the use of antibiotics in animal feed and the high rates of staphylococci bacteria now showing up in U.S. supermarkets. According to study results, some 47 percent of the meat and poultry samples in the study were contaminated with *Staphylococcus aureus* (Trumbull, 2011). Of even greater concern was the fact that more than half the bacteria were resistant to at least three antibiotics, according to the group's findings.

In 2010, the Food and Drug Administration (FDA) recommended that U.S. animal growers begin phasing in limits on the use of "medically important antimicrobial drugs," given to animals to promote growth (Trumbull, 2011). The limits would help preserve the effectiveness of drugs as therapies for humans and animals, according to the director of the FDA's Center for Veterinary Medicine (FDA, 2010). The World Health Organization has recommended a worldwide phase-out of feeding antibiotics to animals to prevent this resistance, and the European Union adopted a similar ban in 2006 (Edwards, 2010).

Unfortunately, in the 1960s, scientists first discovered some strains of staphylococci were becoming resistant to antibiotics. One strain, known as methicillin-resistant *Staphylococcus aureus* (MRSA) has developed resistance to many common antibiotics. MRSA infections now occur increasingly in institutional settings such as hospitals and nursing homes and also in community settings such as schools, colleges, and in the general public. Major pharmaceutical companies have been working to develop increasingly strong antibiotics to deal with this resistant strain.

There are other serious infections also caused by *Staphylococcus aureus,* including toxic shock syndrome and scalded skin syndrome. Symptoms of toxic shock syndrome include a severe headache, high fever, and sore throat. Symptoms can appear suddenly, and if not treated quickly the illness can lead to kidney, liver, or muscle damage. Scalded skin syndrome begins as a localized skin infection and is most common in newborns and young children. A vivid red rash forms with large blisters that burst and leave the skin looking burnt.

Staph infections are most often caused by direct contact between the bacteria and open sores or wounds, cuts, scrapes, insect bites, or body fluids. Warning signs of infection include pain or swelling, skin abscesses, and enlarged lymph nodes in the neck, armpit, or groin. Diagnosis of an infection is made by testing fluids from sores or other body fluids such as urine or blood. Treatment then depends on the severity of the staph infection and its location.

*Sharon Zoumbaris*

*See also* Antibiotics; Food and Drug Administration (FDA); Methicillin-Resistant Staphylococcus Aureus (MRSA).

## References

Edwards, Shane. "Replace Tainted Meat with Healthy Vegetables." *The Post-Standard* (Syracuse, NY), April 22, 2010: A13.

FDA (Food and Drug Administration). "FDA Issues Draft Guidance on the Judicious Use of Medically Important Antimicrobials in Food-Producing Animals." June 28, 2010. www.fda.gov/newsevents/newsroom/pressannouncements/ucm217464.htm.

NIH (National Institutes of Health). *MRSA: Methicillin-resistant Staphylococcus aureus.* February 16, 2011. www.nlm.nih.gov/medlineplus.mrsa.html. "Study Warns of Tainted Meat." *New York Times,* April 16, 2011: A15.

Trumbull, Mark. "Staph in Meat: Are U.S. Cattle and Poultry Over-Drugged?" *The Christian Science Monitor,* April 16, 2011.

## STEROIDS

More properly designated as anabolic-androgenic steroids (AAS) because of their bodybuilding (anabolic) and masculinizing (androgenic) effects, steroids (refers to the class of drugs) are synthetic versions of the male sex hormone testosterone that are illicitly used by, among others, athletes in order to enhance their physical performance and appearance. Legitimate medical uses of anabolic steroids include some hormone problems in men, late puberty and muscle loss from some diseases including AIDS (Acquired Immune Deficiency Syndrome), and cancer.

AAS, unlike other drugs, do not trigger increases in neurotransmitter dopamine, which is responsible for the "high" that often accompanies substance abuse behaviors. However, studies have shown that long-term use of AAS does eventually have an impact on brain chemicals such as dopamine and serotonin and can seriously affect the mood and behavior of the user. Researchers have reported that users may suffer from paranoid jealousy, extreme irritability, delusions, and extreme mood swings including manic-like symptoms that could lead to violence. Other important health problems from abuse of AAS include heart problems (including heart attacks), liver disease (including cancer), and, especially for adolescents, stunted growth due to premature bone maturation and accelerated puberty.

Though they have been banned by the International Olympic Committee since 1975 and prohibited by nearly every sporting organization, they are nonetheless taken by a significant, though ultimately unknown, number of athletes in a variety of sports, with weightlifting, cycling, football, and baseball being among the most prominent. Athletes who take steroids tend to use AAS in stacks and cycles, going well beyond the level of steroids that might be medically prescribed. This practice leads some steroid users to have many problems, including psychological addiction, physiological withdrawal issues, and a bevy of adverse side effects.

AAS were created in the mid-1930s, shortly after testosterone was first isolated by scientists. It is unclear when the illicit use of

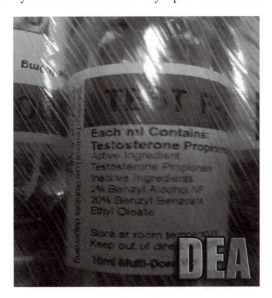

The Drug Enforcement Agency confiscated vials of anabolic steroids during Operation Raw Deal in 2007. There are many recognized health risks associated with the long-term use or large doses of these drugs. (Drug Enforcement Agency)

steroids truly began, but the first reports of such usage date back to 1954 and describe male and female Russian athletes, and weightlifters, particularly, taking AAS in order to increase their weight and muscle strength. Steroid use among American athletes also first took place within the world of weightlifting, with the York Barbell Club in York, Pennsylvania, emerging as the site of much experimentation in the late 1950s and early 1960s. Hoping to help Americans fare better against their steroid-using Russian competitors, Dr. John Ziegler developed Dianabol—a steroid designed to be less androgenic than other AAS—and administered it, along with amphetamines, to American Olympic weightlifters.

Competitive weightlifters' use of AAS was hardly the only example of the Cold War being reflected in international athletics, as American Olympians in a variety of sports took steroids in the 1950s. Many of the athletes on steroids in this era felt that AAS were a kind of wonder drug, while others likely took them because they felt they simply could not compete with athletes who were on steroids. In response to this phenomenon, the International Olympic Committee began to ban drug use among athletes in 1968. The prohibition covered some 20 stimulants and narcotics, but steroids were not among the banned substances. The omission of AAS from the list was not an indication that steroid use was minor among Olympians, for steroid use by American athletes was fairly widespread at the 1968 Mexico City Games. Instead, the International Olympic Committee did not ban steroids because no reliable test for AAS existed at that point. In addition, science was as yet unsure of the precise amounts and ratios of steroids that naturally occur in the body, thus making AAS detection even more difficult.

It is probably safe to assume that AAS use factored significantly in Olympic competitions up until the mid-1970s, when the detection of exogenous testosterone in urine became scientifically possible. The International Olympic Committee consequently banned AAS in 1975. The 1976 Olympic Games in Montreal were the first to feature athletes being tested for steroids, and numerous competitors were disqualified from it and subsequent Olympiads or stripped of the medals they unfairly won. In what is perhaps the most famous case of this, Canadian sprinter Ben Johnson had his gold medal taken away after testing positive for an AAS at the 1988 Summer Olympic Games in Seoul, South Korea. Despite catching Johnson, the International Olympic Committee was widely seen as insufficiently policing its athletes' use of steroids. A decade later, it agreed to implement the antidoping rules and regulations of the independent World Anti-Doping Agency, which was created in the aftermath of a 1998 drug-use scandal that rocked the Tour de France.

The Olympics are hardly the only athletic competition to have been tainted by the illicit use of steroids. AAS use had become an institutionalized staple in professional football by 1963, when the San Diego Chargers distributed oral steroids for players to take at their team meals. The origin of this practice may be traced to the team's strength coach, Alvin Roy, who had been affiliated with United States' weightlifting team. Baseball, too, has a checkered history with AAS, and it is generally believed that steroids made their way into the game some time in the mid- to late 1960s. Steroids became a far more significant element on the diamond in the last two decades, and it is now common to refer to a "steroid age" in baseball's history. Discussion of AAS in baseball came to the forefront when sluggers Mark McGwire and Sammy Sosa both surpassed the game's long-standing, single-season home-run record. In the course of their much publicized pursuit of the record, McGwire admitted to using androstenedione, a muscle-building supplement that was legal at the time but has subsequently been banned by Major League Baseball, the World Anti-Doping Agency, and other sports organizations.

In 2003, baseball banned steroid use and began testing for it, and 5.77 percent of 1,438 anonymous urine samples tested positive for AAS. In 2005, Congress held hearings investigating the use of AAS amongst baseball players, and McGwire stated that the game had a steroid problem, though he refused to answer questions about his own drug use. In the wake of these hearings, Major League Baseball Commissioner Bud Selig hired, in March 2006, former Maine Senator George Mitchell to launch an independent investigation into steroid use in the sport. The resulting Mitchell Report, which was released on December 13, 2007, implicated 86 players.

In addition to the aforementioned Congressional hearings, the government became involved in the issue of steroids and sports as a result of its investigation of the Bay Area Laboratory Co-Operative (BALCO), which begun in August 2002 and focused on the alleged money laundering and illegal distribution of steroids and other performance-enhancing drugs by BALCO's founder, Victor Conte. Internal Revenue Service agents subsequently linked BALCO to a number of high-profile athletes, including baseball home-run king Barry Bonds and Olympic sprinter Marion Jones. Such high-profile cases seem to have done little to diminish the athletic world's interest in AAS, however, as athletes in a variety of sports continue searching for an illicit medical edge.

Even with all the negative publicity generated by athletes who confess to AAS use, the National Institute on Drug Abuse (NIDA), which is part of the National Institutes of Health (NIH), continues to monitor use among U.S. high school students through an annual survey. The Monitoring the Future survey is used to assess drug use among the nation's 8th-, 10th-, and 12th-grade students. Their latest figures show that 2.5 percent of 12th-grade males, versus 0.6 percent of 12th-grade females, reported steroid use. The NIDA survey showed that steroid use among 12th-grade males has consistently been higher than among females or other-aged males.

*Howard Padwa and Jacob Cunningham*

*See also* Food and Drug Administration (FDA); Human Chorionic Gonadotropin (HCG).

## References

"After Years of Denials and Evasions, Mark McGwire, the Home-Run King, Admitted to Steroid Use." *National Review* 62 no. 2 (February 8, 2010): 16.

NIDA (National Institute on Drug Abuse). *NIDA InfoFacts: Steroids.* Revised July 2009. www.drugabuse.gov/infofacts/steroids.html.

Radomski, Kirk with David Fisher. *Bases Loaded: The Inside Story of the Steroid Era in Baseball by the Central Figure in the Mitchell Report.* New York: Hudson Street Press, 2009.

Rosen, Daniel M. *Dope: A History of Performance Enhancement in Sports from the Nineteenth Century to Today.* Westport, CT: Praeger, 2008.

Taylor, William N. *Anabolic Steroids and the Athlete.* Jefferson, NC: McFarland & Company, Inc., 2002

Taylor, William N. *Macho Medicine: A History of the Anabolic Steroid Epidemic.* Jefferson, NC: McFarland & Company, Inc., 1991.

Walder. Gary I. "Doping in Sports: Steroids and Supplements." *World Almanac and Book of Facts.* Pleasantville, NY: World Almanac Books, 2005.

Wadler, Gary I., and Brian Hainline. *Drugs and the Athlete.* Philadelphia: F.A. Davis Company, 1989.

Westreich, Laurence M. "Anabolic Androgenic Steroid Use: Pharmacology, Prevalence, and Psychiatric Aspects." *Psychiatric Times* 25, no. 1 (January 2008): 47–53.

Yesalis, Charles E., ed. *Anabolic Steroids in Sport and Exercise.* Champaign, IL: Human Kinetics Publishers, 1993.

## STRESS

"I am stressed out!"

How many times have you said this or heard someone else say it? It is a common enough complaint that can be elicited by a variety of life events or situations, but it is usually provoked by an accumulation of emotional responses to individual stressors. Imagine the opportunities during a typical work or school day: you oversleep and are late for work or class, you have a disappointing performance review or test score, your work environment is noisy and distracting, your work load requires too much effort with too little resources, and so forth. Combine these with difficulties in your personal life, and you are likely to reach the "stressed out" tipping point. Is being "stressed out" simply a way of expressing frustration when things don't go our way, or is there something more going in both in body and mind?

**Fight or Flight**   Being stressed is actually the result of a complex interaction between our thoughts and emotions, our brains, and our environment. When our perception of situations or events in our environment or our own imagination leads us to feelings of anger, discouragement, anxiety, or fear, our bodies experience the physical symptoms of stress. These physical feelings are an indication of physiological changes occurring. When we are stressed, chemicals are coursing through our blood stream, urgently calling for fighting or fleeing.

These chemicals are not simply tiny Paul-Revere cells; they cause a cascading effect throughout our bodies that affects our heart, our immune system, digestive system, reproductive system, and growth. If we remain in this state of alarm for a long period of time, the aforementioned systems can become damaged or diseased.

**Understanding Stress Factors**   If bridges or rockets could talk, they might tell us that they too are stressed out. In fact, our contemporary understanding of stress began through engineering and the advent of the industrial revolution

(Cooper & Dewe, 2004). The concepts of "stress" and "strain" were applied to structures to better understand how much weight they could safely manage. Strain that exceeded a structure's ability to adequately distribute the weight load would collapse. The Tacoma Narrows Bridge, nicknamed "Galloping Gertie," provides an excellent illustration of the application of stress and strain. In 1940, the suspension bridge that spanned Puget Sound in Washington was completed, but engineers noted that the surface of the bridge had a distinct "bounce" that concerned them (Washington State Department of Transportation, 2010).

Such movement was neither typical nor desirable with a bridge. In November of 1940, their concern was more than justified when the bridge began to twist while being buffeted by high winds. Shortly thereafter, the bridge began a violent oscillating movement that earned it its nickname of Galloping Gertie. Since the structure was already given to bouncing under ordinary conditions, the strong winds pushed the bridge past its ability to compensate for the movement, and it collapsed. Fortunately, no one was hurt.

A more tragic illustration of machine stress occurred with the loss of both the Challenger space shuttle in January of 1986 and the Columbia space shuttle in February of 2003. Both disasters can be attributed to two kinds of stress: machine stress, where failure resulted from critical structural breaches, and the organizational stress that lead to launch decisions in the face of abnormally increased risk. In attempting to understand the events leading to the Challenger disaster, the detailed *Report of the Presidential Commission on the Space Shuttle Challenger Accident* noted how multiple changes prior to shuttle launches "put significant stress on the flight preparation process by diverting resources from higher priority problems" (NASA, 1986, 172).

***Balance*** While humans are *not* machines, the engineering analogy from the industrial revolution provided a metaphor for understanding how humans, like machines, can suffer damage from everyday use (Cooper & Dewe, 2004). One of the benefits of this metaphor is the understanding of balance. Balance is the first key concept in understanding stress. People, bridges, and organizations have an innate sense of their optimal level of functioning and strive to maintain it. Whenever something pushes them past their normal level of balance, they experience stress, either physically or (with humans) psychologically. The physiological systems in human beings are delicately balanced and regulated by a host of chemical, electrical, and mechanical systems that may become easily unbalanced. What may appear to be discrete conditions like elevated blood pressure or blood glucose levels can have dangerous systemic effects on the human body. Like the tightrope walker who braves great heights to demonstrate his uncanny ability to remain balanced (and therefore unharmed), so do the physiological systems of the human body.

***Duration*** A second key concept involves duration. The length of time an individual is exposed to a stressor often determines how well he or she adapts. The title of Robert Sapolsky's book on stress concisely summarizes this: *Why Zebras Don't Get Ulcers* (2004). Sapolsky's point is that zebras are equipped to cope with the acute stress of being hunted. When confronted by a hungry lioness, the zebra's fight-or-fight response is activated. The zebra either escapes and the stressor is removed, or it doesn't escape and the zebra is removed. The stress response doesn't linger. With human beings, however, "the stress-response can become more damaging than the stressor itself, especially when the stress is purely psychological" (Sapolsky, 2004, p. 13). In other words, while zebras don't get ulcers, humans do.

Sapolsky (2004) identified two types of stressors: physical and psychosocial. Acute physical stressors typically involve immediate threats to your physical health or well-being. Examples include being outside without a jacket in cold weather, breaking a bone, or a 24-hour virus. Chronic physical stressors are sustained over a period of time. An assembly line worker who is exposed to unregulated noise or who must perform monotonous tasks repetitively will experience chronic stress. Similar imbalances occur as when faced with an acute stressor, but the body doesn't have the opportunity to recover with repeated exposure.

Psychosocial stressors refer to circumstances or events involving either interpersonal stress (an unreasonable supervisor or a disagreeable neighbor) or psychological stress (worry over a burdensome mortgage or fear of being laid off); the stress is provoked by how we think about these circumstances or events. Psychosocial stressors can be either acute, like when that disagreeable neighbor lets his dog squat in your yard, or chronic, like dealing with an aging and infirm parent. Certain professions and jobs have an unusual amount of chronic stress, including those in the military; police officers and firefighters; health care professionals; those who specialize in therapy to victims or perpetrators of violent crime; and others. Unrelieved or repeated stress in dangerous situations, such as is experienced in wars, often leads to post-traumatic stress syndrome, and in severe cases, suicide.

*Perception*    The role of psychosocial stressors introduces the third key concept: perception. In many cases, our perception of our situation or circumstances determines the extent of the stress we experience. Sometimes it is essential that we perceive things as being stressors. Recognizing the dangers of a snarling dog or an out-of-control roller skater help us avoid physical stressors.

However, psychosocial stressors most often result from how we perceive a potentially stress-inducing event or set of circumstances. Consider, for example, students preparing to take a final exam. Leon spent the last several days studying for the exam, while Cyril waited until the night before. While Leon should be the calmer of the two, Cyril's perception of his grasp of the material (whether his perception is accurate or not) may make the final exam only a mild stressor for him. Leon, more of the skittish type, may experience the final exam as a significant stressor, despite his preparation. Matheny and Riordan (1992) noted that perceptions of helplessness, for example, provoke stress, while perceptions of mastery or control moderate stress.

**Inducing Stress**    Aldwin (2007) categorized two transactions that can induce stress: the transaction between mind and brain, and the transaction between person and environment. The mind–brain transaction illustrates how our perceptions about events or circumstances can be perceived as threatening, which then evokes the stress response. When the stress response is evoked, the delicate physiological balance that keeps us functioning optimally is threatened.

The person–environment transaction involves the extent to which the individual is functioning within an optimal environment. The notion of person–environment fit has been of particular interest to industrial/organizational psychologists, who see "goodness of fit" as an important consideration in work motivation (Latham, 2007). Latham (2007) noted that personal characteristics, such as needs, values, or biological predispositions, interact with the environment and play a role in the development of stress. An environment that is congruent with the individual's needs and values permits the individual to function optimally, while an environment that is incongruent with the individual's needs or values is stressful.

**Responses to Stress**   What happens to us when we are stressed? Let's revisit the snarling dog. Assume you are strolling along the sidewalk and turn the corner, only to find yourself confronted by a fearsome-looking dog. In the instant it takes for you appraise the situation as dangerous, your sympathetic nervous system goes into action, arousing what Walter Cannon in 1939 (cited in Aldwin, 2007) originally termed the "fight-or-flight response." The sympathetic nervous system arouses the various physiological systems that you need to cope with the snarling dog, releasing the chemicals your body needs to mobilize itself: epinephrine (or adrenaline) and norepinephrine.

As a result, your cardiovascular system is aroused, increasing blood pressure, heart rate, and respiration. Additionally, your pupils dilate, glucose is released into the blood stream to provide energy, the blood stream thickens in case of injury, and gastrointestinal activity, reproduction, and growth are inhibited. In explaining the benefit of inhibiting these systems, Sapolsky (2004) noted that "there isn't enough time to derive the energetic benefits of the slow process of digestion, so why waste the energy on it? You have better things to do than digest breakfast when you are trying to avoid being someone's lunch" (p. 11).

Clow (2001) differentiated the activity of the sympathetic nervous system in response to stress into two response systems: the sympathetic adrenal medullary (SAM) response and the hypothalamus-pituitary-adrenal (HPA) axis response. The response systems are activated based on the severity and duration of the stressor. You may notice that both systems have the term "adrenal" in them. This refers to the adrenal glands, which sit above the kidneys. One of their important functions is to release epinephrine into the blood stream, where it "has widespread and rapid effects on physiological systems" (Clow, 2001, p. 51). The epinephrine released by SAM response rapidly increases cardiovascular activity, which in turn carries oxygen to the parts of the body most in need of it to cope with the stressor. The blood vessels that transport the oxygen-rich blood become narrowed, increasing the pressure on the sides of the vessels to more forcefully and quickly transport the blood.

Clow (2001) likened the activation of the SAM response system to lighting a match. "Lighting a match is easy, has an instant effect and the effect doesn't last long" (p. 53). Conversely, the hypothalamus-pituitary-adrenal (HPA) axis response is like lighting a fire; "lighting a fire takes a lot more effort and its effects last much longer" (p. 53). The HPA axis response begins with the hypothalamus, which releases a chemical messenger to the pituitary, which in turn releases a chemical messenger to the adrenal glands. The adrenal glands release glucocorticoids, a steroidal hormone that functions like epinephrine and norepinephrine but remains in the system for much longer (Sapolsky, 2004).

Research by Taylor, Klein, et al. (2000) expanded the traditional notion of fight-or-flight. Taylor et al. (2000) suggested that women are more likely to act out of an impulse to maintain attachment and provide nurturing, an impulse the researchers call tend-and-befriend. The hormone oxytocin, along with female reproductive hormones, is thought to provide the neurochemical basis for this affiliative response. More recently, Taylor, Saphire-Bernstein, and Seeman (2010) found that vasopressin in men functions similarly as a measurement of relationship quality; they concluded that "plasma oxytocin in women and plasma vasopressin in men may be biomarkers of distressed pair-bond relationships" (p. 3) inducing an affiliative response. So the snarling dog provokes both the SAM and HPA axis to respond.

Epinephrine, norepinephrine, and glucocorticoids equip the body to either fight or flee the dog. Once the dog is wrestled to the ground and hog-tied or (more likely) left behind in a cloud of dust, the parasympathetic nervous system begins to bring the heightened systems back to normal. The parasympathetic nervous system counterbalances the reactivity of the sympathetic nervous system, permitting our bodies to return to the optimal balance it requires. A spell on a shady park bench with a decaf latte and a buttered scone would be in order. But what happens to our bodies when the snarling dog becomes an unreasonable supervisor? We can't very well wrestle our boss to the ground, so the acute fight-or-flight impulse becomes chronic.

**Chronic Stress**  Chronic stress spells trouble for the cardiovascular system (Clow, 2001; Sapolsky, 2004). The increased blood pressure that is needed for speeding blood to the systems that needs it to fight or flee becomes chronic hypertension. Hypertension, or high blood pressure, is dangerous because of the damage it does to blood vessels. The increased velocity of the blood during stress damages the smooth inner lining of the blood vessel. In response, the body uses a kind of natural bandage to cover the ruptures. Additionally, fatty deposits manage to find the cracks and crevices and stick there.

The result is a build-up of plaque, which reduces the circumference of the blood vessel; the clinical term for this is atherosclerosis. The more occluded the blood vessel becomes, the less blood flows through it. It can become completely blocked either by continual build-up of plaque or when a blood clot loosens and lodges in the narrowed opening of the blood vessel. The result is a heart attack or stroke. Another danger is claudication, which is pain in the legs and chest due to inadequate blood flow during moderate levels of exertion. High blood pressure can also damage the heart muscle itself, thickening it so that it becomes less efficient. This increases the risk of an irregular heartbeat, which in turn increases the risk of sudden cardiac arrest (Sapolsky, 2004).

Stress research pioneer Hans Selye conceptualized the body's response to chronic stress as adaptive disease (Selye, 1978). The activation of the SAM and HPA axis responses also lead to the inhibition of several other physiological systems. The immune system is one of these systems. Although stressors of short duration can elevate the immune system (Aldwin, 2007), the glucocorticoids released by the HPA axis response inhibits the activity of the more aggressive of the two types of cells (T cells) that fight pathogens while leaving the less aggressive cells (B cells) uninhibited. This imbalance leads to a variety of errors. With the inhibition of T cells, pathogens that should be attacked, like cancer cells, are left alone; harmless cells, like dander from a (snarling) dog, are misperceived as pathogens and attacked, and an allergic response results. Another immune-system error involves "friendly fire." The immune system mistakes its own cells for pathogens and attacks, resulting in autoimmune disorders like Type 1 diabetes and lupus (Sapolsky, 2004).

As we mentioned earlier, digestion is a process that requires time and resources. When we are under stress, digestion is one of those processes that can be inhibited. This isn't problematic when the stressor is acute; however, chronic stress puts the digestive system in a constant state of disruption, potentially leading to a variety of gastrointestinal problems, including irritable bowel syndrome (IBS), gastroesophageal reflux disease (GERD), or peptic ulcers. Researchers have found ample support for the link between stress and gastrointestinal illness through experiments with laboratory animals (Caso, Leza, & Menchen, 2008). Lab rats were immobilized and subject either to cold water immersion or mild foot shocks. These stressors produced gastrointestinal inflammation and other digestive irregularities indicative of disease.

Stressed rats infected with the *Helicobacter pylori* (*H. pylori*) virus, a virus related to the development of ulcers (Sapolsky, 2004) showed more gastrointestinal damage than noninfected rats subject to the same stressors (Caso et al., 2008). Rats are not alone in responding to stress with gastrointestinal problems. A study comparing the stress response and coping resources of both IBS and GERD patients, Orzechowska and colleagues (2008) found no significant difference between the two groups on various psychological factors related to stress.

However, as the intensity of negative emotions increased, so did the severity of symptoms associated with both IBS and GERD. Because there was no significant difference between the two groups on psychological variables related to stress, the authors concluded that their research "may confirm the hypothesis that stress is a non-specific reaction of an organism" (Orzechowska et al., 2008, p. 213).

**Children and Stress** Stress is also a factor in childhood growth and development. When infants do not develop normally, and there appears to be no physical cause for this developmental delay, pediatricians refer to this as non-organic failure to thrive. This phenomenon emerged during the 1930s in the United States as hospitals became strict about minimizing the risk of infection among infants, leading to a minimal amount of handling. This, coupled with the prevailing attitude that cuddling infants would somehow be bad for them, lead to infants being isolated. While hygienic practices improved, the survival rate of hospitalized children, infants were still at risk. At Chicago's Memorial Hospital, for example, "babies were dying seven times faster than the older children" (Blum, 2002, p. 44).

Psychiatrist René Spitz spent four months observing children in a foundling home. While conditions at the home appeared optimal for survival—very clean, ample food and medical care—the children were rarely touched. At the beginning of Spitz's tenure at the foundling home, there were 88 children under three; when he left, 23 had died from infection (Blum, 2002). Spitz's contention was that "isolation from human touch and affection . . . was destroying the children's ability to fight infection" (Blum, 2002, p. 51).

Several more contemporary studies have suggested that the family environment in general and caregiver attachment in particular are major contributors to the infant's failure to thrive (Crittenden, 1987; Gorman, Leifer, & Grossman, 1993; Ward, Kessler, & Altman, 1993). Under stress, natural human growth processes are inhibited (Sapolsky, 2004). Infants in stressful familial situations are therefore at risk. Crittenden (1987) found evidence that nonorganic failure to thrive is related not only to maternal deprivation but also to family conflict. Crittenden observed that the entire family appeared to be affected by the instability, "displaying other psychosomatic manifestations of stress" (1987, p. 51).

Another research finding suggests that failure to thrive is associated with mother–child attachments that are characterized by anxiety, fear, and an inability to cope with stress (Ward et al., 1993). Additionally, Ward and colleagues (1993) found that those infants were being raised in stressful social environments. Another contributor to failure to thrive appears to be the mother's own experience as an infant (Gorman et al., 1993). These mothers were more likely to report unstable relationships with their caregivers and a childhood characterized by crisis. As mothers themselves, they "reported feeling more depressed, reported more negative life stress, had less optimal social networks, and had a more negative perception of their babies" (Gorman, 1993, p. 327).

**Personality**  Stress can also have a negative impact on the psyche. As far back as 1881, the American physician George Beard noted that suffers of "nervous exhaustion" had a predisposition, or a diathesis, toward it. Like a predisposition toward tuberculosis, people with a nervous temperament are predisposed to nervous exhaustion. Once predisposed, any environmental stress had the potential to activate the diathesis. This is one explanation for the onset of depression (Monroe & Simons, 1991). A biological predisposition is not the only factor in the onset of depression. Brown and Harris (1978, cited in Jones and Bright, 2001) found that women who experienced negative life events and lacked a supportive social network were more likely to develop depression.

Personality is another factor in the predisposition toward stress and depression. In general, people whose personalities can be characterized as expressing negative affectivity (Watson & Clark, 1984) have a more difficult time coping with stress. Even when not confronted by an overt stressor, individuals with this characteristic will nevertheless experience some level of distress. Additionally, several personality theories associate negative affectivity to neuroticism (Jones & Bright, 2001). People who are high in neuroticism have chronic levels of instability, which can include anxiety, depression, hostility, self-consciousness, poor impulse control, and poor coping strategies when confronted with stress (Costa & Widiger, 2002).

The so-called Type A personality—the harried executive juggling multiple phone calls and barking out orders—has been popularly linked with stress. Originally, the Type A person was called the coronary-prone personality because two cardiologists, Friedman and Rosenman (1959, cited in Cooper & Dewe, 2004) began to notice a common pattern of behaviors among their patients. These patients were ambitious, competitive, and driven, with a tendency toward anger and hostility. Subsequent research has found that not all aspects of the on the Type A personality are harmful. The one variable that does appear harmful, however, is the Type A's tendency toward anger and hostility (Sapolsky, 2004). How does being angry put you at risk for heart disease? Sapolsky (2004) noted that Type A people who react with hostility are more likely to react with intensity to social stressors others would find only mildly upsetting. The intense reaction ignites the stress response with all its attendant damage to the cardiovascular system. "For the Type A, life is full of menacing stressors that demand vigilant coping responses of a particularly hostile nature" (Sapolsky, 2004, p. 327).

The common denominator with both negative affectivity and the Type A personality involves the perception of threat. This perception activates the HPA axis stress response that permits us to fight or flee. However, it would be incorrect to assume that all stress is merely a product of our perception. As Aldwin (2007) noted, one of the transactions that provokes stress is the transaction between person and environment. This has been amply researched primarily in literature dealing with the person–environment fit (P-E fit) theory and organizational stress (Edwards, Caplan, & Harrison, 2000).

The essence of the P-E fit theory is that stress results when there is a misfit between the person and the environment. The misfit occurs when either the environment is unable to provide for the perceived needs of the person, or the person does not have the resources to meet the demands of the environment (Edwards et al., 2000). When either of these conditions is sustained, the individual is at risk for developing stress-related illness, and the organization is at risk for compromising the quality and productivity of its output. It is logical to generalize the P-E fit theory of organizational stress to other life domains, and research in nonwork settings appears to support the findings of work-related research (Michalos, 1985, cited in Edwards et al., 2000).

One benefit of the P-E fit theory is that it doesn't locate the source of all stress in our heads. There are objective conditions that are stressful, and our sustained stress response to those conditions can make us sick. One of these conditions is a lack of control, where the choices available to workers on the job are constrained by conditions or policies (Maslach, 2000). How can we cope both with our own perception of stressors and an environment that pushes our ability to maintain our balance? Matheny and Riordan (1992) offered four strategies: (1) get an accurate appraisal of both your stressors and your resources, (2) decide to either live with the stressor or get rid of it, (3) change the way you think about stress and stressors, and (4) reduce your body's level of arousal.

**Appraisal Coping and Benefits of Stress**    Making an appraisal of our stressors goes hand-in-hand with perception. When we perceive anything as a stressor, we appraise it to be threatening either to our physical health or our sense of well-being. Many people appraise public speaking as a threat to their sense of well-being because of the potential for embarrassment and shame, neither of which will directly cause physical harm. Lazarus and Folkman (1984, cited in Aldwin, 2007) divided appraisals into five categories: stressors that are appraised as harmful, stressors that are appraised as threatening, stressors that are appraised as challenging, stressors that are appraised as causing loss, and stressors that are appraised as benign.

One of the best ways to accurately appraise a stressor is to monitor what you say to yourself about it. Often, without being aware of it, we say things to ourselves like, "I'll never get through this" or "I just can't cope." More often than not, these are inaccurate assessments of the stressors. If we think we'll never get through something, does that mean we'll die? These absolute statements may be a reflection of the intensity of the emotion we feel about the stressor, but it is nevertheless wrong. We usually do get through things, sometimes not well, but we get through things; we cope, perhaps not always well, but we do employ some coping strategy to help manage the stressor.

Seligman (2006) noted that helplessness and depression often emerge when we appraise stressors as being permanent, pervasive, hopeless, and somehow our fault. Imagine, for example, a work situation where your supervisor micromanages you and offers very little support. Appraising this as never-ending and undermining every part of your life—even the nonworking parts—is very likely to bring about hopelessness. Believing it's your fault, even if you have evidence to the contrary, only makes the situation worse.

However, a more accurate appraisal might be that this is temporary (as you look for another job), specific to your work life and not to family, church, or social life. This more accurate appraisal is more hopeful. These appraisals alone increase the level of resources you have available to you. Additionally, you can recall how you may have managed similar stressors in the past, identifying successful strategies and avoiding past mistakes. Moreover, you can deflate catastrophic thinking by asking yourself, "What's the worst that can happen?" (Matheny & Riordan, 1992).

Deciding to eliminate a stressor is contingent on whether it is reasonable to think it can be eliminated. Seeking another job or seeking a transfer can eliminate a stressful job. However, a chronic illness like type 1 diabetes or asthma cannot be eliminated. This ongoing stressor requires a change in the way we think about it. It is possible to think differently about a chronic stressor without lapsing into naïve cheerfulness (which will create new stress because people will want to slap you silly).

Positively reframing a chronic stressor as a challenge, as an opportunity to shift focus to other priorities, or as a means of achieving spiritual growth are all reasonable approaches to living with a chronic stressor. Since much stress is based on our perception of stressors, thinking differently about stress itself is also helpful. It is irrational to believe that stress can be eliminated. In fact, some degree of stress is beneficial, because it can stretch us to develop additional coping skills and provide opportunities for new successes, which in turn bolsters our confidence in handling stress in the future. Stress is often a factor in athletic and other competitive endeavors and can push people to accomplish more and produce better performances.

Since stress expresses itself in physiological arousal, it is helpful to sustain lifestyle practices that moderate it. Proper sleep hygiene is essential for stress management. Sleep deprivation is itself a stressor and can trigger similar physiological changes that other stressors provoke. Aerobic exercise has been shown to be a buffer against stress. Meditation is believed to activate the part of the brain that is related to muscular relaxation, and it is particularly helpful for people of faith to meditate with spiritual words or phrases consistent with their faith tradition (Benson, 1975, 1984, cited in Matheny & Riordan, 1992).

Stress is a phenomenon that is nearly universal. It is difficult to imagine anything that cannot be pushed beyond its ability to recover without distress or damage. Human beings differ from bridges and space shuttles in our ability to cope with stress by managing how we think about our stressors. "Galloping Gertie" the suspension bridge had no opportunity to reframe the high winds that eventually led to her catastrophic failure. We, however, are uniquely equipped with the cognitive capacity to decide what things in our environment pose a threat and how we are going to think about them. This cognitive flexibility provides a key weapon in the battle against stress. While we cannot think away run-away taxi cabs or prowling campground bears, we can think accurately and intentionally about those less urgent stressors that we encounter day to day. Such accuracy in how we appraise stressors may someday make the difference between heartburn and a heart attack.

*Kevin J. Eames*

*See also* Depression; Psychosomatic Health Care; Psychotherapy.

## References

Aldwin, C. W. *Stress, Coping, and Development: An Integrative Perspective.* 2nd ed. New York: The Guilford Press, 2007.

Beard, G. M. *American Nervousness, Its Causes and Consequences. BiblioLife.* 1881/2008.

Benson, H. *Beyond the Relaxation Response.* New York: Berkley, 1984.

Benson, H. *The Relaxation Response.* New York: Morrow, 1975.

Blum, D. *Love at Good Park.* Cambridge, MA: Perseus Publishing, 2002.

Brown, G. W., and T. O. Harris. *Social Origins of Depression.* London: Tavistock Publications, 1978.

Caso, J. R., J. C. Leza, and L. Menchen. "The Effects of Physical and Psychological Stress on the Gastrointestinal Tract: Lessons from Animal Models." *Current Molecular Medicine* 8, no. 4 (June 2008): 299–312.

Clow, A. "The Physiology of Stress." In *Stress: Myth, Theory, and Research,* edited by F. Jones and J. Bright, 47–61. Harlow, England: Pearson, 2001.

Cooper, C.L., and P. Dewe. *Stress: A Brief History.* Malden, MA: Blackwell Publishing Ltd., 2004.

Costa, P.T., Jr., and T.A. Widiger. "Introduction: Personality Disorders and the Five-factor Model of Personality." In *Personality Disorders and the Five-factor Model of Personality.* 2nd ed., edited by P.T. Costa Jr. and T.A. Widiger, 3–14. Washington, DC: American Psychological Association, 2002.

Crittenden, P. "Non-organic Failure-to-thrive: Deprivation or Distortion?" *Infant Mental Health Journal* 8, no. 1 (Spring 1987): 51–64.

Edwards, J.R., R.D. Caplan, and R.V. Harrison. "Person-environment Fit Theory: Conceptual Foundations, Empirical Evidence, and Directions for Future Research." In *Theories of Organizational Stress,* edited by C.L. Cooper, 28–67. Oxford: Oxford University Press, 2000.

Friedman, M., and R.H. Rosenman. "Association of Specific Overt Behavior Pattern with Blood and Cardiovascular Findings." *Journal of the American Medical Association* 169, no. 12 (1959): 1286–96.

Gorman, J., M. Leifer, and G. Grossman. "Nonorganic Failure to Thrive: Maternal History and Current Maternal Functioning." *Journal of Clinical Child Psychology* 1993: 327–336.

Jones, F., and J. Bright. *Stress: Myth, Theory, Research.* Harlow, England: Pearson Education Ltd., 2001.

Latham, G.P. *Work Motivation: History, Theory, Research, and Practice.* Thousand Oaks, CA: Sage, 2007.

Lazarus, R.S., and S. Folkman. *Stress, Appraisal, and Coping.* New York: Springer, 1984.

Maslach, C. "A Multidimensional Theory of Burnout." In *Organizational Theories of Stress,* edited by C.L. Cooper, 68–85. Oxford: Oxford University Press, 2000.

Matheny, K.B., and R.J. Riordan. *Stress and Strategies for Lifestyle Management.* Atlanta, GA: Georgia State University Press, 1992.

Michalos, A.C. "Multiple Discrepancies Theory." *Social Indicators Research* 16 (1985): 347–413.

Monroe, S.M., and A.D. Simons. "Diathesis-stress Theories in the Context of Life Stress Research: Implications for the Depressive Disorders." *Psychological Bulletin* 110, no. 3 (November 1991): 406–25.

NASA. *Report of the Presidential Commission on the Space Shuttle Challenger Accident.* June 6, 1986. http://history.nasa.gov/rogersrep/v1ch8.htm.

Orzechowska, A., A. Talarowska, M. Wysokiński, K. Zboralski, and W. Gruszczyński. "Psychological Factors in the Course of Gastroesophageal Reflux Disease and Irritable Bowel Syndrome." *Gastroenetrologia Polska* 15, no. 4 (2008): 213–17.

Sapolsky, Robert. *Why Zebras Don't Get Ulcers.* New York: Henry Holt and Company, 2004.

Seligman, M.E.P. *Learned Optimism.* New York, NY: Vintage, 1992/2006.

Selye, H. *The Stress of Life.* New York: McGraw-Hill, 1978.

Taylor, S.E., L.C. Klein, B.P. Lewis, T.L. Gruenewald, R.A.R. Gurung, and J.A. Updegraff. "Biobehavioral Responses to Stress in Females: Tend-and-Befriend, not Fight-or-Flight." *Psychological Review* 2000: 411–29.

Taylor, S.E., S. Saphire-Bernstein, and T. Seeman. "Are Plasma Oxytocin in Women and Plasma Vasopressin in Men Biomarkers of Distressed Pair-Bond Relationships?" *Psychological Science* 20 (2010): 3–7.

Ward, M.J., D.B. Kessler, and S. Altman. "Infant-Mother Attachment in Children with Failure to Thrive." *Infant Mental Health Journal* 14, no. 3 (1993): 208–20.

Washington State Department of Transportation. *Tacoma Narrows Bridge Connections.* 2010. www.wsdot.wa.gov/TNBhistory/Connections/connections3.htm.

Watson, D., and J. W. Pennebaker. "Health Complaints, Stress, and Distress: Exploring the Central Role of Negative Affectivity." *Psychological Review* 96, no. 2 (1989): 234–54.

Watson, D., and L.A. Clark. "Negative Affectivity: The Disposition to Experience Aversive Emotional States." *Psychological Bulletin* 96, no. 3 (1984): 465–90.

## SUICIDE

Suicide is intentional, self-inflected death and is one of the leading causes of death in the world. Women and men of all ages, ethnicities, and socioeconomic backgrounds commit suicide. Since the beginning of recorded history, people have taken their own lives.

People who attempt suicide may differ in their motives and in their determination to end their lives. In his classic book *Deaths of Man,* published in 1973, Edwin Shneidman identified four kinds of people who attempt suicide. Death seekers unambiguously intend to end their lives. As Shneidman described, they may waver in their intent over hours or days, but in the moment of the attempt, they are determined and single-minded, and thus choose a suicide method that is almost certain to result in death.

Death initiators are also certain that they wish to die. Their suicidal act is based in the belief that they are going to die before long anyway, perhaps within days, weeks, or months, and they are expediting the process. Death initiators are often elderly or very ill. Death ignorers believe that taking their own lives will lead to a different and better existence rather than merely the end of their current existence. For instance, they may believe that by committing suicide they will be reunited in the spiritual world with a deceased loved one. Many child suicides are of this type, but adult suicides may also fit into this category. Death darers have mixed feelings about death. They are in pain and wish to die but are not single-minded in this wish, even at the moment of the attempt. They tend to have complex motives for their attempt, including a wish to die, a wish to express anger toward someone else, a desire to make someone feel guilty, or a desire to get attention. Their attempt reveals their ambivalence. Overall, death darers choose methods that may not be lethal, and they may contact another person (e.g., call someone on the phone) immediately prior to or during the attempt.

As is demonstrated by these different types of people who attempt suicide, suicide may be motivated by different reasons or may be based in various ways of thinking. Researchers have identified different types of immediate circumstances or ongoing life conditions that can trigger suicidal behavior. First, underlying psychological disorders are clearly tied to many suicide attempts. As psychiatrist Howard Sudak reported in his 2009 review of suicide, 60 percent to 70 percent of people who commit suicide suffer from significant depression, and 10 percent suffer from schizophrenia. Suicidal thoughts are a common symptom of depression, and, thus, treating depression is likely to decrease suicide risk.

As reported by psychiatrist Zoltan Rihmer and colleagues, a program in Sweden successfully reduced the suicide rate in a community by training physicians to identify and treat depression in its early stages. In schizophrenia, suicide is most frequently linked to demoralization, despair, fears of further decline in one's own mental and psychological functioning, or frustration over one's low quality living circumstances, such as homelessness. Thus, if the quality of life of people who are diagnosed with schizophrenia can be improved—even if particular symptoms, such as delusions and hallucinations, are not effectively treated—perhaps some suicides among schizophrenic patients can be prevented.

Suicide attempts often occur with alcohol or other drug use. In a French sample of suicide attempters, Michel Lejoyeux and colleagues found that 40 percent drank alcohol prior to the attempt. Use of other kinds of drugs may also be linked to suicide attempts. The exact role that the use of alcohol or other drugs has in the suicide attempts is unclear. Ingesting the drug may decrease one's ability to problem solve, increase feelings of aggression, decrease fear of a suicide attempt, or some combination of these. Other explanations are also possible.

Changes in mood frequently occur prior to a suicide attempt. The most common mood change is increased sadness. Other feelings that may increase include anxiety, anger, and shame. Suicidologist Edwin Shneidman described a type of generalized psychological pain that he calls "psychache." Psychache seems unbearable and intolerable to the person; possibly, the only end to psychache would be death. Suicide attempts are also often preceded by feelings of hopelessness, feelings as if the current life circumstances and ways of thinking and feeling will never end.

Stressful events often precede a suicide attempt. Immediate stressors that can trigger an event include loss of a loved one through death, divorce, or abandonment; loss of a job; stress of combat; or involvement in a natural or human-made disaster such as an earthquake, hurricane, or mass shooting. Chronic stress may also lead to suicide attempts, such as the long-term stress associated with serious illness or living in a physically or emotionally abusive environment, such as may happen with abused children, abused spouses, or prison inmates. Additionally, particular occupations are associated with elevated suicide rates; these occupations may be experienced as especially stressful. These occupations are psychiatrist, psychologist, physician, nurse, dentist, lawyer, police officer, farmer, and unskilled laborer.

Sometimes suicidal behaviors increase in a community or society when another or others attempt or commit suicide. When famous people such as actors, artists, and political figures attempt or commit suicide, suicide attempts and completions increase. For instance, when Marilyn Monroe committed suicide in 1963, the suicide rate increased in the United States the following week. Additionally, when a suicide occurs in a workplace or school, other suicides may follow in that workplace or school. When this contagion effect is known, workplaces and schools often intervene, making additional counseling services available to employees and students when a suicide occurs.

In addition to attempting to uncover triggers that may lead to suicidal behavior, scholars have endeavored to understand deeper, underlying reasons about why people commit suicide. At least three theoretical positions predominate: biological, psychodynamic, and sociocultural. Biological factors may underlie suicide. Suicidal behavior runs in families. For instance, the famous suicide in 1961 of American novelist Ernest Hemingway was followed 35 years later by the suicide of his granddaughter, actress and model Margaux Hemingway. A biological factor that has received research support involves a neurotransmitter, or chemical messenger in the brain.

Specifically, suicidal behavior is often associated with low activity of the neurotransmitter serotonin. Low activity of serotonin is also associated with depression. However, it appears that the depression itself is not a sufficient explanation for suicidal behavior. As discussed in a review article by John Mann and Diane Currier published in 2010, low serotonin activity occurs among suicidal individuals who have never suffered from depression. Since low sero-

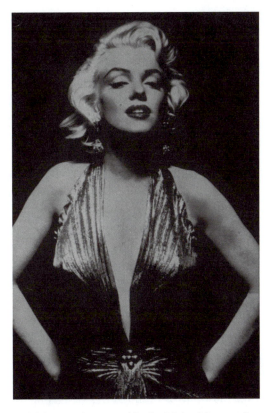

Suicide rates increased in the United States after Marilyn Monroe committed suicide in 1963. The National Institutes of Mental Health statistics show suicide is among the leading causes of death in the United States. (AP/Wide World Photos)

tonin activity may be a causal factor in suicidal behavior that is independent of the causal factor of depression, what is it about low serotonin that may lead to suicidal behavior? The leading theory is that low serotonin activity may be associated with aggression and impulsive behavior.

According to the psychodynamic view originally associated with Sigmund Freud and proposed in the early 1900s, psychological factors best explain suicide. Freud said that suicide is associated with depression. In the cases of depression that most concerned Freud, and that he believed were the majority of depression cases, an individual had lost a loved one through death or abandonment. The loss leads the depressed individual to "introject" or internalize characteristics of the lost one in order to keep the person close.

At the same time, the depressed person feels intense anger toward the loved one (even if the loved one died). The anger is directed inward, toward the introjected loved one. The anger may become so intense as to be murderous (or in this case, suicidal), leading to destructive behavior including suicide. Consistent with Freudian theory, as discussed earlier in this article, depression often underlies suicidal behavior. Additionally, research has supported another component of Freud's explanation. In a study published in 1982, Kenneth Adam and colleagues found that losing a parent at an early age doubles the risk of suicide attempt at some point in one's lifetime.

A classic perspective on suicide is Emile Durkheim's sociocultural view, originally proposed in 1892. According to Durkheim, suicide risk is directly related to individuals' connections to social groups. These groups include family, community groups, and religious groups. There are three types of suicides: egoistic, anomic, and altruistic. Egoistic suicides occur among individuals who are disconnected and isolated from society by choice. They are not socialized into the society, and are not interested in the rules of society. They have rejected society. If many people like this exist in a particular society, the suicide rate will be elevated. Anomic suicides occur among those who have a need for connection and for whom that need is not met. Society has not given these individuals stable and satisfying social connections, such as family, community groups, or religion, and the individual is left feeling alienated and that life has no meaning.

The third type, the most different from the other two, is altruistic suicide. Individuals who engage in these acts are exceptionally well-connected socially. They will sacrifice their lives for the good of their society. Examples include the Japanese kamikaze pilots of World War II and soldiers who throw themselves on top of grenades in order to save their comrades. In all three types of suicide, Durkheim's explanation focused most on societal factors as causes of suicidal behavior.

Related to the sociocultural view, suicide rates vary between countries and within subcultures in countries. For instance, the World Health Organization reports very high suicide rates—more than 20 per 100,000 people per year—in some countries, including Japan, Russia, Hungary, Belarus, Estonia, Lithuania, Ukraine, Sri Lanka, and Kazakhstan. A few countries have very low rates by comparison—fewer than 5 per 100,000, including Greece, Egypt, Albania, Armenia, Bahrain, Brazil, Guatemala, and Venezuela. The rates in both the United States and Canada are about 12 per 100,000. Benjamin Saddock and Virginia Saddock have argued that religious beliefs may provide a partial explanation for these differing rates. Countries that are predominantly Catholic, Muslim, or Jewish tend to have low rates. Additionally, people who are very religious commit suicide less frequently.

As reported by Howard Sudak, suicide rates differ for women and men, worldwide. Although women attempt suicide more often than do men, men's attempts are more lethal, resulting in a rate for men that is three times the rate for women. Men's more lethal methods include shooting or hanging themselves. Conversely, a common method among women, drug overdose, is much less likely to result in death. In the United States, suicide rates vary by race. Among five racial groups studied, Native Americans have the highest suicide rate. The rate of European Americans, which is 12 per 100,000, is almost twice the rate of African Americans, Asian Americans, or Hispanic Americans. The rate among Native Americans may be explained by extreme poverty and high rates of alcoholism. Religiosity and other cultural values may play protective roles for African Americans and Hispanic Americans.

Lastly, suicide rates vary by age in the United States. The highest rate is among people over age 65 years, that is, 19 out of 100,000 persons. Many of these suicides appear to be related to poor health and feelings of hopelessness associated with poor health. Additionally, older people have lost friends and family to death, resulting in losses of support and companionship. In the United States, aging tends to be associated with a loss of status. In subcultures in which the elderly receive more respect and status, such as among Native Americans, suicide rates are relatively low.

Clearly, preventing suicide is a concern for mental health professionals. The first suicide prevention program in the United States was established in Los Angeles in 1955. Today, hundreds of suicide prevention centers exist throughout the United States. Additionally, there are hundreds of suicide hotlines in the United States. The counselors at these centers and working for these hotlines and other mental health centers, hospital emergency rooms, and pastoral centers are trained to offer crisis intervention to individuals in need. Crisis intervention involves establishing rapport with the person in need, understanding the client's problem and assessing suicide potential, then encouraging the client to become aware of all of his or her resources (e.g., personal characteristics, social support availability) and developing a plan to help the client make changes in his or her life.

According to many experts, including Howard Sudak, an effective way to prevent suicide is to treat the underlying condition, for instance, depression (present in the majority of cases of suicide), alcohol addiction, or schizophrenia. In depressed individuals, cognitive-behavioral therapy has been found to decrease suicidal behavior. In individuals diagnosed with schizophrenia, the medication clozapine has been found to decrease suicidal behavior. Sudak stated that future research on suicide should include investigating other treatments utilizing rigorous research designs. For instance, antidepressant medications should be investigated thoroughly, as should various types of psychotherapy. Additionally, as new biological treatments for depression (e.g., deep-brain stimulation and vagal nerve stimulation) are researched for their effectiveness in decreasing depression, their effects on suicidal behavior should also be studied.

*Gretchen M. Reevy*

*See also* Depression; Psychotherapy; Stress; World Health Organization (WHO).

## References

Adam, Kenneth S., Anthony Bouckoms, and David Streiner. "Parental Loss and Family Stability in Attempted Suicide." *Archives of General Psychiatry* 39, no. 9 (1982): 1081–85.

Comer, Ronald J. *Abnormal Psychology.* New York: Worth, 2010.

Durkheim, Emile. *Suicide.* New York: Free Press. 1951. Originally published 1892.

Heisel, Marnin J. "Suicide." In *Clinical Handbook of Schizophrenia* edited by Kim. T. Mueser and Dilip V. Jeste, 491–504. New York: Guilford Press, 2008.

Lejoyeux, Michel, Francois Huet, Micheline Claudon, Anika Fichelle, Enrique Casalino, and Valerie Lequen. "Characteristics of Suicide Attempts Preceded by Alcohol Consumption." *Archives of Suicide Research* 12, no. 1 (January 2008): 30–8.

Mann, John J., and Diane M. Currier. "Stress, Genetics and Epigenetic Effects on the Neurobiology of Suicidal Behavior and Depression." *European Psychiatry* 25, no. 5 (2010): 268–71.

Rihmer, Zoltan, Wolfgang Rutz, and Hans Pihlgren. "Depression and Suicide in Gotland. An Intensive Study of All Suicides before and after a Depression-training Programme for General Practitioners." *Journal of Affective Disorders* 35 (1995): 147–52.

Sadock, Benjamin J., and Virginia A. Sadock. *Synopsis of Psychiatry: Behavioral Sciences/ Clinical Psychiatry.* Philadelphia: Wolters Kluwer/Lippincott Williams & Wilkins, 2007.

Shneidman, Edwin S. *Comprehending Suicide: Landmarks in 20th Century Suicidology.* Washington, DC: American Psychological Association, 2001.

Shneidman, Edwin S. *Deaths of Man.* Lanham, MD: Jason Aronson, 1973.

Sudak, Howard S. "Suicide." In *Kaplan & Sadock's Comprehensive Textbook of Psychiatry,* edited by Benjamin J. Sadock, Virginia A. Sadock, and Pedro Ruiz, 2717–32. Baltimore: Lippincott, Williams, and Wilkins, 2009.

## SUPPLEMENTS. *See* DIETARY SUPPLEMENTS

# *T*

## TAI CHI

Tai Chi, an ancient Chinese form of martial art, is practiced by many for purposes ranging from achieving wellness to enhancing artistic and athletic performance. It involves slow flowing movements, deep breathing, relaxation, and meditation. Tai chi is a form of Qigong, a practice that dates back 2,500 years according to some accounts. Qigong was and still is used for healing purposes and involves controlled breathing along with movement exercises.

Important components of tai chi are yin and yang and chi, or energy. Yin and yang refers to opposing forces that rely on each other to exist but must do so in harmony. Traditional Chinese medical practitioners believe that sickness is a result of imbalances within the body. Tai chi and other forms of Qigong seek to correct these energy imbalances through movement. Once there is harmony, vital chi can flow normally.

There are three main types of tai chi practiced in the United States today: yang, wu, and tai chi chih. The yang style requires maintaining a wide stance with bent knees during most of its 24 movements. In its traditional form it contains 108 movements. This form is more physically demanding than the other two. The wu style consists of 24 movements in its short form and 100 movements in its traditional form. It is milder than the yang style because participants can use a narrower stance. The tai chi chih style, which has 20 movements, also uses a higher stance, but less weight gets transferred from one leg to the other.

Additional movements in tai chi occur with the arms and hands. They can also include twisting at the waist and turning the body around. Referred to as "forms," these movements are frequently named after animals and phenomena seen in nature.

Western medicine increasingly acknowledges the role of many traditional Chinese approaches to healing. In academic medical centers across the country, researchers are examining the effects of tai chi on various types of diseases and conditions. For example, during research conducted at Tufts University and

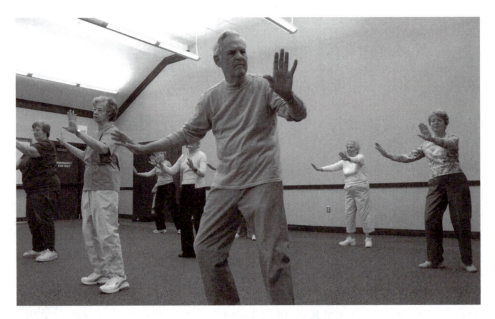

Elderly adults practice Tai Chi. Research has revealed health benefits that accompany the practice of Tai Chi. Tai Chi has become increasingly popular with elderly Americans thanks to research that has revealed health benefits including a reduction in arthritis pain and increased physical mobility associated with its practice. (AP/Wide World Photos)

published in the *New England Journal of Medicine,* tai chi appeared to offer some therapeutic benefit to patients with fibromyalgia. Fibromyalgia is a musculoskeletal disorder that results in severe pain for those who have the condition. Other illnesses that tai chi purports to improve include high blood pressure, heart disease, depression, and cancer. However, researchers caution that more studies are needed over a longer period of time and with larger numbers of study participants to determine whether tai chi results in true healing.

In 2008, the National Institutes of Health released a survey showing that Americans spent billions of dollars on complementary and alternative medicine. This included $4.1 billion on activities like yoga, tai chi and Qigong. Tai chi has long played a role in helping performers enhance their skills. Actors use tai chi to develop greater awareness of their bodies and how they move as they perform. In sports, athletes use the ancient art to develop a competitive edge.

*Abena Foreman-Trice*

*See also* Fibromyalgia; Qigong; Traditional Chinese Medicine; Yoga.

### References

MedicineNet. "Tai Chi." September 1, 2010. www.medicinenet.com/tai_chi/article.htm.
National Institutes of Health, National Center for Complementary and Alternative Medicine. "The Use of Complementary and Alternative Medicine in the United States: Cost Data." July 2009. http://nccam.nih.gov/news/camstats/costs/NHIS_costdata.pdf.

T'ai Chi: The International Magazine of Tai Chi Chuan. "Qigong: An Ancient Way to Balance Mind and Body." n.d. www.tai-chi.com/info_detail.php?id=16.

Wayne, Chenchen, Christopher H. Schmid, Ramel Rones, Robert Kalish, JanethYinh,DonL.Goldenberg,Yoojin Lee, and Timothy McAlindon, "A Randomized Trial of Tai Chi for Fibromyalgia." *New England Journal of Medicine* 363 (2010): 743–54.

## TANNING

Tanning refers to the natural or artificial process of darkening one's skin color. Typically, tanned skin is achieved via sun exposure, but, in recent years, tanning beds that deliver ultraviolet rays or booths that cover users with a topical spray that mimics a natural tan have become increasingly popular. Indoor tanning with UV radiation lamps or beds has been linked to the three main types of skin cancer: basal cell carcinoma, squamous cell carcinoma, and melanoma, the most dangerous form of skin cancer.

The debate about altering one's skin color has been going on for centuries; in some cultures, darkened skin color and cosmetic use were seen as markers of wealth and attractiveness, while in others, darkened skin was seen as primitive and uncivilized. In 18th-century Europe and America, cosmetic skin whiteners and home remedies to cure accidental tans were popular. As the Industrial Revolution took hold, however, Western notions about skin color began to change. In Europe, as the working class headed indoors to do factory work, the

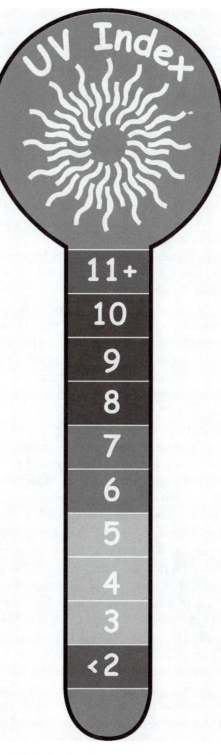

The EPA index for sun exposure to UV radiation offers numbers on the strength of the sun's rays. (Environmental Protection Agency)

wealthy started associating darkened skin with leisure time and wealth. This new association did not take hold in America until the early 20th century because Victorian propriety forbade skimpy bathing costumes and daywear and looked down upon any alteration of one's skin color.

By the turn of the 20th century, however, new ideas surfaced about leisure time, skin color, and appropriate dress and behavior for women. In particular, women of the 1910s and 1920s began challenging female stereotypes and limitations by putting off marriage and childbearing, donning skimpier clothing (including bathing costumes and dresses that showed off arms, legs, and chests), and wearing cosmetics, which had previously been associated with oversexualized women. These changes, coupled with the accidental tan of European fashion icon Coco Chanel in the early 1920s, paved the way for the rising popularity of tanning in America. Advertisers and other social conduits began associating tanning with health, personal and national strength, female beauty, and female liberation. Advertisements for skin products began focusing on how the products enhanced a tan; this was a departure from ads prior to the 1920s that promoted products that preserved white skin.

As tanning's popularity grew, advertisers from the 1930s to the 1960s promoted obvious products, like tinted face powder and nylons, as well as unobvious products like silverware, by drawing connections between a tan and patriotism, anticommunism, and an acceptance of civil rights activity and the feminist movement. During the 20th century, most products and advertisements related to tanning targeted women, though advertisements for alcohol and car makers, vacation spots, and even a few cosmetic preparations like Man Tan, a 1950s tinted cosmetic, encouraged tanning for men.

Despite a discussion of the health risks of tanning, which began in the 1960s, Americans continued associating tans with leisure time, wealth, beauty, and health through the end of the 20th century; accordingly, advertisers and producers continued promoting tans. "Several times a week, Jaclyn, 22, drives to a tanning bed lined with 100-watt UV bulbs for 15 minutes. It's a routine she's been loyal to since her senior year in high school. 'I hate being pale,' she says. 'It makes me feel ghostly and sick. I look healthier with a tan.' But what about the potential effects on her skin—the age spots, the wrinkles, the *cancer?* 'By the time I have to worry about that, they'll have something to fix it'" ("Tanning Junkie," 2009). Because of tanning's reputation for giving good health, Americans started looking for easier and faster ways to get sun exposure. Tanning beds (machines using artificially produced ultraviolet rays to tan users' skin) were introduced in the 1930s. These beds were originally advertised to tubercular Americans, for whom sun exposure was considered healing, and even as a home appliance for adventurous sorts, but by the 1970s, tanning beds were available to the general public in commercial tanning salons. Through the 1980s and 1990s, tanning salons sprung up across the nation, offering Americans quick and intense tans. When scientists made connections between skin cancer and outdoor sun exposure, tanning bed manufacturers promoted beds as safe alternatives. But through the 1990s, studies consistently demonstrated higher risks of skin cancer among tanning bed users because of the intensity of ultraviolet exposure in tanning beds. Despite the risk, there is currently still a large culture of Americans, particularly young women, who use tanning beds.

In the 1960s, many Americans became aware of the strong links between sun-tanning and skin cancer, among other less serious maladies like wrinkles. Though literature connecting tanning with skin cancer began showing up in popular magazines as early as 1941, it was not until the early 1960s that a serious challenge to tanning's popularity emerged. And though advertisers continued to encourage tanning to sell products, the late 1960s and early 1970s saw the emergence of increasing studies and reports about the dangers of tanning as well as the introduction of alternative products, such as leg creams and other cosmetic substitutes that gave the appearance of a tan. Similarly, sunscreen became widely popular, particularly after the sun protection factor (SPF) rating system was implemented in the 1970s. And yet, Americans continued to ignore the warnings of physicians and prescriptive literature and tan, often with low SPF sunscreen or no sunscreen at all; the association of a tan with good health and beauty was too strong to reverse overnight. It took a concerted effort by scientists, doctors, and others from the 1980s to the present day, armed with frightening statistics about skin cancer mortality rates, to get the word out and convince more Americans to either use stronger sunscreen or avoid sun exposure altogether.

In the 21st century, Americans seem more informed about the risks associated with suntanning. There is copious literature about the risks of sun exposure and the problems associated with darkening one's skin. The positive associations tied to tanning, however, continue to hold strong in the national psyche. As a result, new products have emerged that can be used to alter one's skin color safely; most notably, self-tanning lotions and booths that spray a topical tanning product have become popular and safe alternatives. Additionally, there is much greater attention to sunscreen and sun safety in popular literature and culture, signaling a slowly developing awareness of the dangers of suntanning and attention to preventative measures. A number of U.S. states have passed legislation regulating indoor tanning facilities in an attempt to reduce risks to consumers. According to figures from the Centers for Disease Control and Prevention, 28 states had implemented state laws dealing with tanning as of 2006 (Mayer et al., 2008).

*Devon Atchison*

*See also* Cancer.

## References

Hansen, Devon. "Shades of Change: Suntanning and the Twentieth Century American Dream." PhD diss., Boston University, 2007.

Mayer, J. A., K. D. Hoerster, L. C. Pichon, D. A. Rubio, S. I. Woodruff, and J. L. Forster. "Enforcement of State Indoor Tanning Laws in the United States." *Prev. Chronic Dis.* 5, no. 4 (2008): www.cdc.gov/pcd/issues/2008/oct/07_0194.htm.

Peiss, Kathy. *Hope in a Jar: The Making of America's Beauty Culture.* New York: Metropolitan Books, 1998.

Segrave, Kerry. *Suntanning in 20th Century America.* Jefferson, NC: McFarland & Company, 2005.

"Tanning Junkie." Oprah Magazine, August 2009, 146. www.oprah.com/style/In-Beauty-Treatment_1/6.

## TARGET HEART RATE

Target heart rate (THR) is a concept used to describe the ideal heart rate reached during exercise (typically aerobic) in order to maximize cardiovascular benefit. Calculated as a proportion of maximum heart rate ($HR_{max}$), individual target heart rates are highly variable, in part due to the large variation in $HR_{max}$ found in the population. THR and $HR_{max}$ are dependent on numerous factors including age, gender, current cardiovascular fitness, and general physical condition.

There are a number of methods used to determine a target heart rate. The key factor in estimating an individual's THR is determining $HR_{max}$. While population level trends in $HR_{max}$ are easily observable, standard deviations tend to be large. In one study of an Olympic rowing team, $HR_{max}$ was found to range from 166 to 208 (Mickelson, 1982). This demonstrates the wide variability in $HR_{max}$, even within relatively homogenous groups. For individuals, $HR_{max}$ is best determined in a controlled laboratory setting, via a cardiac stress test. However, this is impractical for most people and therefore, many formulae have been proposed to estimate $HR_{max}$.

The most commonly cited formula is $\mathbf{HR_{max} = 220 - age}$. This formula, while easy to use and commonly cited, is not actually very accurate. Originally proposed in 1970, this formula was never intended to be used by the general population for determining exercise regimes (Kolata, 2001). A 2002 study by Roberg and Landwehr concluded that there is no currently known formula that predicts maximum heart rate with an acceptably small standard error. However, the authors noted that if a formula were to be used, the least objectionable (though it still has a large standard error) is

$$\mathbf{HR_{max} = 205.8 - (0.685) \, (age)}$$

Ideally, an individual's THR is found via a series of tests in a controlled environment. However, this is not practical and in practice, THR is most commonly calculated as approximately 60 percent to 80 percent of an individual's $HR_{max}$, although the exact percentages vary slightly by source. For example, the American Heart Association gives a broad 50 percent to 85 percent range (American Heart Association, n.d.), while the Mayo Clinic suggests a tighter 70 percent to 85 percent range (Mayo Clinic, 2007). The most common way to calculate these ranges is to directly multiply $HR_{max}$ by the target intensity. For example, 80 percent intensity would be calculated as $\mathbf{THR_{80\%} = (HR_{max}) \, (0.80)}$. Thus, an individual with a $HR_{max}$ of 200 bpm would have a THR of 120 to 160 bpm (assuming 60%–80%). This calculation's popularity owes to its ease of use, although an alternate method, known as the Karvonen method, is actually more accurate (Davis & Convertino, 1975). The Karvonen method takes the percentage intensity as a percentage of the difference between an individual's $HR_{max}$ and resting heart rate ($HR_{rest}$). Again using 80 percent intensity, the calculation would be

$$THR_{80\%} = HR_{rest} + (HR_{max} - HR_{rest}) (0.80)$$

Therefore, using the Karvonen method, an individual with a $HR_{max}$ of 200 bpm and a $HR_{rest}$ of 60 bpm would have a THR of 144 to 172 bpm.

While it is clear that these formulas have large standard deviations, there is no expert consensus on whether THR estimates based on formulas should be used in planning exercise. Ultimately, the fact remains that using these formulae for estimating THR and $HR_{max}$ remains popular, it is important to be cognizant of their flaws and use caution in relying on them to guide one's exercise.

*David Chen*

*See also* Aerobic Exercise; Exercise; Heart Health.

### References

American Heart Association. "Target Heart Rates." n.d. www.heart.org/HEARTORG/GettingHealthy/PhysicalActivity/Target-Heart-Rates_UCM_434341_Article.jsp#Tt7WPnNhK0o.

Davis, James A., and Victor A. Convertino. "A Comparison of Heart Rate Methods for Predicting Endurance Training Intensity." *Medicine and Science in Sports* 7, no. 4 (1975): 295–8.

Kolata, Gina. "Maximum Heart Rate Theory Is Challenged." *The New York Times,* April 24, 2001.

Mayo Clinic. "Tool: Target Heart Rate Calculator." October 28, 2010. www.mayoclinic.com/health/target-heart-rate/SM00083.

Mickelson, Timothy C., and Frederick C. Hagerman. "Anaerobic Threshold Measurements of Elite Oarsmen." *Medicine and Science in Sports and Exercise* 14, no. 6 (1982): 440–4.

Robergs, Robert A., and Landwehr, Roberto. "The Surprising History of the '$HR_{max}$ = 220 – Age' Equation." *Journal of Exercise Physiology* 5, no. 2 (2002): 1–10.

## THERAPEUTIC TOUCH

Therapeutic Touch (TT) is a so-called energy healing method that involves placing the healer's hands slightly above a patient's body without actually making physical contact (Krieger, 1975). The name itself can be misleading, since TT does not normally involve touching a patient and traditionally entails the healer working approximately 2 to 6 inches away from the patient's body (Herdtner, 2000). TT supposedly can manipulate the human energy field in a number of ways, such as by transferring the healer's own energy into the patient or by removing blockages to energy flow within the patient. It is speculated that this might induce states of relaxation as well as stimulate immune and other healing activities in the patient's body. According to this tradition, the human energy field is an open process that continuously flows and communicates with other human energy fields (Denison, 2004). The main assumption behind TT is that practitioners can learn to detect and change the human energy field of others, revealing an ability to heal that is considered natural and within everyone's capability to learn. Many studies, however, have failed to measure substantial benefits from this therapy.

**Origins**  TT was introduced in 1972 by Dolores Krieger, a nursing instructor at New York University, and Dora Kunz, an energy healer, who together developed this approach at a spiritual retreat center called Pumpkin Hollow, in New York, with the intent to teach it mainly to nurses interested in learning to supplement their more conventional healing work (Therapeutic Touch, 2010). However, TT has roots in many ancient healing traditions, such as the Biblical laying on of hands, even though it does not endorse any specific religion or operate from any specific spiritual doctrine. In fact, Krieger claimed that belief in TT's efficacy is not required for a patient to benefit from its effects.

TT is an extension of Kunz's supposedly lifelong ability to see and sense the human energy field, along with her claimed ability to help heal others using the energy field. TT also originated from a nursing theory created by Rogers (1970), now referred to as Rogers' Science of Unitary Human Beings (Herdtner, 2000). According to Rogers, human beings are energy fields that are continuously open, have no boundaries, and are constantly in a mutual exchange with what he called "environmental fields." Rogers theorized that these energy fields are "wholes" that can be identified by patterns. Although these patterns cannot be directly observed, Rogers suggested that the manifestations of these patterns can be observed through the mutual exchange of the human field and the environmental field. In addition, TT fits with the themes of interpersonal caring and patient empowerment emphasized within the nursing profession. TT incorporates Roger's view that the patient is an important part of the healing process and should be the primary decision maker in promoting effective health changes. It also arose as an alternative to mainstream medical approaches that were seen to emphasize a dehumanizing model of medical treatment, valuing technology more than caring.

In contrast to an authoritarian approach to medical care in which the doctor is viewed as the expert and the patient only as a passive recipient of medical services, TT encourages nurses and patients to interact in caring ways (Herdtner, 2000). Krieger (1993) stated the following: "A basic recognition upon which Therapeutic Touch was developed initially was exactly that in the final analysis, it is the client who heals himself. The healer or therapist, in this view, acts as a human energy support system until the healee's own immunological system is robust enough to take over" (Krieger, 1993). TT quickly gained widespread popularity among the nursing community and became more broadly popular in the 1970s. It is still taught within many nursing schools, practiced in many hospitals, and there are an estimated 47,000 health professionals in more than 80 countries trained in TT (Straneva, 2000). TT training is also endorsed by various professional groups, such as the American Holistic Nurses Association (2010).

**Research on Effectiveness** Studies examining the effectiveness of TT in general have mixed results. Krieger argued that TT is effective in managing pain and anxiety as well as in promoting wound healing, while others state that numerous case studies have shown it to be effective (Denison, 2004). In terms of possible mechanisms, Krieger considered hemoglobin levels to be a possible marker of well-being, as a molecule in the blood carrying oxygen to all the body's cells, and reported that following a TT session, a significant number of patients showed higher hemoglobin levels. Other studies have found TT to be effective in decreasing anxiety in dementia patients (Doherty, Wright, Aveyard, & Sykes, 2006) and in fibromyalgia patients (Denison, 2004). TT has also been found to reduce pain associated with migraine headaches (Lothian, 1993) and promote wound healing and pain management (Straneva, 2000).

Not all studies have supported the effectiveness of TT. One particularly noteworthy study was done by Emily Rosa, an 11-year-old girl who was the youngest to ever publish a paper within the *Journal of the American Medical Association* (Rosa, Rosa, Sarner, & Barrett, 1998). She recruited 21 TT practitioners to test whether or not they could accurately detect the human energy field. To accomplish this, she had practitioners stand on one side of a cardboard screen, while she stood on the other. Practitioners were instructed to place their hands through holes in the screen, while Emily randomly placed her hands in front of the practitioners. After many replications, results of the study showed that only 44 percent of the practitioners were able to accurately detect her energy field, which was slightly worse than chance.

In other studies, Olsen, Sneed, Bonnadonna, Ratliff, and Dias (1992) used TT to treat victims suffering from a hurricane disaster and found that it was not effective in reducing stress, while Hughes, Meize-Grochowski, and Harris (1996) did not find significant reduction in anxiety among adolescent psychiatric patients receiving TT. Many other studies have shown inconclusive results, leading some critics to refer to TT as "quackery," especially for its lacking both an objective and theoretical basis (e.g., Rayner, 1999).

Although the existing studies on TT are inconclusive, in a broader context there is a growing body of research that highlights the importance of touch. Particularly noteworthy is Field's work at the University of Miami School of Medicine (Touch Research Institute, 2010), where over 100 studies have shown the positive effects of various massage therapies involving touch. Some of these significant findings suggest that touch is effective in enhancing growth in premature infants, decreasing pain in fibromyalgia, enhancing immune function in HIV and cancer patients, increasing pulmonary function in asthma, and decreasing glucose levels in diabetes, to name just a few of its benefits. It is important to note, however, that therapeutic touch practice does not actually involve physical contact, such as these various massage approaches, so extrapolating from the massage research to TT is only speculation.

The question remains, does TT heal, and, if so, through what mechanisms? Is there an actual energy field that a TT healer can sense in patients and then manipulate to result in healing? Alternatively, could the fact that a TT healer spends time and bestows concentrated attention on patients, especially within nursing settings during times when patients are suffering from difficult illnesses and might feel especially alone and vulnerable in the face of invasive and complicated technologies, be enough to account for any healing, perceived or real?

*Cheryl Fracasso and Harris Friedman*

*See also* Fibromyalgia; Human Immunodeficiency Virus (HIV); Stress.

### References

American Holistic Nurses Association (2010). "AHNA Endorsed Programs." www.ahna. org/Education/EndorsedPrograms/tabid/1207/Default.aspx.

Denison, B. "Touch the Pain Away: New Research on Therapeutic Touch and Persons with Fibromyalgia Syndrome." *Holistic Nurse Practice* 18, no. 3 (2004): 142–51.

Doherty, D., S. Wright, B. Aveyard, and M. Sykes. "Therapeutic Touch and Dementia Care: An Ongoing Journey." *Nursing Older People* 18, no. 11 (2006): 27–30.

Herdtner, S. "Using Therapeutic Touch in Nursing Practice." *Orthopaedic Nursing* 19, no. 5 (2000): 77–82.

Hughes, E.E., R. Meize Grochowski, and C.N.D Harris. "Therapeutic Touch with Adolescent Psychiatric Patients." *Journal of Holistic Nursing* 14 (1996): 6–23.

Krieger, D. "Therapeutic Touch: The Imprimatur of Nursing." *The American Journal of Nursing* 75, no. 5 (1975): 784–87.

Krieger, D. *Accepting Your Power to Heal: The Personal Practice of Therapeutic Touch.* New York: Bear & Company, 1993.

Lothian, J.A. "A Modern Version of the Laying on of Hands. Can Aid in Relaxation During Labor—and beyond: Therapeutic Touch." *Childbirth Instructor* 32 (1993): 34–6.

Olsen, M., N. Sneed, R. Bonadonna, J. Ratliff, and J. Dias. "Therapeutic Touch and Post-Hurricane Hugo Stress." *Journal of Holistic Nursing* 10 (1992): 120–36.

Rayner, C. "A Patient's Eye View of Quality." *British Medical Journal* 319 (1999): 525.

Rogers, M.E. *An Introduction to the Theoretical Basis of Nursing.* Philadelphia: E. A. Davis, 1970.

Rosa, L., E. Rosa, L. Sarner, and S. Barrett. "A Close Look at Therapeutic Touch." *Journal of the American Medical Association* 279, no. 13 (1998): 1005–10.

Straneva, J.A. "Therapeutic Touch Coming of Age." *Holistic Nursing Practice* 14, no. 3 (2000): 1–13.

Therapeutic Touch. "Therapeutic Touch Defined." 2010. www.therapeutictouch.org/what_is_tt.html.

Touch Research Institute. "History of the Touch Research Institute. 2010.www6.miami.edu/touch-research/About.html.

## TRADITIONAL CHINESE MEDICINE

Chinese medicine, also known as Traditional Chinese Medicine (TCM), is a medical system developed thousands of years ago in China. This system diagnoses and treats patients using a unique form of analysis for diagnosis and herbs and other

Chinese practices for treatment. Sometimes erroneously referred to only as acupuncture, TCM also includes the treatment modalities of Chinese herbal medicine, Qigong (a meditation style), Tui Na (Chinese massage), and dietary therapy as well as acupuncture. In contrast, scientific Western medicine is largely based on an approach that focuses on the body and not on the mind or spirit. Western medicine works to identify and treat molecular abnormalities that cause disease, and treatment uses drugs and/or surgery.

Being an ancient discipline, TCM evolved without the advent of modern science. Therefore, diagnosis is made, in part, by observing the human body as it relates to the natural world around it. It is holistic in nature, meaning anything that affects one part of the body necessarily affects other systems within the body. A headache, for instance, is not seen as an isolated event. Rather, it is merely a symptom related to a deeper cause, whether emotional, energetic, or physical in nature. Treatment focuses on the root cause of a disorder. If the root is addressed and corrected, the symptom will not be able to manifest.

**Slow Medicine**   Using an analogy, TCM could be considered "slow medicine" when compared to modern medicine, which could be called "fast medicine." Rather than using drugs to fix an isolated problem, TCM looks to balance the individual and return health from the inside out. Once harmony is restored, the symptom can no longer exist because the body is in balance. However, achieving balance takes time. Acupuncture, Chinese herbal medicine, and dietary modification may take weeks or even months to take effect, hence, the label "slow medicine." However, once balance and harmony is restored, the result is long lasting because the reason for the disorder has been addressed.

For example, a person may take ibuprofen to remedy the symptom of a headache. This works quickly but does nothing to address the question of why the

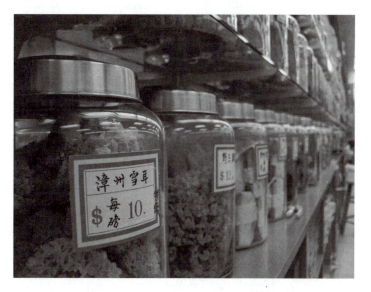

Jars containing herbs used in traditional Chinese medicine line the shelves in this store in Chinatown, San Francisco. (iStockPhoto)

person gets repeated headaches in the first place. TCM looks to ascertain the reason behind the headaches, which may have its roots in any number of the body's systems. This takes time, but once the body is assessed, the reason behind the headaches is determined and a treatment protocol is implemented, balance is restored and the headaches stop.

Chinese medicine is believed to have begun approximately 5,000 years ago. Since much of Chinese medicine came before the advent of modern science, demons, spirits, and ghosts were used periodically as explanations for some of the observed phenomena in ancient times. When Chiang Kai-shek and the Kuomintang came to power in China in the late 1920s, acupuncture and Chinese medicine were characterized as old school and ancient, and leaders wanted it replaced by the more modern Western medicine. After World War II and the Communist party coming to power, the national view changed. Party leader Chairman Mao said Chinese medicine was the people's medicine, being both cheap and readily available to all, and he elevated it to its previously honored status. However, being of a nonreligious nature, he decreed that any mention of demons and spirits be left out of the teachings of Chinese medicine. Thus began the distillation of what is now known as Traditional Chinese Medicine, or TCM, and what is the version of Chinese medicine currently being taught in the teaching colleges throughout China and the world.

**Basic Concepts** To have a basic understanding of TCM, one must entertain certain concepts that are foreign to the minds of many westerners but are central both to Chinese thought and TCM. The concepts of yin and yang, chi, the meridian system, premodern causes of disease, and Five Element theory must be discussed before beginning to explore and understand TCM.

Yin and yang are concepts central to the workings of TCM. They should be seen as one interconnected entity rather than opposites, as one could not exist without the other. The original meaning for the Chinese character of yang was the sunny side of the slope. Yang is therefore likened to characteristics such as male, heat, brightness, upward and outward, and the sun. Yin, on the other hand, originally meant the shady side of a slope (Kaptchuk, 1983). Yin is likened to the characteristics of female, cold, darkness, downward and inward, and the moon. Yin and yang are two poles of one whole, two aspects that cannot exist without the other. As depicted in the ubiquitous symbol, yin constantly transforms into yang and yang into yin. Within yin there is necessarily an element of yang, hence the dot in the symbol, and visa versa. While something may be characterized as yang (the flower of a plant), it is only yang when compared to something more yin (the root of the same plant). Something can be either yin or yang, depending on what it is compared to. A hot tub would be yang when compared to a tepid bath but yin when compared to a vat of bubbling oil. One way TCM looks at the human body is the relationship between yin and yang. For example, a person with a red face, a booming voice, and a boisterous nature would be considered a yang-type person, especially when compared to a frail, soft-spoken, pale-faced person, who would be considered yin type.

While yin and yang may be the basis of TCM, the concept of chi can be seen as its driving force. The idea of chi runs deep in many Asian cultures. Often translated as "vital energy," "vital force," or "life force," chi is a difficult concept to translate with a few words. It is often described as the energy that animates the different forms in the world, or the energy inherent in all things. Einstein's famous equation, $E = mc^2$, would seem to support this idea, as his equation states that energy exists within all forms of mass.

Another western concept that may help give a better understanding of chi is the famous Star Wars idea of "the force." Many people postulate that the idea for the force had origins in eastern thought. In fact, when Obi Wan Kenobi states, "The force is what gives a Jedi his power, it is an energy field created by all living things. It surrounds us, penetrates us, and binds the galaxy together," he could easily be giving a definition of chi. To carry the Star Wars analogy further, the dark side and the light side of the force are but two aspects of a single entity. An excellent example of the yin-yang dynamic in action is when Anakin Skywalker (good, light) transforms into Darth Vader (dark, evil), morphing from one side to the other. This so-called force, or power, of chi can be seen as its yang aspect. The yin aspect of chi is centered more on intellect, consciousness and spirit.

Chi courses through the body via meridians. The meridian system is an invisible network of channels and conduits through which the chi flows. The ancient medical text, *The Huang Di Nei Jing,* states, "The function of the channels (meridians) is to transport the Qi and blood and circulate Yin and Yang to nourish the body" (Ni, 1995). There are 14 main meridians named primarily after organs and many smaller branches of these main meridians. While the meridians are named after organs and their pathways flow through the organs, they are separate from the organs themselves. It is into specific points on the meridians that acupuncture needles are placed. Acupuncture is said to regulate the flow of chi in the body, thus restoring balance and harmony to it.

As TCM predates modern science, viruses, bacteria and other microscopic organisms were not seen as causes of disease. Rather, the causes of disease are known as the six pernicious influences and the seven emotions.

**Influences and Emotions** The six pernicious influences are wind, heat, cold, dampness, dryness, and summer heat. These must be seen as analogies rather that absolutes. A viral infection with symptoms of fever and a sore throat would be seen as a combination of wind and heat—wind because of the swift onset of disease, and heat for the fever and hot, raw throat. A viral infection with symptoms of chills and a clear runny nose would be seen and a combination of wind and cold. Dampness could be seen as analogous to phlegm. Dryness is a symptom of dryness. Summer heat is analogous to heatstroke.

The seven emotions are joy, fear, anger, sadness, worry, fright, and grief. Sometimes a variation of these seven is listed, which highlights the fact that these seven are only examples of the multitude of human emotions. The key is that emotions, both positive and negative, affect the workings of the human body.

Just as the ancient Greeks attributed four humors to the human condition, Chinese medicine assigns five humors to the human condition. These are water, wind, fire, earth, and metal. Each element is related to a certain organ, a certain emotion, a certain flavor, a certain smell, and so forth. The interplay between the elements is observed in nature and reflected back in the human condition. While a balanced human experiences the multitude of emotions, an excess of a particular emotion can negatively affect the body. The Five Element theory relates to the seven emotions and the body's organs in the following manner. Anger causes chi to rise and is related to the liver. Joy scatters chi and is related to the heart. Worry, also seen as pensiveness or rumination, knots chi and is related to the spleen. Sadness and grief weakens chi and are related to the lungs. Fear and fright are both related to the kidneys. Fear causes chi to descend and right causes chi to become chaotic (Ni, 1995).

TCM takes the Five Element interplay into account when assessing a patient. One particular style of Chinese medicine is known as Five-Element Acupuncture. This particular style was popularized by J.R. Worsley of England. In Five-Element Acupuncture, the dynamic and interplay between the elements is the main diagnostic criteria. Five-Element Acupuncture pays particular attention to the emotional and spiritual well-being of a person. The color of a person's face, their smell, the sound of their voice, and their predominant emotion and how these relate to the interplay between the five elements is the main diagnostic criteria. The energy of a particular element usually predominates in an individual. This element is central to the diagnosis and is known as the causative factor.

**The Four Examinations**   In TCM, diagnosis and assessment of the body, as it relates to yin, yang, and the health of its chi, is done by assessment. Traditionally, TCM uses what is called the Four Examinations. These are looking, listening, asking, and touching.

"Looking" refers to a visual examination of the patient. A practitioner looks to see if there is a spark in a patient's eye and assesses the nature of his or her facial color. In TCM, the tongue is examined. Its shape, color, coating, and size all reflect certain harmony or disharmony within the body.

"Listening," which also includes smelling, applies to the tenor and force of a person's voice as well as a person's smell. For instance, if a person's voice turns weepy when speaking about a particular event, it might indicate an imbalance in the metal element, which relates to the lungs.

"Asking" refers to a practitioner's questioning of a patient to ascertain the health and wellness of the different systems within the body. A practitioner may ask about a patient's energy level, appetite, digestive health, feelings of fever or chills, quality of sleep, and the predominance of a certain emotion or any number of other health-related items. For women, the regularity, intensity, and quality of the menses are of particular importance. If a patient's primary complaint is pain related, the practitioner will ask questions about the pain; where does it hurt, how intense is the pain, and, about the nature of the pain, is it dull, sharp, stabbing or of a different quality.

"Touching" refers primarily to pulse taking. Pulse taking is integral to the art of Chinese medicine. It is said there are 28 different types of pulses. Rate, rhythm, depth, and strength are some of the parameters assessed. Chinese medicine also looks at the quality of the pulse. This is a subjective assessment that takes many years to learn. The subjective pulse can be classified as wiry (like a violin string), tense (wiry with a quiver), slippery (like one's hand is in a bowl of pearls), or choppy (like a knife being pulled along bamboo). Each of these qualities reflects the harmony, or lack thereof, within the body. A pulse could be rapid, strong, and slippery at the same time.

Once all the information from the Four Examinations is gathered, the practitioner synthesizes the information into a working diagnosis. In TCM, as taught in the teaching colleges of China, the primary diagnostic method is called the Eight Principles. The Eight Principles are yin/yang, internal/external, excess/deficiency, and hot/cold. The body is assessed according to these principles. Is the body yin type (pale face, weak voice) or yang in type (red in the face, loud voice), hot (fever) or cold (chills)? Is the problem one of an excess nature (high blood pressure) or deficient nature (lethargy), of internal origin (ulcer) or external origin (common cold)?

These parameters are then applied to the organ system. For instance, the lungs may be too yin (phlegmy) or too yang (dry). The problem may be one of an internal origin (shortness of breath) or external origin (cough with fever). The problem could be excess type (strong, phlegmy cough) or a deficient type (weak, feeble cough). The nature of the phlegm could be hot (green phlegm) or cold (pale phlegm). If the patient has a cough of recent onset with copious, green phlegm, she might be diagnosed with and external attack of wind/heat with phlegm attacking the lungs.

Once a diagnosis is established, a practitioner may choose between any of the modalities that comprise TCM. Using our prior diagnosis of an external invasion of wind/heat with phlegm affecting the lungs, a practitioner may choose to use acupuncture, Chinese herbal medicine, diet and exercise therapy, or any combination of modalities within the scope of TCM. For instance, a practitioner might choose acupuncture points such as Lung 7, Large Intestine 11, and Stomach 40 to clear the wind/heat and reduce phlegm. An herbal formula named Chrysanthemum and Mulberry might be chosen to address the cough. The patient might be advised to avoid dairy products, as they can exacerbate a phlegm condition. Once the patient has recovered from the illness, the practitioner might recommend a treatment protocol to address why the patient gets sick frequently. This would entail an in-depth assessment of the individual and diagnosis based on the Eight Principles. Treatment would then include one or more of the modalities common to TCM. Among the treatment modalities used in TCM, acupuncture and Chinese herbal medicine are the most commonly used.

**Treatment** Acupuncture is the insertion of fine needles into specific points on the body. The exact mechanism of how it works is not sufficiently explained by western science. However, according to the principles of Chinese medicine, acupuncture regulates the flow of chi within the body. The needle can be seen as a fulcrum, off which the body can more easily lever and regulate its chi flow. Pain is seen as a blockage of the chi flow. This can be likened to a stream being blocked by a beaver dam. The flow of the stream is slowed, and the outlying areas become swampy and mucky. So is the body's chi flow interrupted. Acupuncture helps reestablish the healthy flow of chi, restoring balance and harmony to the body and thus relieving pain.

Chinese herbal medicine can be administered alone or along with acupuncture. The Chinese herbal medicine pharmacopeia contains well over 1,000 substances, most of which are plants but a few of which are animal and mineral substances. Each herb is classified as to its energy (hot or cold), its taste (sweet, sour, bitter, salty, or acrid), the meridian it affects, and its functions. The herb ginseng, for example, is warming to the body, its flavor is sweet and slightly bitter, it enters the Lung and Spleen meridians and strongly strengthens chi. Generally, Chinese herbs are administered as part of a formula, which usually consists of six or more individual herbs. Certain herbs are formulated together because they work well for a specific problem or diagnosis. Traditionally, these herbs are boiled for about an hour and then ingested as a tea throughout the day. Nowadays, these formulas are also prepared in a variety of ways, including pills, powdered extracts, and alcohol- or glycerin-based tinctures.

While the root of the medicine is ancient, Chinese medicine is always evolving and adapting. Throughout its long history, this form of medicine has withstood the scrutiny of time, and new theories have been developed, written about, and tested. These principles became enfolded into the knowledge base of what is Chinese medicine. To this day, Chinese medicine adapts to modern conditions. For instance, acupuncture is frequently used in fertility clinics to improve the chances of conception with in vitro fertilization. Studies in the late-20th century showed an increased percentage of successful conception with the inclusion of a particular acupuncture protocol. Since that time, it has been adopted by fertility clinics throughout the west. Acupuncture is also used in cancer clinics, refugee camps, and Olympic training centers. According to the World Health Organization, acupuncture is effective in treating a myriad of conditions, including low back pain, sciatica, headaches, morning sickness, labor induction, allergic rhinitis, depression, and rheumatoid arthritis, to name a few.

In the United States, Chinese medicine practitioners are trained at colleges of Chinese medicine that are located throughout the country. These colleges are generally four year, 2,400 hour courses. Once graduated from a school, practitioners are certified by passing for a national board exam. The exam, administered by the National Commission for the Certification of Acupuncturists (NCCA) has been adopted by most states and serves as a standard for students, even in states with their own exam, such as California. Once passed, graduates are registered by the state in which they choose to practice. Licensing for qualified practitioners is now available in 36 states and in the District of Columbia.

**Training and Certification** The Accreditation Commission for Acupuncture and Oriental Medicine (ACAOM) is the national accrediting agency recognized by the U.S. Department of Education to accredit master's level programs in the acupuncture and Oriental medicine profession. As an independent body, ACAOM accredits master's degree and master's level acupuncture and Oriental medicine programs. There are currently over 60 schools and colleges with accredited or candidacy status with the ACAOM.

Information about accredited programs is also available from the Council of Colleges of Acupuncture and Oriental Medicine, which has brochures and catalogues of accredited schools in the U.S. and in other countries. Requirements vary among countries. For example, in Canada, the provinces of British Columbia, Alberta, and Quebec have licensing requirements. In Australia, the regulations vary by state, and there is no government regulation of acupuncture in the United Kingdom.

When choosing an acupuncturist, it is important to look for the initials LAc, DiplAc or D.O.M., which means the individual is fully qualified and has passed the national board exam. Licensed Acupuncturists, LAc, are required to have a minimum of 1,800 to 2,400 hours or more of educational and clinical training, depending on individual state requirements. In most states they must also be certified with the NCCAOM. The DiplAc signifies completion of a diploma program at schools certified by the ACAOM and usually includes three academic years of study. The D.O.M. is the doctor of Oriental medicine degree, and it indicates additional training beyond state licensure to practice acupuncture.

TCM faces growing regulatory challenges in the Untied States and Europe over the use of various imported mixtures and compounds. In 2009, these TCM exports were valued at 1.46 billion U.S. dollars according to the Ministry of Commerce of the People's Republic of China ("Exports," 2010). With so much at stake for both the United States and China, the U.S. Pharmacopeial Convention (USP) and other international standards-setting organizations are working with government regulatory agencies to develop standards for ingredients historically used in TCM. Regulation in the United States is important because these compounds could be classified as a drug when used for treating or preventing diseases rather than as a dietary supplement, as they are now, when used to maintain health. TMC products were classified as dietary supplements with few exceptions, following passage of the Dietary Supplement Health and Education Act of 1994. This classification meant they were not subject to Food and Drug Administration (FDA) testing before they were allowed to be sold.

All dietary supplements in the United States are required to have labels that contain the supplement facts; directions of use; and the name of the manufacturer, distributor, or importer. In an ongoing effort to standardize TMC herbal exports from China, many TMC medicinal prescriptions with fixed combinations of herbs are now being formulated into tablets, pills, and liquids known as Chinese patent medicines (CPM). The CPM have gained wide acceptance in Asia as well as in other parts of the world as TCM also grows in popularity. The first Chinese-made pill to treat cardiovascular conditions is expected to be marketed in the United States as early as 2013 and has passed several crucial FDA drug trials ("Chinese Patent Traditional Medicines," 2010). The pill is composed of herbal extracts and has already been approved in Canada, Russia, Vietnam, and some African countries.

*David Teitler*

*See also* Acupuncture; Dietary Supplements; Qigong; Tai Chi.

### References

"Acupuncture Is an Important Component of Traditional Chinese Medicine." *Women's Health Update* June 1, 2010.

"Ancient Chinese Medicine May Help Chemotherapy Patients: Study." *Xinhau News Agency,* August 18, 2010. General Reference Center Gold.

Beinfield, Harriet, and Efrem Korngold. *Between Heaven and Earth: A Guide to Chinese Medicine.* New York: Ballantine Books, 1992.

"Chinese Patent Traditional Medicine First Time Passes U.S. FDA Crucial Clinical Trials." *Xinhua News Agency,* August 7, 2010. General Reference Center Gold.

Deadman, Peter, Mazin Al-Khafaji, and Kevin Baker. *A Manual of Acupuncture.* Oxfordshire, England: Journal of Chinese Medicine Publications, 2007.

"Exports of Traditional Chinese Medicine Reach 1.46 Billion U.S. Dollars." *States News Service,* August 9, 2010. General Reference Center Gold.

Griffiths, James C. "Traditional Chinese Medicines and Western Regulatory Paradigms: Traditional Chinese Medicine Is Widely Used but Questions Persist Regarding Its Regulatory Status." *Pharmaceutical Technology* 33, no. 7 (July 2009): 64.

Hsu, H. Y., Y. P. Chen, S. J. Shen, C. S. Hsu, C. C. Chen, and H. C. Chang. *Oriental Material Medica, a Concise Guide.* Long Beach, CA: Oriental Healing Arts Institute, 1986.

Kaptchuk, Ted. J. *The Web that Has no Weaver: Understanding Chinese Medicine.* New York: Congdon & Weed, 1983.

Maciocia, Giovanni. *The Foundations of Chinese Medicine: A Comprehensive Text for Acupuncturists and Herbalists.* 2nd ed. New York: Churchill Livingstone, 2005.

Ni, Maoshing. *The Yellow Emperor's Classic of Medicine: A New Translation of the Neijing Suwen with Commentary.* Boston: Shambhala, 1995.

Unschuld, Paul U. *Huang Di Nei Jing Su Wen: Nature, Knowledge, Imagery in an Ancient Chinese Medical Text.* Berkeley: University of California Press, 2003.

Worsley, J. R. *Traditional Acupuncture: Traditional Diagnosis.* Taos, NM: Redwing Book Co., 1990.

## TRANS FATS

Trans fats are as common as packaged cookies, cakes, pies, or other sweets. Scientifically they are monounsaturated or polyunsaturated fatty acids made when vegetable oil is hydrogenated. During this process, hydrogen is added to unsaturated fatty acids and heated to a very high temperature. This results in partially hydrogenated oil when the oil hardens at room temperature. This creates a more stable food and gives it a longer shelf life, along with a nice, creamy feel when eaten, which is important for manufacturers of processed foods, who relied on it heavily, until recent years. Shortening and oleo are the most recognizable forms of partially hydrogenated oil. The problem is, trans fats are bad for us.

In 2006, the U.S. Food and Drug Administration (FDA) added trans fat to the nutrition label requirements established by the National Labeling and Education Act (NLEA) of 1990. Then, in July 2008, food legislation required that fat content of greater than five grams be listed in one-gram increments, less than five grams could be listed in half-gram increments, and lower than a half of a gram could be listed as containing no grams of fat. Critics of trans fats continue to call for the FDA to revise its labeling rules and require that food labels reflect any trans fat content, even amounts below a half of a gram.

While most fried foods and commercially baked goods until recently contained at least some trans fats, manufacturers have now experimented using other fats in an attempt to meet the new guidelines. Of course, a small amount of trans fat occurs naturally in some animal products, such as in lamb, beef, milk, butter, and cheese. While U.S. consumers eat more saturated fat than trans fat on average, and neither is considered healthy, it is the trans fat that has received the bulk of criticism from legislators and nutritionists who want to ban its use completely.

In fact, California became the first state in the nation to ban trans fats in all restaurant food as of 2010. This followed the lead of similar legislation passed in 2006 in New York City, which at that time banned artificial trans fats from restaurants, school cafeterias, pushcarts, and almost every other food-service operation in the city. Philadelphia did the same. Major businesses like Walmart and McDonald's were also paying attention to the legislation against trans fats and have slowly gotten away from trans fats. A study funded by the National Institutes of Health, and released by the University of Minnesota's School of Public Health, showed that major American fast food chains including McDonald's, Burger King, and Wendy's have significantly decreased the amount of trans fats in their French fries, and at the same time they have not raised the levels of saturated fats to compensate.

Walmart also launched a major initiative in 2011 to reformulate thousands of items by 2015 to remove all remaining industrially produced trans fats, as well as reducing sodium content by 25 percent and added sugar content by 10 percent. Walmart executives said they hoped to build on First Lady Michelle Obama's "Lets Move" campaign by making healthy food choices more convenient and affordable to U.S. families ("Walmart," 2011).

The company's announcement earned the praise of Center for Science in the Public Interest (CSPI), whose executive director, Michael F. Jacobson, called the news an opportunity to virtually eliminate artificial trans fat in packaged foods and help push food manufacturers to cut the sodium content as well. He added those two moves by Walmart could save thousands of lives each year from heart disease or stroke (Jacobson, 2011). It was the CSPI that asked the FDA in 1993 to require that companies list trans fats on the Nutrition Facts labels. The CSPI has continued to lobby against trans fats since that time.

Despite their poor image, fats aren't all bad. Some fats are needed for good health to help the body absorb fat-soluble vitamins. Fats contain saturated or

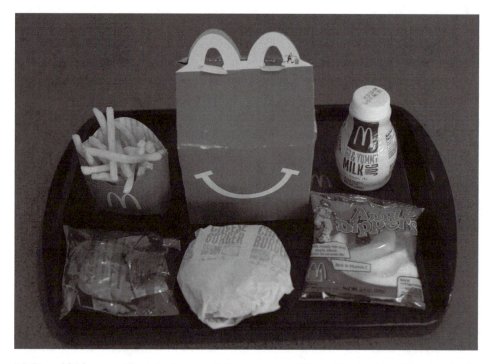

McDonald's has significantly decreased the amount of trans fats in their French fries in response to consumers' demands for trans fat–free foods. (AP/Wide World Photos)

unsaturated fatty acids, two of which are essential and must be included in the diet for a person to be healthy. Those two are linoleic and linolenic acid, and they are found in plant foods. The saturated fats are found in red meat; butter; whole milk; poultry; and coconut, palm, and tropical oils. These fats are high in cholesterol and are known to increase blood cholesterol levels.

There are also good fats; the monounsaturated fats, which include olive oil, canola oil, and peanut oils and which can also be found in avocados and nuts. Polyunsaturated fats, unlike monounsaturated fats, which begin to solidify if chilled, remain liquid no matter the temperature, include omega-3 fatty acids, which are considered especially healthy. The polyunsaturated fats can be found in walnuts, corn, sunflower, soy, and vegetable oils.

In the case of trans fats, scientists suggest that, gram for gram, trans fats are twice as damaging to health as saturated fat. Studies have shown that trans fat raises LDL cholesterol in a similar way to saturated fat and also raises blood triglyceride levels. When the increased LDL gets inside the arteries, it can cause inflammation and prevent the normal healing responses and can lead to insulin resistance, diabetes, and heart attack. It is thought that trans fats depress the protective high-density lipoproteins (HDL), otherwise known as the "good" cholesterol, which helps prevent heart attacks. Trans fats also effect triglycerides and make blood platelets stickier than usual, which raises the possibility they will form clots throughout the bloodstream. The World Health Organization has done its own analysis of the effects of trans fats and recommended ending the use of trans fat by food manufacturers and called for a reduced consumption to no more than 1 percent of dietary intake per day (Nishida & Uauy, 2009).

Due to label requirements in the United States, consumers should read labels to avoid trans fats. Other things that are important to avoid include partially hydrogenated oil, shortening, and oil blend. Some foods are being reformulated to meet the changing requirements; for example, tub margarines may be trans-fat free, but stick margarine is not. Also, look for trans fat in unlikely places, such as snack bars, condiments, icing, and other processed foods. When checking labels, the lower the partially hydrogenated oil or shortening appears in the list of ingredients, the less of it will be in the food. Just because labels say "0 grams trans fat," check the ingredients list for those telltale words. Remember, labels can round down to 0 if there is less than half a gram of trans fat—however, that is only per serving. Thus eating more than 1 serving means eating more grams of trans fat. The problem is not in having an occasional serving of a processed baked good, the problem lies in daily food choices that rely on processed, packaged foods rather than fresh fruits, vegetables, or whole grains.

*Sharon Zoumbaris*

*See also* Cholesterol; Fats; Food and Drug Administration (FDA); Heart Health.

## References

Jacobson, Michael F. "Walmart to Require Elimination of Artificial Trans, Reduction of Sodium & Added Sugars." January 20, 2011. *Center for Science in the Public Interest.* www.cspinet.org/new/201101201.html.

"Major Fast Food Chains Have Reduced Trans Fats; McDonald's, Burger King and Wendy's Sizzle Increasingly Fewer Fries in the Unhealthful Fats, Study Shows." *Consumer Health News.* July 16, 2010. www.businessweek.com/lifestyle/content/healthday/641171.html.

Nishida C., and R. Uauy. "WHO Scientific Update on Health Consequences of Trans Fatty Acids." *European Journal of Clinical Nutrition* 63 (2009): S1–S4. doi: 10.1038/ejcn.2009.13. www.nature.com/ejcn.

Severson, Kim. "Trans Fat Fight Claims Butter as a Victim." *The New York Times,* March 7, 2007, F1.

Springen, Karen. "Chew the (Trans) Fat." *Newsweek,* July 21, 2003, 62.

"Trans Fat." *Centers for Disease Control and Prevention* (CDC). April 14, 2010. www.cdc.gov/nutrition/everyone/basics/fat/transfat.html.

"Walmart Launches Major Initiative to Make Food Healthier and Healthier Food More Affordable." *Walmart Corporate.* January 20, 2011. http://walmartstores.com/pressroom/news/10514.aspx.

# U

## U.S. DEPARTMENT OF AGRICULTURE (USDA)

The U.S. Department of Agriculture (USDA), one of the largest federal agencies, oversees the federal government's role in administering farms, farm life, and agriculture in general. The USDA also protects the public through its system of food inspection, and it assists citizens through distribution of commodities.

The USDA is a diverse organization with components that perform a multitude of functions stemming from the production of food. For example, the USDA has a research component. It is part of the distribution system in that it administers the food stamp program and also distributes foods to schools. It has been mandated to develop programs that encourage sustainability as well as being tasked with preserving the natural resources of the country in the form of grasslands and protection of the national forests. Finally, the USDA is tasked with encouraging and supporting the agricultural economy, protecting markets, and participating in the world economic marketplace.

In 1839, Congress created the Agricultural Division as a division of the Patent Office. Its original mandate was to research and collect agricultural statistics for the Patent Office, and its original budget was $1,000. It took President Abraham Lincoln to create the Department of Agriculture as a free-standing agency in 1862. Lincoln's Department of Agriculture was not a cabinet-level agency, and as in many states today, it was headed by a commissioner.

This was politically significant, because the country was primarily agricultural at this time. On creating this new agency, Lincoln said that it was the "people's department." By 1889, President Grover Cleveland determined that the Department of Agriculture should become a cabinet-level agency.

Because the country was based on agricultural roots, the need to improve agricultural practices and continue to provide enough food for the country was in the collective mind of Congress in 1887. Congress enacted the Hatch Act, which established agricultural experiment stations. These state-based stations could be tailored to the needs of each state. In the early 20th century, there was a movement to eat well and educate the public about healthy eating. So in 1906, Congress enacted the Food and Drug Act, which included a mandate to the USDA to begin educating the citizenry regarding the preparation and proper handling of food.

The educational role of the USDA was furthered by the passage of the Smith-Lever Act of 1914. This act created the cooperative extension service, with an office in every state, which teaches about agriculture and home economics. This gives the USDA a platform in every state.

The USDA is responsible for regulations that monitor and control the slaughtering industry. These include the regulations regarding the handling and slaughtering of animals and keeping of the meat. As the country was becoming more urban and meat was not bought directly from farmers but was beginning to be shipped around the country, the meat-packing industry and butchery practices were creating conditions that allowed for the growth of lethal pathogens. With the USDA rules stemming from the Meat Inspection Acts of 1890 and 1891, there was a new emphasis on proper handling and enforcement.

The USDA provided crucial services to farmers and consumers to ensure that food production continued during the Great Depression of the 1930s. The USDA launched the National Victory Garden Program during World War II. This program encouraged families to grow fruits and vegetables in backyard garden plots so that commercial farmers could spend their resources on producing food for troops. Also during the war, the USDA established price controls and a system for food rationing.

Throughout its history, the USDA has endured allegations of discrimination leveled by African American farmers who have claimed that they were not allowed access to USDA programs, such as loan guarantees and educational programs. In 1999, a lawsuit that was brought against the USDA alleging discrimination against African American farmers was settled.

Approximately 2 percent of Americans work in agriculture. The USDA continues to aid farmers through its special programs that emphasize the life of the farmer and growing. It establishes rules and regulations regarding food safety and nutrition; meat, poultry and egg product safety; water safety programs in rural areas; and food-borne hazards research.

The agency also is charged with operating federal antihunger programs, housing, telecommunications, and drinking-water programs; loan programs create new jobs and other possible improvement of rural life, such as better living conditions, increased access to utilities and less isolation and the inclusion of rural areas into the mainstream of America. Because such a small proportion of the population works in agriculture, the USDA has an increased role in ensuring that there is no hunger, so it spends more than half of its resources on food distribution—food stamps, school breakfast and lunch programs, and distribution of commodities to the poor and elderly.

The USDA has established goals to remain a viable, important, and necessary agency in the pantheon of agencies in the cabinet. As the world of agriculture continues to change rapidly, the agency must remain flexible and meet the needs of the country. It has identified five areas that establish its mission.

The first part of its mission is to increase opportunities in the international marketplace. This means that the USDA must create new markets. This is a political and marketing process, because it requires the USDA to participate in international trade organizations, remain aware of restrictions and requirements of other countries, and provide financial and educational support for U.S. farmers so that they can take advantage of these opportunities. This includes loan programs and the continuation of crop insurance, which allows farmers to feel comfortable with the risk of growing and producing new foods. The basic commodities must also remain in production, however, so managing the current food supply is also part of its mission.

Second, the USDA wants to ensure the continuity of farm life. With the diminishing numbers of people in the agricultural industry, there is concern that the industry will become totally commercial and leave no family farms. In order to ensure biodiversity and maintain rural life, the USDA is involved in lending funds and has loan guarantee programs that can finance rural community improvements. The Rural Utilities Service Agency, a part of the USDA, assists in rural infrastructure projects.

By creating programs that ensure food safety with regard to meat, poultry, and eggs, the USDA is completing one of its missions. It is also charged with the reduction in the number of farm-related insects and other pests and with the prevention of animal disease and food-borne illness. All of these goals can be met by regular inspections, the enforcement of regulations, and the education of farmers and producers.

Another goal is the eradication of hunger and diseases caused by malnutrition. The flip side of this goal is to ensure that those with sufficient means do not overeat, which can lead to eating disorders and obesity-related illnesses.

Finally, the USDA wishes to ensure biodiversity in agriculture, maintain healthy forests and grasslands by good management techniques on public lands, and coordinate with private land holders. The USDA has control over the Health Forest Initiative as well as the Natural Resources Conservation Service. Managing soil is the key to healthy agriculture and is part of the purview of the USDA.

To accomplish these tasks, the USDA works with other federal government agencies, corporations and agencies in the private sector, researchers and scientists at private companies and universities, as well as foreign governments. The USDA has 17 agencies and 12 offices.

*William C. Smith and Elizabeth M. Williams*

*See also* Food and Drug Administration (FDA); National School Lunch Program (NSLP).

## References

"A Condensed History of American Agriculture 1776–1999." n.d. www.usda.gov/news/pubs/99arp/timeline.pdf.
"History of the U.S. Department of Agriculture." www.usda.gov.

Information for Laws and Regulations. n.d. www.usda.gov/wps/portal/!ut/p/_s.7_0_A/7_0_
    1OB?navtype=SU&navid=LAWS_REGS.
"USDA's Role in Nutrition Education and Evaluation." *Food Review* 18, no. 1 (January–April
    1996): 41.

## U.S. DEPARTMENT OF HEALTH AND HUMAN SERVICES (HHS)

A relatively new cabinet department founded in 1979, the Department of Health and Human Services (HHS) was created by splitting what was formerly the Department of Health, Education, and Welfare (created in 1953 during the term of President Dwight D. Eisenhower) into Health and Human Services and the Department of Education. The portfolio of HHS contains the public health of the United States and maintaining the welfare of the citizenry. Although the Social Security Administration was originally a part of HHS, that function was transformed into an independent agency in 1995. Today, HHS has the administration of the U.S. Public Health Service and the Family Support Administration.

The HHS is responsible for many health-related programs. It also is responsible, along with the Food and Drug Administration and the U.S. Department of Agriculture (USDA), for food safety. The Food Safety Working Group, which advises the president and the executive branch on matters of food safety, is made up the representatives from the USDA and the HHS. This group has recommended, for example, that the Office of Homeland Security (HS), which has jurisdiction over imports into the United States, put into place food security and safety measures that will ensure the importation of healthy and safe food. This resulted in the creation of the Commercial Targeting and Analysis Center for Import Safety by HS. Although it is administered by HS, the Center is run in cooperation with the USDA's Food Safety and Inspection Service, the Environmental Protection Agency, the Food and Drug Administration, and others agencies, whose experts are available when needed.

The HHS is responsible for all aspects of public health, which include diseases. But it also includes illness caused by food-borne pathogens, lifestyle diseases like obesity, mental and emotional conditions that are related to food such as anorexia nervosa and bulimia nervosa, as well as such public health problems as Type 2 diabetes, gout, and alcoholism.

A part of HHS is the U.S. Public Health Service Commissioned Corps. This is the uniformed branch of the Public Health Service headed by the Surgeon General. The Corps is made up of only commissioned officers who are generally considered noncombatants. They can be assigned to the armed forces, however, by the president. The Corps members wear a uniform that is like the Navy uniform with the special Public Health Service insignia. The Corps began its existence as first the Marine Hospital Fund and then the Marine Hospital Service in 1871. Corps members originally help with the health of merchant marines but came to enforce other public health-related matters such as quarantines.

Since 2000, the Surgeons General have addressed the public health issue of obesity. In 2001, the Surgeon General issued a Call to Action, calling attention to the public health problem that obesity represented and asking for the government to act toward preventing the condition. The call to action listed a number of recommendations for lifestyle changes and activities that could be adopted by schools. Having the Surgeon General identify a public health problem gives that problem a high priority in the eyes of the public as well as in the public health community.

In 2010, the Secretary of HHS, the Surgeon General, and First Lady Michelle Obama announced an initiative to combat obesity in both adults and children. There is a role for HHS and the Surgeon General in advising other agencies of government as to how those agencies can support the initiative, as well as producing guidelines and recommendations for schools, parents, and all citizens; collecting statistical information regarding obesity and its complications; and disseminating that information to citizens.

The Centers for Disease Control and Prevention (CDC) is another agency that operates under the aegis of HHS. Despite the public position of HHS and the Surgeon General, the CDC has stated that while obesity continues to be high and a public health problem, it appears to have leveled off in 2003 to 2004. The CDC has yet not determined the reason that the incidences of obesity did not continue to grow. The CDC has also conducted studies of the health costs attributed to obesity. They estimated that in 1998, when the study was conducted, that $78.5 billion of health costs could be attributed to obesity-related illnesses. About half of those costs were borne by the Medicare and Medicaid systems.

The CDC has published a number of studies that indicate that obesity is a larger problem for those in poverty or those at risk for poverty. This circumstance was recognized by Michelle Obama in her initiative against obesity. This is important not only as a public health issue but also as a social welfare issue. Social welfare issues are also administered by HHS.

The Centers for Medicare & Medicaid Services (CMS) are administered under HHS. The Social Security Administration, however, determines eligibility for Medicare and produces the checks for payment of Medicare-covered expenses. Similarly, the CMS administers the Medicaid program. Unlike Medicare, which operates as a federal system, each state administers its own Medicaid program. These programs are not identical and can reflect the cultural and political differences of each state. It is the responsibility of CMS to ensure that the states comply with federal Medicaid regulations and requirements. Both of these programs are enabled by the Social Security Act of 1965. The HHS, through its Office of the Inspector General (OIG), investigates Medicare fraud. It has a large enforcement branch that investigates criminal activity. Besides regular training as criminal investigators and officers, the OIG officers receive training in forensic accounting and other special training to uncover fraud and abuse in both the Medicare and Medicaid systems. The OIG operates in cooperation with state law enforcement in investigating Medicaid fraud and abuse. HHS, through the OIG, also is tasked under the Child Support Recovery Act with investigating the intentional avoidance of paying child support in all states and the District of Columbia.

*Elizabeth M. Williams*

*See also* Centers for Disease Control and Prevention (CDC); Environmental Protection Agency (EPA); Food and Drug Administration (FDA); Medicaid; Medicare; U.S. Department of Agriculture (USDA).

### References

Department of Health and Human Services. www.hhs.gov.

United States Food and Drug Administration. "FDA Strategic Priorities 2011–2015." April 20, 2011. www.fda.gov/AboutFDA/ReportsManualsForms/Reports/ucm227527.htm.

The White House Press Office. "President Obama Signs Healthy, Hunger-Free Kids Act of 2010 into Law." December 13, 2010. www.whitehouse.gov/the-press-office/2010/12/13/president-obama-signs-healthy-hunger-free-kids-act-2010-law.

# V

## VACCINATIONS

Vaccines may be among the greatest medical achievements of all time. A vaccine is a preparation, typically injected (although other routes of delivery exist), that stimulates the body's immune system to provide resistance or outright immunity to a given disease. In brief, the body's immune system is designed to "remember" diseases it has encountered before in order to mount a quick and effective response if the disease is encountered again. Vaccines typically contain an agent that looks like the disease of interest. When injected, they trigger the immune-system response. Then, the body remembers the disease and signals the individual's immune system to eliminate the pathogen if exposed to it again in the future.

Vaccines are available for a wide range of diseases that once devastated world populations. Although too numerous to list in their entirety, some of the more commonly given vaccines include polio, tetanus, diphtheria, measles, mumps, and tuberculosis.

Of course, not all disease can be prevented by vaccines. The immune memory produced by a vaccine or previous infection is not always sufficient to fend off illness due to the nature of the disease. For instance, the development of a vaccine for Human Immunodeficiency Virus (HIV) continues to elude researchers at least in part because HIV mutates too rapidly, making the immune memory ineffective.

Prior to the discovery of vaccination, preventing serious smallpox infection relied on the process of inoculation, a practice thought to have originated in India or China well before the 15th century (Radetsky, 1999). While vaccination involves exposing a patient to a weakened or altered form of the disease, inoculation actually exposes an individual to the disease itself. As an example, inoculation might take smallpox residue from an infected individual and rub it into a skin wound on a patient's arm. This would typically produce a milder form of the disease than if the patient were exposed to the disease via the respiratory route. Their exposure would immunize the patient against future smallpox exposure.

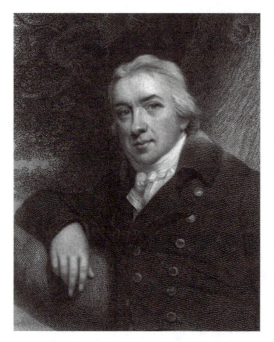

Edward Jenner (1749–1823) was an English physician who discovered the first vaccine for smallpox. (Jupiterimages)

Unfortunately, exposure to the live, active disease was still a significant hazard, which is why the discovery of vaccination by Edward Jenner in 1796 was so important.

Although anecdotal reports suggest Jenner may not have been the first individual to vaccinate, he is generally credited with discovering vaccination because his work led to its widespread understanding and application. Sometime in the early 1790s, Jenner noticed that milkmaids who had contracted cowpox did not develop smallpox. In 1796, Jenner tested his theory by deliberately exposing his gardener's son to cowpox (Radetsky, 1999). The boy developed a mild fever but no serious illness. Afterwards, Jenner exposed him to smallpox and observed that the boy did not contract smallpox. Jenner repeated this with several other subjects and observed the same pattern. He presented his findings to the Royal Society. From there, the practice of vaccination spread, and eventually vaccination was chosen over inoculation with the actual smallpox virus.

While Jenner is credited with first discovering vaccination, it was Louie Pasteur, in the 1870s, who expanded the notion of vaccination to other diseases. Even though Jenner's smallpox vaccine worked because cowpox was a naturally occurring, weaker "version" of smallpox, the concept was not possible to expand to other diseases. Pasteur then demonstrated via chicken cholera and anthrax that the actual pathogen could be artificially weakened and given as a vaccine. This opened the field of vaccines to a plethora of diseases (Stern, 2005).

Since that time, vaccines have been developed for over a dozen diseases as well as other compounds, such as toxins. Vaccines have successfully reduced many diseases to levels far below the prevaccination era, making many diseases, such as measles, now extremely rare in the United States and in other countries with high vaccination rates.

The greatest vaccine success story to date is the eradication of smallpox, the first disease a vaccine was developed to prevent. Due to an aggressive international campaign to vaccinate individuals against smallpox during the early and middle 20th century, smallpox was officially declared eliminated in 1980, thus ending the threat of one of the most deadly diseases in human history. There is now a global effort underway to eradicate polio using many of the same strategies.

The move to eradicate polio has been fairly successful so far, with the World Health Organization (WHO) declaring in 2006 that polio remains endemic in only four countries: India, Pakistan, Afghanistan, and Nigeria. Researchers continue to focus on developing new vaccines and improving vaccination rates with known vaccines.

Vaccines work by stimulating the immune system to remember the disease, and, in turn, the immune system includes memory T and memory B cells that can live for decades. That ability of T and B memory cells allows an individual to retain immunological memory throughout most of his or her life. However, the life span of immunological memory can vary with the individual, with the specific disease, and with the type of vaccine.

Vaccines can be loosely divided into categories based on what is used to stimulate the immune system (NIAID, 2011). Closest to the original vaccines are live-attenuated vaccines. These contain a weakened form of the actual pathogen; for example, a virus may have a key gene in its replication cycle inactivated. While these vaccines are often the most effective in producing immune memory, they are also the riskiest, because the pathogen is still, to some extent, functional. Next are killed/inactivated vaccines, which contain the whole pathogen but are completely inactive. Finally, there are vaccines that contain only a particular subunit of the pathogen, such as a key protein or other marker.

Along with these three main types of vaccines, there are others, such as toxoid vaccines like tetanus, which do not target the actual bacteria. Instead, they target the toxin that it produces. Finally, there are other, less common, sometimes experimental forms of delivering vaccines that are used in specific diseases, or those being tested and evaluated for future use.

In general, almost everyone should get certain vaccines such as for measles, mumps, and rubella (MMR) and hepatitis B. In the United States, the Advisory Committee on Immunization Practices (ACIP) has established a recommended vaccine schedule for individuals in the United States based on vaccine and age (CDC, 2011). The precise vaccines recommended may vary from country to country, depending on diseases that are endemic there and the judgment of the local health authorities. For example, the tuberculosis vaccine, BCG, is routinely given in many countries but not the United States. Instead, American vaccines routinely include measles, mumps, and rubella (MMR), diphtheria and tetanus toxoids and acellular pertussis (DTaP), Haemophilus influenzae type b (Hib), rotavirus (Rota), and others. Since these vaccines are a public-school requirement, vaccine coverage rates are extremely high in the United States. Some vaccines are good for life, whereas others require occasional "booster" shots to retain their memory. Influenza evolves every season, which means a new vaccine is developed each year, and individuals are advised to reimmunize themselves annually.

There are other vaccines given on a situational basis. For instance, individuals in the United States do not typically receive the yellow fever vaccine. However, if individuals expect to travel to a country where yellow fever is endemic, they are advised by the State Department to get vaccinated. Aside from travel, individuals in specialized occupations may receive applicable vaccines. For example, an animal-control expert would typically receive a rabies vaccine, even though rabies is not recommended for the general public unless an infection is suspected.

While vaccination is extremely important, there are circumstances that arise when a person should not receive a certain vaccine. This usually occurs if the individual has a documented history of an adverse reaction to a particular ingredient in that vaccine or other medical issues to be considered. For a great majority of people, vaccination is important and advisable unless specifically instructed otherwise by a physician.

Vaccines are considered very safe; still, reactions do occur. The majority of these are mild and include fever, pain, and swelling at the injection site. These reactions do not require hospitalization. However, in rare cases, allergic reactions and other serious reactions have been documented, including anaphylactic shock. It is important to emphasize that deadly reactions are exceedingly rare and scientists and physicians strongly support the benefits of vaccination as a choice that far outweighs the risks.

Vaccines can also be controversial, as was illustrated by the 1999 paper published in the *Lancet* (Wakefield, 1999) that claimed a link between the MMR vaccine and autism. Although the study has been discredited and the original paper withdrawn, numerous follow-up studies found no increased risk of autism from the MMR vaccine (Doja, 2006). Yet, many Americans continue to believe that the MMR vaccine increases the risk for autism and, consequently, they refuse to vaccinate their children. This has become a public health concern, as vaccination rates dropped significantly following the 1998 report, which lead to a rise in cases of measles, mumps, and rubella.

Vaccines hold a special place in medical treatment as one of the most important medical developments ever. Vaccine research is ongoing as scientists look for cheaper, safer alternatives to existing vaccines and strive to develop new vaccines. One disease receiving a lot of attention is HIV, which has so far eluded vaccine development, even as numerous trials attempt to find one.

Vaccines also show potential in combating diseases not commonly thought of as vaccine-preventable, such as dental carries or cavities. Another exciting development in the field of vaccine research is the potential for vaccines to be used in noninfectious disease, such as cancer. These so-called cancer vaccines exist and have been developed to target viruses that lead to cancer rather than targeting the individual cancerous cells. Researchers are working to find a vaccine that triggers the body's immune system to recognize cancerous cells and may one day be able to vaccinate individuals against particular types of cancer. Although such research is still in preliminary stages, scientists suggest that their early research is promising.

Vaccines have already eliminated one of human history's worst diseases, small pox, and are on the verge of eliminating polio. Vaccines are one of public health's greatest tools against infectious disease and will continue to play a critical role in the future of human health and medical care.

*David Chen*

*See also* Dental Health; Immunization; Pandemics; Pasteur, Louis.

# Recommended Immunizations

2010 Recommended Immunizations for Children from Birth Through 18 years old approved by the Centers for Disease Control and Prevention (CDC), the American Academy of Pediatrics, and the American Academy of Family Physicians.

## Key

| | |
|---|---|
| DTaP | Diphtheria, Tetanus, Pertussis |
| HepA | Hepatitis A (2 doses) |
| HepB | Hepatitis B |
| Hib | Haemophilus influenzae, type b |
| HPV | Human Papillomavirus |
| IPV | Inactivated Poliovirus |
| MCV4 | Meningococcus |
| MMR | Measles, Mumps, Rubella |
| PCV | Pneumococcus |
| RV | Rotavirus |
| Varicella | Chicken pox |

## Age

| | |
|---|---|
| Birth to 2 months | HepB (1st dose) |
| 2 to 4 months | IPV |
| 2 to 6 months | Rotavirus, DTaP, Hib, PCV |
| 6 months | Influenza vaccine (begin yearly vaccination) |
| 6 to 18 months | HepB (2nd and 3rd doses), IPV |
| 12 to 15 months | MMR, PCV, Varicella (1st dose) |
| 12 to 23 months | HepA (2 doses) |
| 15 to 18 months | DTaP |
| 4 to 6 years | DTaP, IPV, MMR, Varicella (2nd dose) |
| 11 to 12 years | DTaP, HPV (3 doses), MCV4 |
| 13 to 18 years | MCV4 (if not given at 11 to 12 years) |

If children miss a shot, there is no need to start over, just return to your primary care physician for the next shot.

*—Sharon Zoumbaris*

---

*The Human papillomavirus (HPV) vaccination was approved by the Food and Drug Administration (FDA) in 2006 to prevent cervical cancer and other conditions caused by the human papillomavirus. It is recommended, but not required, for girls age 11 or 12, with catch-up vaccination at ages 13 through 26 years. However, the vaccine should ideally be administered before potential exposure to HPV through sexual activity. Females who are sexually active can still be vaccinated, and HPV4 may be administered to males ages 9 through 26 years, to reduce their likelihood of acquiring genital warts.

## References

CDC (Centers for Disease Control and Prevention). "Advisory Committee on Immunization Practices (ACIP)." October 26, 2011. www.cdc.gov/vaccines/recs/acip/default.htm.

Doja, Asif, and Wendy Roberts. "Immunizations and Autism: A Review of the Literature." *Canadian Journal of Neurological Sciences* 33, no. 4 (2006): 341–46.

NIAID (National Institute of Allergy and Infectious Disease). "Types of Vaccines." April 19, 2011. www.niaid.nih.gov/topics/vaccines/understanding/pages/typesvaccines.aspx.

Radetsky, Michael. "Smallpox: A History of Its Rise and Fall." *Pediatric Infectious Disease* 18, no. 2 (1999): 85–93.

Stern, Alexandra, and Howard Markel. "The History of Vaccines and Immunization: Familiar Patterns, New Challenges." *Health Affairs* 24, no. 3 (2005): 611–21.

Wakefield, Andrew J. "MMR Vaccination and Autism." *The Lancet* 354, no. 9182 (1999): 949–50.

WHO (World Health Organization). "Polio Endemic Countries Hit All-Time Low of Four." February 1, 2006. www.who.int/mediacentre/news/releases/2006/pr05/en/index.html.

## VEGANS. *See* VEGETARIANS

## VEGETABLES

Many Americans have a love affair with their food, as long as it's fast, fried, and loaded with fat. Vegetables, on the other hand, are crisp, colorful, and low in calories, at least they are low as long as they are not fried or covered with cheese. Vegetables are also loaded with phytochemicals, nutrients, fiber, minerals, and vitamins.

Studies have shown that a diet rich in vegetables and fruit can help reduce the risk of high blood pressure or hypertension, heart disease, stroke, and may reduce the risk of some kinds of cancer. Yet, even though Americans know all this about vegetables, statistics show that the majority of them do not eat the recommended five servings per day. In fact, according to 2009 statistics from the Centers for Disease Control and Prevention (CDC), just over 20 percent of Americans achieved the recommended five or more servings of fruit and vegetables, and almost 5 percent ate just one serving or none each day (CDC, 2011).

That figure is surprising since American grocery stores routinely carry as many as 70 different types of fresh vegetables and fruits. To most people, the definition of a vegetable is an edible plant. In actuality, each different vegetable comes from a specific part of each plant, parts that include the flowers, seeds, leaves, stems, roots, and bulbs. Examples of flowers commonly eaten include broccoli, cauliflower, and artichokes. Vegetables that are the seeds of the plants include corn, peas, and many beans. Americans eat many leaves, including spinach, lettuces, mustard greens, and collard greens. Stem vegetables include celery and rhubarb as well as asparagus and bamboo shoots. Root vegetables include potatoes, carrots, beets, radishes, and turnips, and familiar bulbs are onions, garlic, and shallots.

There are several plants that have been long considered to be vegetables but that are actually fruit. Those include tomatoes, eggplant, and bell peppers. Vegetables can be eaten raw or cooked, although some are only edible when cooked, such as rhubarb. Most Americans consider vegetables as side dishes or use them in casseroles or stews. Vegetarians, vegans, and those who follow a macrobiotic diet may consumer more vegetables than the average American.

Many root vegetables are harvested in the fall and can be stored in a cool, dark place to last through the winter. However, during storage, vegetables can lose moisture and their vitamin content can degrade. Nutritionists recommend storing vegetables in the refrigerator for as little time as possible before eating.

Nutritionists suggest that the best way to get a variety of fruits and vegetables is to use the colors as a guide. Those with the deepest, richest colors contain the most powerful phytochemicals, and a healthy diet should look like a rainbow with greens, yellows, oranges, reds, purples, and blues. In fact, literature, such as the *Wisconsin National Nutrition Month,* emphasizes vegetable colors. The theme for their March 2011 nutrition celebration was "Eat Right with Color" and focused on fruits and vegetables and their diverse colors and how those colors correspond to nutrients such as fiber, folate, potassium, and vitamins A and C.

A variety of factors contribute to Americans' poor consumption of vegetables, from the low cost and availability of fast food to the growing number of urban

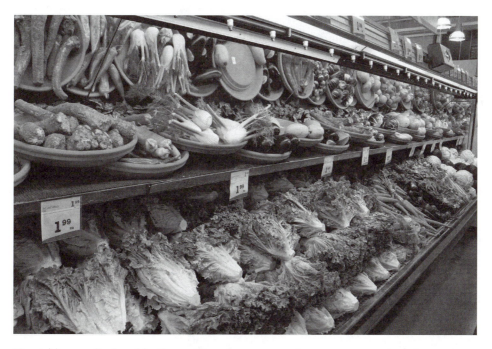

Vegetables are displayed in the produce department of a grocery store. American grocery stores typically carry around 70 different types of fruits and vegetables. (iStockPhoto)

"food deserts." Cities like South Los Angeles are considered food deserts, a term adopted by social policy planners in the 1990s to describe low-income areas with little or no access to affordable, healthy food, including fresh vegetables and fruit. In a study funded by the National Institutes of Health (NIH), results showed that neighborhood food environments do influence fruit and vegetable intake, and the presence of a convenience store in a neighborhood was linked to almost two fewer daily servings of vegetables or fruits among some ethnic groups (Zenk et al., 2009).

With national obesity rates continuing to climb, especially among children and teens, government nutrition programs are working to get more fresh vegetables and fruits into youngster's diets. One way to encourage kids to eat more fruits and vegetables may be as simple as better presentation. A Cornell University group conducted a study that put fruit in brightly colored bowls and found that it was eaten twice as fast as fruit in dull racks or trays. The researchers also discovered that kids bought triple the amount of salad if the salad bar was closer to the cash register (Just & Wansink, 2009).

Nutrition educators suggest that another way to interest children in fruits and vegetables is to involve them in preparation of the food. Have the children select the items at the grocery store or go to a farmer's market. When children help prepare the food and serve it, nutritionists say youngsters have an easier time accepting new foods, even spinach.

*Sharon Zoumbaris*

*See also* Fiber; National Institutes of Health; Vegetarians.

### References

CDC (Centers for Disease Control and Prevention). "What Is Your Average Frequency of Fruit and Vegetable Consumption per Day?" http://apps.nccd.cdc.gov/5ADay Surveillance.
"Fruits and Vegetables." *Harvard Special Health Report* 14, no. 17 (Annual 2008): 14 (3). www.health.harvard.edu.
Just, David R., and Brian Wansink. "Smarter Lunchrooms: Using Behavioral Economics to Improve Meal Selection." *Choices: The Magazine of Food, Farm and Resource Issues* 24, no. 3 (3rd Quarter 2009): 24 (3).
Schmitt, Barton D. *Your Child's Health*. New York: Bantam, 2005.
Zenk, S. N., L. L. Lachance, A. J. Schulz, G. Mentz, S. Kannan, and W. Ridella. "Neighborhood Retail Food Environment and Fruit and Vegetable Intake in a Multiethnic Urban Population." *American Journal of Health Promotion* 23, no. 4 (March–April, 2009): 255–64.

## VEGETARIANS

"Vegetarian" is a blanket term for a person whose diet omits animal products. However, there are many definitions and categories, from the very stringent to the most lenient. It's important to remember that vegetarianism is a personal choice and is best defined by each individual and his or her specific dietary needs. In the most basic sense, a vegetarian is a person who does not eat meat, poultry, fish, or any kind of animal product. Vegetarians eat fruits, vegetables, legumes, grains, soy, seeds, and nuts. The number of vegetarians in the United States varies widely, depending on which organization is doing the survey.

Subclassifications include vegans, lacto-vegetarians, ovo-vegetarians, pollo-vegetarians, pesca-vegetarians, and lacto-ovo-vegetarians. The lacto-vegetarian has a diet that includes dairy foods but not eggs. The reverse is the ovo-vegetarian, who eats eggs but no dairy. Both lacto- and ovo-vegetarians do not eat meat, poultry, or fish products. The lacto-ovo-vegetarian consumes milk, cheese, yogurt, and eggs but not meat, fish, or poultry. This designation is the easiest eating style in terms of menu planning, and usually offers the largest variety of choices for those dining in sit-down or fast food restaurants. Most vegetarians in the United States are lacto-ovo-vegetarians, according to the American Dietetic Association (ADA).

A pollo-vegetarian eats a diet similar to that of a lacto-ovo-vegetarian, but also includes poultry among food selections. The pesca-vegetarian mimics the lacto-ovo eating habits but includes fish and seafood. The strictest category is the vegan, who avoids all animal products, including hidden items such as gelatin, beef and chicken stocks, lard, and, for many vegans, honey. A vegan diet includes vegetables, fruits, grains, legumes, nuts, and seeds. Many vegans also avoid products such as wool, leather, silk, and cosmetics and soaps made from animals.

Well-known vegetarians in history include Leonardo da Vinci, Albert Einstein, Benjamin Franklin, Charles Darwin, Thomas Edison, George Bernard Shaw, Leo Tolstoy, Henry David Thoreau, Mahatma Gandhi, and Clara Barton; who all abstained from eating meat. Famous contemporary vegetarians include Chelsea Clinton, Jonathan Safran Foer, Herschel Walker, Forest Whitaker, Brad Pitt, Madonna, and Paul McCartney. Former President Bill Clinton discussed in a 2011 interview that, to further improve his heart health after undergoing a quadruple bypass and angioplasty, he has been on a vegan diet (Martin, 2011).

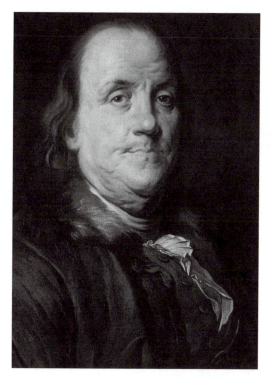

Benjamin Franklin, who achieved worldwide renown as a writer, scientist, statesman, and diplomat, was also a vegetarian. (National Archives)

**The Diet and Health Connection**   Many nutritionists and doctors acknowledge the health benefits of a plant-based diet when compared to a meat-based diet high in cholesterol and saturated fat. Research shows that, on the whole, vegetarians eat a more healthy diet than nonvegetarians and consume about two to three times as much fiber as their meat-eating counterparts. And a diet high in fiber can actually lower the chances of developing certain cancers, particularly colon cancer, according to the National Cancer Institute.

Studies by mainstream organizations from the World Health Organization (WHO) to the American Dietetic Association (ADA) and the American Cancer Society (ACS) confirm that a vegetarian diet can improve health. A report by the American Institute on Cancer Research (AICR) and the World Cancer Research Fund (WCRF), released in November 2007, showed a link between colon cancer and processed meats such as hot dogs and salami—a link they suggested was as strong as the connection between lung cancer and cigarettes. The AICR report was based on five years of analysis by teams of independent researchers, international experts, and peer reviewers who examined more than 7,000 health studies.

The AICR recommendations for cancer prevention were clear: "Eat more of a variety of vegetables, fruits, whole grains and legumes such as beans," and "Limit consumption of red meats (such as beef, pork, and lamb) and avoid processed meats" (AICR, 2007). In fact, medical costs linked to eating meat are estimated to be $30 billion to $60 billion per year, based upon the higher prevalence of cancer as well as obesity, hypertension, heart disease, diabetes, gallstones, and foodborne illnesses among meat eaters when compared with vegetarians (Horsman & Flowers, 2007, p. 37). The American Cancer Society (ACS) released its own recommendation, suggesting that a diet high in vegetables and fruits and low in animal fat and meat provides a reduced risk of some of the most common cancers. The society's guidelines for cancer prevention include a similar recommendation to eat a diet "with an emphasis on plant sources" (ACS, 2007).

**What Do Vegetarians Eat?**   A vegetarian diet does not have to be bland, brown, and boring. The plant kingdom is a multicolored world of crunchy, chewy, creamy, and meaty textures. From portobello mushrooms to polenta, from summer corn to seitan, there are wonderful tastes to try. Gourmet cuisine is also part of the vegetarian experience, with foods like roasted pepper and tomato soup; fassolada, a Greek bean soup; and mango raita, a fruity yogurt sauce. Nutritionists say the biggest mistake new converts make is to fill up on fattening foods such as cheese, French fries, pizza, avocados, and nuts. They say the best diet is rich in fiber and complex carbohydrates and low in fat—consider apples, oranges, bananas, bagels, popcorn, pretzels, bean tacos or burritos, salads, frozen juice bars, smoothies, or rice cakes. Other good meal choices include noncream soups and salads.

Good nutrition for vegetarians and vegans is not difficult to achieve. Basically, nutrients are divided into five groups: proteins, carbohydrates, fats, vitamins, and minerals. A meatless diet does not automatically lead to protein deficiency.

Remember, it wasn't until the 20th century that meat was a common protein source.

*Proteins*   People require some 20 amino acids for optimum health; 11 of those are manufactured by our bodies, but the other 9 must come from the foods we eat. All the required amino acids can come from plant foods or can be manufactured by the human body. People need protein to maintain healthy skin, bones, muscles, and organs. Many plant foods, such as soy, are protein rich and also provide protective phytochemicals. Beans, peas, and lentils are richer in magnesium and lower in sulfur amino acids than meat, which means they cause the body to excrete less calcium. Legumes provide iron, zinc, a number of B vitamins, and lots of fiber.

Where can the average American go to find out what constitutes appropriate nutrient levels of vitamins, minerals, carbohydrates, proteins, and fats? The Recommended Dietary Allowance (RDA) was established by the U.S. Department of Agriculture (USDA) to provide nutrition guidelines for Americans. Recently, the RDA was replaced by the Dietary Reference Intake (DRI), which includes four different reference values and offers more flexible numbers based on activity level, age, and other factors. According to the USDA, the DRI for protein is 0.8 grams of protein per kilogram of body weight (g/kg)—about 45 grams for an average woman and 55 grams for an average man. This includes a margin to account for individual variations and applies to vegetarians and meat eaters alike. Recommended intake levels during pregnancy, lactation, and infancy through adolescence differ slightly.

Although some protein is necessary, high intakes of protein can be harmful—particularly animal protein, which studies show can contribute to heart disease, stroke, and colorectal cancer. Animal proteins are associated with cholesterol and saturated fat, whereas plant foods are cholesterol-free and most are low in saturated fat. The protein in common vegetarian foods ranges from 18 grams of protein in one cup of cooked lentils or black, navy, kidney, or pinto beans to 28 grams of protein in one cup of cooked soybeans. In comparison, a fast-food hamburger patty made of a quarter pound of beef has 19 grams of protein, and a chicken leg has 15 grams.

*Carbohydrates*   There are three types of carbohydrates: monosaccharides, or simple sugars; disaccharides, composed of two monosaccharides; and polysaccharides, also known as complex carbohydrates, or starches. Carbohydrates are an important source of energy for the brain, central nervous system, and muscle cells. They are found in sugars, fruits, vegetables, cereals, and grains. Carbohydrates are also broken down into two other categories on nutrition labels: fiber and sugar. The simple sugars provide energy but lack fiber, vitamins, or minerals. The complex carbohydrates, or starches, contain lots of fiber, vitamins, and minerals and are naturally low in fat. Many types of grains are good sources of complex carbohydrates, and whole grains such as brown rice and whole wheat provide particularly rich nutrients and fiber.

All carbohydrates are eventually broken down into sugars in the body. The difference between complex carbohydrates and simple sugars is that complex carbohydrates are broken down gradually and provide energy over a longer period of time. The fiber in these foods is important. Fiber provides health benefits by preventing constipation as well as lowering the risk of diabetes and heart disease. But all carbohydrates are not created equal. Nutritionists caution that the monosaccharides, or simple sugars, present a nutritional problem on two fronts. First, filling up on high-sugar foods such as soft drinks, cookies, sweets, and fruit drinks can contribute to weight gain. Second, simple-sugar foods contain very few vitamins or minerals and can lead to poor health if they are continuously eaten instead of more nutritious foods. Someone with a diet of 2,000 calories per day should eat about 300 grams of carbohydrates. A slice of whole wheat bread has 20 grams of carbohydrates, a medium baked potato has some 51 grams, an apple has 21 grams, and a tablespoon of sugar about 12 grams.

*Fats*   Despite their poor image, fats aren't all bad. Some fat is needed to supply energy and help the body absorb the fat-soluble vitamins, A, D, E, and K. Fats contain saturated or unsaturated fatty acids, two of which—linoleic and linolenic acid—are essential and must be provided in the diet. Luckily, both those fatty acids are widely found in plant foods. When choosing fats, the best options for vegetarians and meat eaters alike are the monounsaturated and polyunsaturated fats, which can lower the risk of heart disease by reducing cholesterol levels.

Monounsaturated fats include olive, canola, and peanut oils and can be found in avocados and most nuts. Polyunsaturated fats come from safflower, corn, sunflower, soy, cottonseed, and vegetable oils. Unlike monounsaturated fats, which begin to solidify when chilled, polyunsaturated fats remain liquid whether at room temperature or in the refrigerator. The polyunsaturated fats called omega-3 fatty acids are especially beneficial and can be found in flaxseeds, flax oil, walnuts, and, in small amounts, in soybean and canola oils.

Saturated fats come from red meat, poultry, butter, and whole milk as well as coconut, palm, and other tropical oils. These fats are also high in cholesterol, and although dietary cholesterol isn't technically a fat, it is known to increase blood cholesterol levels, as does saturated fat. The human body produces cholesterol during the process of cell building, and cholesterol can leave behind fatty deposits or plaques in arteries. When the plaques build up, they reduce blood flow and increase the risk of a heart attack or stroke.

The U.S. Surgeon General, the National Academy of Sciences, the American Heart Association, the American Dietetic Association, the USDA, and the U.S. Department of Health and Human Services (HHS) all recommend keeping dietary fat intake at 30 percent or less of total calories. Fat is measured in grams, so for someone eating a diet of 2,000 calories per day, daily fat intake should be 65 grams or less, preferably coming from monounsaturated or polyunsaturated sources. The 2005 *Dietary Guidelines for Americans* also strongly recommends consuming less than 10 percent of daily calories from saturated fats and keeping trans-fat consumption as low as possible.

*Vitamins*   Vitamins are a key area where many Americans fall nutritionally short, and vegetarians—who eat a rainbow of fruits and vegetables rich in vitamins, minerals, and fiber—have a nutritional advantage. Vitamin A, or beta carotene, can be found in yellow, red, or orange vegetables such as carrots and to-matoes, fruits such as apricots and peaches, and leafy green vegetables. B vitamins are important for the health of the nervous system and play a role in the metab-olism of carbohydrates, fats, and proteins. B vitamins are water-soluble and are not stored in the body, so they need to be supplied daily by a healthy diet. Good sources of B vitamins, except for B12, include whole-grain cereals, wheat germ, nuts, seeds, yeasts, and green vegetables.

Vitamin B12 deficiencies are rare. The vitamin is found in meat, dairy, and eggs, so vegetarians and vegans need to monitor their intake to make sure they get enough. Many veggie burgers, soy products, and breakfast cereals are fortified with B12. Even though little is needed, B12 plays important roles in the produc-tion of DNA and RNA, in making red blood cells, and in keeping the nervous system operating.

Fruits, especially citrus fruits such as oranges and lemons, are great sources of vitamin C, also known as ascorbic acid. Vegetables including broccoli, pota-toes, and tomatoes contain vitamin C, as do strawberries, kiwifruit, and canta-loupe. Vitamin C helps to fight disease and infection, aids the repair of tissue, and acts as an antioxidant. The recommended amount of vitamin C for healthy people is 60 milligrams per day. Taking extra vitamin C as treatment for a cold is a common practice; however, research on the benefits of these megadoses remains inconclusive.

Healthy bones depend on calcium, but calcium needs vitamin D to be ab-sorbed into the body. Vitamin D is also important for building and maintaining muscles. Known as the sunshine vitamin, vitamin D is made in the body when sunlight hits the skin. So 15 minutes or less of sunshine three times a week can provide enough of the vitamin for a healthy adult. Vitamin D is also found in for-tified soy beverages, orange juice, and cereals.

The term "vitamin E" describes a family of eight antioxidants—alpha, beta, gamma, and delta tocopherol and alpha, beta, gamma, and delta tocotrienol. Alpha-tocopherol ($\alpha$-tocopherol) is the most active form in the human body, and is the form of vitamin E found in the largest quantities in the blood and tissue. Because vitamin E is fat-soluble, it is generally found in rich foods such as avo-cado, nuts, olives, and vegetable oils, and also in spinach and other green leafy vegetables. The results of studies on the use of vitamin E in the treatment and prevention of several diseases, particularly in cancer and heart disease, are still inconclusive.

Vitamin K is known as the clotting vitamin; without it blood would not clot. This fat-soluble vitamin is stored in fatty tissue and is found in spinach and other green leafy vegetables, cabbage, cauliflower, soybeans, and cereals. It is also made by the bacteria that line the gastrointestinal tract. Vitamin K deficiency is very rare.

Misuse of vegetarian eating has also been associated with eating disorders like anorexia and bulimia. Those who choose to be vegetarian should be doing it cor-rectly and with the right motivation rather than trying to camouflage an eating disorder. Teenagers are particularly susceptible to this. A report in the *Archives of*

*Pediatric Adolescent Medicine* in August 1997 looked at how some teens hid eating disorders behind the healthy façade of vegetarianism. The study reported that although vegetarian teens ate more fruits and vegetables than their meat-eating peers did, they were also twice as likely to diet frequently. The meatless teens were also four times as likely to diet intensively and eight times as likely to abuse laxatives. According to the study, this was the first population-based look at eating disorders and their connections to vegetarianism.

The authors of the report suggested that due to the increased social acceptance of vegetarian diets, teens who adopt a meatless diet should be evaluated carefully by their parents and health care professionals. Excessive dieting, binge eating, intentional vomiting, and laxative abuse are more obvious red-flag behaviors associated with anorexia and bulimia, and teens, as well as adults, may try to hide them by changing to a vegetarian diet. This is not to say that every teen who decides to go vegetarian is going to develop an eating disorder, but when it is pursued to extremes, there is potential for serious problems.

*Marjolijn Bijlefeld and Sharon Zoumbaris*

*See also* Amino Acids; Carbohydrates; Eating Disorders; Fats; Proteins; Vitamins.

## References

ACS (American Cancer Society). "Cancer Prevention and Early Detection: Facts and Figures, 2007." 2007. www.cancer.org/docroot/STT/content/STT_1x_Cancer_Prevention_and_Early_Detection_Facts__Figures_2007.asp.

AICR (American Institute for Cancer Research.) "Recommendations for Cancer Prevention." 2007. http://preventcancer.aicr.org/site/PageServer?pagename=recommendations_home.

Bode, Janet. *Food Fight: A Guide to Eating Disorders for Pre-Teens and Their Parents.* New York: Simon and Schuster, 1997.

Horsman, Jennifer, and Jamie Flowers. *Please Don't Eat the Animals: All the Reasons You Need to Be a Vegetarian.* Sanger, CA: Wood Dancer Press, 2007.

Katzen, Mollie. *Vegetable Heaven.* New York: Hyperion, 1997.

Krizmanic, Judy. *A Teen's Guide to Going Vegetarian.* New York: Viking and Puffin Books, 1994.

Lappé, Frances Moore. *Diet for a Small Planet.* 20th anniversary ed. New York: Ballantine Books, 1991.

Lavelle, Marianne, and Kent Graber. "Fixing the Food Crisis," *U.S. News and World Report,* May 19, 2008: 36–42.

Martin, David S. "From Omnivore to Vegan: The Dietary Education of Bill Clinton." *CNN.com.* August 18, 2011. www.cnn.com/2011/HEALTH/08/18/bill.clinton.diet.vegan/index.html.

Neumark-Sztainer, Dianne, Mary Story, Michael D. Resnick, and Robert W. Blum. "Adolescent Vegetarians: A Behavioral Profile of a School-Based Population in Minnesota." *Archives of Pediatrics and Adolescent Medicine* 151, no. 8 (August 1997): 833.

Pollan, Michael. *The Omnivore's Dilemma: A Natural History of Four Meals.* New York: Penguin Group, 2006.

## VIRTUAL HOSPITAL

Since the advent of the Internet, medical information has become increasingly available to health care providers and consumers alike. However, this body of literature is massive, often contradictory, and, consequently, overwhelming. With this in mind, several members of the University of Iowa Health Sciences community created the Virtual Hospital in 1992. The Virtual Library is an online digital library of authoritative multimedia health sciences information, largely contributed by the faculty and staff from the University of Iowa's (UI) Roy J. and Lucille A. Carver College of Medicine and UI Hospitals and Clinics.

While UI's Virtual Hospital was one of just a few sites of its kind in 1992, in the past two decades comparable websites have emerged, including the Virtual Naval Hospital, which is specifically geared toward military and naval medicine. Furthermore, in 2006, several segments of the Virtual Hospital began breaking away to create their own entities, including the Virtual Pediatric Hospital and Anatomy Atlases.

The virtual hospital project was executed with two goals in mind: (1) "to create a new paradigm for academic publishing," enabling authors to keep ownership of their content and (2) To further the broader University mission of educating patients and families about their health by organizing a source of quality, peer reviewed health information, which could be accessed rapidly and conveniently (D'Alessandro et al., 1998, p. 554). Since its inception, the Virtual Hospital has been referenced by millions of Internet users.

When the Virtual Hospital launched in 1992, it contained only three virtual textbooks. However, in just six short years, it grew into a Web database of 120 textbooks and booklets from 159 authors in 29 departments in four colleges on the UI Health Sciences campus, and it is continuously being added to. To supplement contributions from the UI Health Sciences community, the Virtual Hospital also contains 200 textbooks and booklets from state and national health care agencies and administrative information from three professional societies. The electronic catalog is organized into information intended for patients and information geared toward health care providers. Materials available for patients include textbooks and booklets on health promotion and disease prevention, disease information, and postvisit and home care instructions.

For providers, textbooks, teaching files, patient simulations, clinical practice guidelines, clinical references, newsletters, lectures, conferences, and continuing education courses have been incorporated. Publications in the Virtual Hospital have been found to be particularly useful, as they often integrate literature with clinical experience and wisdom. Furthermore, the information covers a broad array of topics, including, but not limited to, anesthesia, cancer, dentistry, neurosurgery, preventative medicine, and pharmacy. Given the wide breadth of content, depth is sometimes limited in certain subject areas. Aware of this, the site often provides links to other appropriate authoritative digital libraries.

The Virtual Hospital promotes active, self-directed learning, allowing people to access information wherever and whenever they need it with relative ease.

Content can be viewed by going to www.uihealthcare.com/vh using a basic Web browser and does not require the use of helper applications or Web-browser plug-ins. Furthermore, the interface is fairly intuitive and user friendly, with each page linking to the digital library home page, online help, search page, outline, and comment form.

Users can also have confidence in the rigor of the materials they view. There is great transparency in authorship. Each page states the author's name, degree and affiliation. In addition, most content is reviewed by departmental peer review boards organized on the UI Health Sciences campus. Users will note each entry is assigned one of three grades of peer review: "Not Peer Reviewed" (content for which no appropriate departmental peer review board exists), "Internally Peer Reviewed" (a peer review board within the University of Iowa Health Sciences campus), and "Externally Peer Reviewed" (a peer review entity outside the University of Iowa Health Sciences campus). Finally, editors periodically review and revise each posting to reflect new health information. The date of the last review is indicated on the entry. The Virtual Hospital and its related sources provide authoritative, free online resources to the consumer and to other health care professionals.

*Laura McLaughlin*

*See also* Online Health Resources.

### References

"Anatomy Atlases: A Digital Library of Anatomy Information." www.anatomyatlases.org/.
D'Alessandro, Michael P., Jeffrey R. Galvin, William E. Erkonen, Teresa A. Choi, David L. Lacey, and Stephana I. Colbert. "The Virtual Hospital: Experiences in Creating and Sustaining a Digital Library." *Bulletin of the Medical Library Association* 86 (1998): 553–63.
University of Iowa Hospitals and Clinics. "Virtual Hospital." August 14, 2009. www.ui healthcare.com/vh/.
"The Virtual Naval Hospital." April 26, 2011. www.vnh.org/.
"The Virtual Pediatric Hospital." n.d. www.virtualpediatrichospital.org/.

## VIRUS

Prior to the 1930s, "virus" was a general term for any microbial agent of infectious disease. Since then, however, the term has been restricted to such agents that pass through filters that retain bacteria and other, larger microbes, appropriately called "filterable viruses." The simple term "virus" is now used.

Viruses are obligate intracellular parasites that can exist as potentially active but inert entities outside of cells. Viruses can infect many animal, plant, and protist cells with effects ranging from unapparent infection to lethality. All virus infections have an entry phase; an intracellular phase of multiplication, integration, or latency formation; a virus release phase; and usually some type of host response. These host responses usually appear as signs and symptoms of the infection. Well-known virus diseases include measles, chicken pox, rabies, hepatitis, the common cold, influenza, yellow fever, and AIDS.

**Initial Entry and Local Virus Multiplication**   All viruses have some structural features in common: a core of nucleic acid (either RNA or DNA) that acts as the viral genome and encodes the viral functions, and a coat of protein that may or may not be surrounded by a lipid membrane. At the cellular level, a virus first must enter the cell, often by adsorption or attachment to a specific receptor on the surface of the target cell. A virus receptor may be a molecule or group of molecules that the cell uses for other purposes; for example, one of the lymphocyte cell recognition molecules is used by the human immunodeficiency virus (HIV) as its attachment and entry site. In some cases, only the viral nucleic acid enters the cell, but in other cases, the entire virus is taken into the cell, and the viral genome is exposed after a process of "uncoating." If virus proteins enter along with the genome, the proteins often regulate expression and replication of the viral genes. Some viral proteins may function to suppress host gene expression to help the virus subvert cellular processes to its own advantage. Some genes of the virus are expressed immediately after infection, and their translation into proteins starts the intracellular virus replication phase. Once a large number of viral genomes have been produced, and a sufficiently large pool of virus structural proteins has accumulated, virus assembly takes place.

**The Virus Release and Viremic Phase**   The cell then ruptures or is lysed from within by specific enzymes. Hundreds to thousands of new infectious virus particles burst forth from each infected cell, each one available to spread the infection. Some viruses, however, do not undergo this lytic cycle but have evolved a symbiotic relationship with the host cell. They integrate their genomes into the host cell chromosome in a "repressed" or latent state by a complex process that differs for RNA- and DNA-containing viruses.

Common routes of infection of animals are through the respiratory tract, the gastrointestinal tract, directly into the blood stream, by sexual contact, or by the bite of an infected insect vector. After the local infection of susceptible cells, the initial viremia (virus in the blood) transports the progeny virus to target cells or tissues in the body where the virus may replicate further, adding more virus to the blood (secondary viremia). Often, the immunological responses of the individual are provoked only by the secondary viremia because the primary viremia may be inadequate in duration or intensity to do so.

**Immunological Responses in the Host**   Most virus infections are asymptomatic or, at most, cause such common and inconsequential symptoms that the infection passes unnoticed. Analysis of the antibodies in normal human serum shows that we have many antiviral antibodies that indicate a history of prior unrecognized encounters with many viruses.

The viremic phase of infection allows the cells of the immune system to respond to the presence of virus. If the virus is sufficiently immunogenic, a primary antibody response occurs in about a week. This response results in the production of long-lasting memory—B cells that can be activated later by subsequent exposure to the same virus to provide a rapid and intense secondary immune response. This immunological memory is the primary reason for lifelong immunity once a person has survived a particular viral infection.

The specific antibodies produced by the primary immune response can combine with the virus in the blood and result in circulating immune complexes that facilitate the destruction and clearance of the virus from the body, but also result in activation of some processes such as the production of fever.

Some viruses that enter into a latent or symbiotic state within the host cell can provoke abnormal cell behavior. Many such viruses carry extra genes that regulate cell division and can result in the malignant transformation of the cell to produce a cancer. These cancer-causing (oncogenic) viruses are a special group of viruses that are of great current interest because of both their special biology and their practical importance.

**Effects on the Host**   The usual outcome of a viral infection is recovery of the organism with long-lasting immunity. After the initial local virus multiplication, viremic phase, and immunological responses, the virus is eliminated from the body. The immune memory cells provide for long-term protection against another infection. If this sort of immunity is produced by deliberate infection, usually with a weakened strain of virus, the process is called "vaccination" (more accurately, immunization). If, however, the immune system is compromised, if the virus replication overwhelms the immune system, or if the virus enters cells or tissues that are hidden from the immune system, the virus may destroy critical tissues or organs and result in illness or death.

The classic mode of prevention of viral diseases is by artificial immunization with whole attenuated viruses or parts of virus particles. This approach was first used in the case of smallpox, when it was observed that infection with viral material from a mild case often resulted in a mild case of smallpox (so-called inoculation, or variolation) that then conveyed lifelong immunity. Later, a related but nonlethal virus, the cowpox virus, was used to induce immunity to smallpox.

Some viruses, after the primary infection, enter into a latent form and remain asymptomatic until later reactivation. The herpes group of viruses is especially prone to such latent infections. Initial infection, for example, with the chicken pox virus (actually a member of the herpes group) produces viremia and generalized skin rash. The virus then latently infects the dorsal root ganglia of the spinal cord and later, at times of lowered immunity, the virus reactivates, producing skin lesions along the distribution of the spinal nerve, resulting in a case of "shingles." Chicken pox and shingles are different manifestations of the varicella-zoster virus. A few viruses (e.g., HIV) are known to replicate at such a low level and to remain relatively benign initially, yet to escape the immune system and establish a true persistent infection.

Host cell proliferation may result from latent virus infections resulting in local, limited growths such as viral warts and the small skin lesions caused by the virus of *molluscum contagiosum*. Other latent infections can lead, in ways not yet fully understood, to malignant diseases such as Burkitt's lymphoma, nasopharyngeal carcinoma, Kaposi's sarcoma, and cervical cancer.

**Virulence and Transmission** Viruses are called virulent if they have a high propensity to cause disease or other evidence of infection. This principle has been widely exploited to produce vaccine strains of viruses. Virulence may be related to the interaction of essential viral functions with related host cellular functions. In certain cases, the virulence genes of the virus can be deleted or modified to make avirulent variants. A virus strain may be virulent for one host species and avirulent for another. Repeated selection for virulence in one host species may select for mutations that render the virus less virulent (attenuated) in another. The transmissibility of the virus is an important factor in the spread of infections and is often a genetic property of a specific viral strain. Highly transmissible strains of the influenza virus and of the common cold virus are much more likely to cause epidemic outbreaks than virus strains of lower transmissibility.

Because viruses are intracellular parasites that depend on many cellular processes for their growth and replication, there are few unique, virus-specific pathways that can be targeted with antiviral drugs without interfering with the uninfected host cells. The very simplicity of viruses and their nearly total dependence on cellular functions have been major reasons why there are few effective antiviral drugs and why viral chemotherapy remains a stubborn challenge.

*William C. Summers*

*See also* Common Cold; Food-borne Illness; Immune System/Lymphatic System; Influenza; Salmonella; Vaccinations.

### References

Acheson, Nicholas H. *Fundamentals of Molecular Virology.* Hoboken, NJ: Wiley, 2007.

Crawford, Dorothy H. *The Invisible Enemy: A Natural History of Viruses.* New York: Oxford University Press, 2002.

Fields, B. N., D.M. Knipe, and P.N. Howley, eds. *Fields' Virology.* 3rd ed. Philadelphia: Lippincott-Raven, 1996.

Henderson, Donald A. *Smallpox: The Death of a Disease: The Inside Story of Eradicating a Worldwide Killer.* Amherst, NY: Prometheus Books, 2009.

Levy, J.A., H. Fraenkel-Conrat, and R.A. Owens, eds. *Virology.* 4th ed. Englewood Cliffs, NJ: Prentice Hall, 1994.

Oldstone, Michael B.A. *Viruses, Plagues, and History.* New York: Oxford University Press, 1998.

## VITAMINS

By definition, everyone needs vitamins. And for many people, taking a multivitamin is a daily routine, a form of nutritional insurance to guard against bad eating habits. In fact, according to industry figures, about half of American adults take a daily multivitamin and adults as a whole spent upwards of $9.2 billion in 2009 on vitamins (Alderman, 2009).

Yet, before Americans pop a pill or take a tablet, they may want to educate themselves on the health and safety issues that vitamins present and on the research that is just beginning to illuminate their long-term effects. The American Dietetic Association (ADA) suggests that vitamins and supplements may be necessary for some people based on their specific circumstances, including pregnant women; nursing mothers; vegans; people with food allergies or food disease, such as celiac disease; people with cancer or bone disease; and senior citizens. What about adults and children who do not fit into these categories? Does everyone really need vitamins and supplements?

The term "vitamin" comes from the Latin word "vita," meaning life, and from the word "amine." Amines were organic compounds that were thought to prevent disease. The "e" on "vitamin" was eventually dropped when it was discovered that not all vitamins contained an amine group. Vitamins fall into two categories: essential and nonessential. The essential vitamins are needed to sustain life and to promote health, but they come from sources outside the human body. The nonessential vitamins are vital to good health, but the body can manufacture them without outside sources.

Vitamins are also classified by their ability to be absorbed in fat or water. Water-soluble vitamins are the eight B vitamins and vitamin C. They must be consumed frequently, because they are not stored, with the exception of some B vitamins. The fat-soluble vitamins—A, D, E, and K—are usually obtained from fat-containing foods and can be stored in the body's fat, which means they do not need to be eaten every day. Vitamin D is the only the fat-soluble vitamin that is manufactured by the body through exposure to sunlight; all the others come from what is eaten. While the fat-soluble vitamins reside in the fatty tissues, meaning they do not need to be consumed every day, they can also build up to dangerous levels and cause problems if they are eaten or taken in excess.

The Food and Drug Administration (FDA) published the first set of nutritional recommendations in 1941, known as the Recommended Dietary Allowances (RDA), to guide Americans on appropriate daily vitamin needs. Since the mid-1990s, the RDA became part of a broader set of guidelines called Reference Daily Intake (RDI), which is used to determine the Percent Daily Value used on all food labels. The Percent Daily Value is a general suggestion based on a 2,000-calorie diet for a healthy adult.

Surprisingly, the 2010 Dietary Guidelines for Americans do not recommend any vitamin supplement for a healthy population consuming a variety of foods. The latest report released by the Dietary Guidelines Advisory Committee suggested that while many Americans understand the importance of good nutrition, they rely on a daily multivitamin pill. The report suggested "nutrient intake should come primarily from foods" ("Nutrient Adequacy," 2010). The committee also stated that as scientists learn more about nutrition and the human body they have come to realize the importance of eating foods in their intact forms rather than relying on pills to meet daily nutrients. The guidelines, updated every five years, were released in August 2010.

By contrast, the Council for Responsible Nutrition (CRN), the Vitamin C Foundation, The National Health Federation (NHF), and the International Society for Orthomolecular Medicine (ISOM) are among those organizations strongly promoting the use of vitamins and other key supplements, and these organizations offer their own evidence of their health benefits. In order to weigh both sides of the argument, it is important to understand the role each vitamin plays in overall health. The vitamins include vitamin A; the eight vitamin B complex group of B1 or thiamine, B2 or riboflavin, B3 or niacin, B6 or pyridoxine, pantothenic acid, biotin, B9 or folic acid, and vitamin B12; vitamin C; vitamin D; vitamin E; and vitamin K.

**Vitamins A to K**   Vitamin A is fat-soluble and comes from animal foods like liver, egg yolks, cream, and butter or from the beta carotene that occurs in green leafy vegetables and yellow fruits and vegetables. Plants do not actually contain vitamin A but they do contain beta carotene, which can be converted to vitamin A in the intestine and then absorbed by the body. Vitamin A affects skeletal growth, skin health, and the wellness of mucous membranes. There is some suggestion by researchers that it can help prevent cataracts and cardiovascular disease, and one of the first signs of a deficiency of this vitamin is "night blindness"—when a person has the decreased ability to see at night. A deficiency of this vitamin can also slow growth, cause skin abnormalities, and increase susceptibility to infection. In severe cases, it can cause death. The Percent Daily Value for vitamin A is 5,000 international units (IU).

Vitamin B1, or thiamine, was the first of the B vitamins to be identified. It plays a key role in the metabolism of carbohydrates and maintains appetite as well as intestinal function. This vitamin also affects the cardiovascular and nervous systems. Good food sources include yeast, legumes, whole grains, nuts, and thiamine-enriched cereal products. Thousands of years ago, the Chinese first described a disease known now as *beriberi,* which is caused by a deficiency of thiamine. Symptoms include nausea, fatigue, and mental confusion, and it affects the nervous and gastrointestinal system. Thiamine is located in the husks or bran of rice and other grains but is removed during the modern milling process. Manufacturers now enrich these grains and add thiamine back to eliminate the problem of deficiency disease. The Percent Daily Value for thiamine is 1.5 milligrams (mg).

Vitamin B2, or riboflavin, is also needed to metabolize carbohydrates as well as fats and proteins. A deficiency can cause skin lesions and sensitivity to light. This vitamin can be found in liver, milk, meat, dark green vegetables, whole grains, and mushrooms. The Percent Daily Value for riboflavin is 1.7 milligrams.

Vitamin B3, or niacin, assists in the release of energy from glucose. Pellagra is a disease caused by a deficiency of niacin, and its symptoms include sunburn-type eruptions on the skin when exposed to sunlight as well as diarrhea, mental confusion, and depression. Large doses of niacin have been prescribed to reduce levels of cholesterol, but over long periods it can cause liver damage. Excellent sources of niacin are found in liver, poultry, meat, tuna, salmon, dried beans, dried peas, and nuts. It is present in whole grains except corn, where the niacin is part of a molecule that cannot be absorbed. Pellagra was once common in areas of the world where the diet consisted of corn and corn products, such as Spain, Mexico, and the southeastern United States. It was discovered that treating corn with an alkaline solution, such as lime water, released the niacin and made it available for the body to absorb. The Percent Daily Value of niacin is 20 milligrams.

Vitamin B6, or pyridoxine, works with the body to allow absorption and metabolism of amino acids, glucose, and fatty acids. It also assists in the formation of red blood cells and the building of body tissue. Liver and organ meats, spinach, avocados, green beans, bananas, whole-grain cereals, and seeds are all good sources of this vitamin. A deficiency of vitamin B6 causes depression, nausea, and vomiting. The Percent Daily Value of B6 is 2 milligrams.

Pantothenic acid, another of the B complex vitamins, is important for the successful metabolism of many substances, including fatty acids, steroids, and carbohydrates. The adrenal gland is an important site of pantothenic acid activity. This vitamin can be found in foods including liver, kidney, eggs, and dairy products and is also manufactured by intestinal bacteria. A deficiency of this vitamin causes anemia. The Percent Daily Value for pantothenic acid is 10 milligrams.

Another B vitamin, biotin, is important for the metabolism of carbohydrates and in the formation of fatty acids. It too is synthesized by intestinal bacteria and is available in egg yolk, tomatoes, yeast, kidney, and liver. A deficiency in this vitamin causes dermatitis, although it is rare. The Percent Daily Value for biotin is 300 micrograms (mcg).

A lack of vitamin B9, or folic acid, has been linked to neural tube defects, a type of birth defect that causes serious brain or neurological disorders such as spina bifida. It can be found in green leafy vegetables, fruits, dried beans, sunflower seeds, and wheat germ. Folic acid's role in the body includes forming hemoglobin and synthesizing proteins. Although it is a water-soluble vitamin, folic acid is stored in the liver and does not need to be eaten daily. Due to the importance of this vitamin, the U.S. government began requiring that it be added to flour, cornmeal, rice, and pasta beginning in 1998 in order to prevent birth defects. The Percent Daily Value for folic acid is 400 micrograms.

Vitamin B12 is the most complex of all the vitamins and is important for healthy nervous-system functioning. This vitamin is available from animal sources including liver, kidneys, meat, fish, eggs, and milk. For vegans or vegetarians who eat few or no animal products, a supplement is suggested to ensure adequate amounts. This B complex vitamin is necessary for folic acid, or vitamin B9, to do its job effectively. The Percent Daily Value for B12 is 6 micrograms.

Vitamin C, one of the most widely recognized of the vitamins, is also known as ascorbic acid. It is needed by the body for the formation and maintenance of collagen, a protein that helps form bones and teeth. Vitamin C also improves the absorption of iron from foods. Citrus fruits, berries, tomatoes, and peppers are excellent sources of vitamin C. A vitamin C deficiency can cause scurvy, a nutritional disease with symptoms that include hemorrhages, loosening of teeth, and bone problems. Large doses of vitamin C are widely believed to improve symptoms of the common cold, but scientists have not found definitive proof of this. There is also controversy over whether vitamin C lessens the risk of heart disease and cancer, and research into this question is ongoing. The Percent Daily Value for vitamin C is 60 milligrams.

Vitamin D is needed to build healthy bones, and it improves the body's ability to retain calcium and phosphorus. It has been called "the sunshine vitamin" and can be manufactured in the body with exposure to as little as a half-hour of sunlight. Vitamin D deficiency causes rickets, a disease with symptoms that include bowlegs, knock-knees, and other bone deformities. This is a fat-soluble vitamin that can be stored in the body. To prevent the disease, the U.S. government requires milk to be fortified with vitamin D. Other prepared foods in recent years also added vitamin D as a supplement. Food sources include egg yolk, liver, and tuna. The Percent Daily Value for this vitamin is 400 international units.

Vitamin E plays a role in the formation of red blood cells as well as muscle and other tissues. It is also involved in immune function and other metabolic processes. Naturally occurring vitamin E exists in eight chemical forms: alpha-, beta-, gamma-, and delta-tocopherol and alpha-, beta-, gamma-, and delta-tocotrienol. The alpha-tocopherol is the only form that is recognized to meet human vitamin requirements. It can be found in vegetable oils, wheat germ, green leafy vegetables, and liver. Scientists suggest it may have an anticoagulant effect on the blood, but research to identify just how strong that effect may be is ongoing. The Percent Daily Value for vitamin E is 30 international units.

Vitamin K is important for the clotting of blood, and anyone suffering from a blood disease can experience some deficiency, although the bacterial synthesis of this vitamin usually provides enough for a healthy adult. Good sources include alfalfa and fish livers as well as leafy green vegetables, egg yolks, soybean oil, and liver. The suggested safe level for adults is 80 micrograms.

**History of Vitamins** Early pioneers in vitamin research included surgeon James Lind, who in 1746 discovered that vitamin C could prevent and cure the disease of scurvy. Lind, an English naval captain and doctor, found that when limes were added to a seaman's diet it kept him from getting the nutritional disease that caused extreme fatigue, nausea, muscle and joint pain, and internal bleeding. In 1897, a Dutch physician named Christian Eijkman sought to understand the causes of another nutritional disease, beriberi. Working with rice, he discovered that an important nutrient was lost when the hulls were removed and the rice was polished. That missing nutrient, thiamine, was not present in the polished grains. His work was followed by Frederick Gowland Hopkins, a British biochemist who was also interested in nutritional deficiency diseases. Hopkins shared the 1929 Nobel Prize in physiology and medicine with Eijkman for their research on vitamins. Hopkins had earlier created diets for experimental animals and concluded there were what he called "accessory food factors" that were essential for human health. His papers on the subject are considered classics in the history of vitamin nutrition.

Hopkins work led others, including biochemist Casimir Funk, to identify the fat-soluble and water-soluble vitamins. Funk published a paper on vitamin deficiency diseases, coined the word "vitamine," and identified four vitamins, including B1, B2, C, and D. Since that time, additional vitamins have been identified, and the relationship between vitamins and disease has been established.

**Vitamins and Health** American consumers are used to turning to the government for information about the safety and effectiveness of products. In their infancy, vitamin and other dietary supplements were chiefly considered preventives against nutritional diseases. Now they are increasingly being taken by Americans to counteract poor nutritional choices. This shift in thinking concerning manufactured vitamins prompted a new law, which amended the 1938 Federal Food, Drug, and Cosmetic Act, and sought to create a regulatory framework for the safety and labeling of vitamins and other dietary supplements. The resulting legislation dramatically changed how vitamins would be handled.

The 1994 the Dietary Supplement Health and Education Act defined vitamins as dietary supplements rather than prescription drugs and shifted the burden of proof of safety away from the manufacturers and onto the FDA. Since 1994 the government has also had to wait for reports of dangerous complications. Even now the FDA must provide overwhelming evidence from clinical trials and reports of harm before they can force a product off the shelves. Manufacturers of prescription drugs, by law, must still prove their products are safe before they are sold to the public.

**Megavitamin Supporters** There are many Americans who believe that megadoses of vitamins and other dietary supplements are a vital to their health. Chief among those was Nobel Prize–winner and biochemist Dr. Linus Pauling, who was an early promoter of megadoses of vitamins and nutrients more than 40 years ago. Pauling is regarded by some as the founder of the science of orthomolecular medicine. He introduced the word "orthomolecular" in the 1960s to describe the use of natural substances, especially nutrients, in treating illness and maintaining good health.

Pauling, who died in 1994, and several colleagues founded the Institute of Orthomolecular Medicine, later renamed the Linus Pauling Institute of Science and Medicine, in Palo Alto, California. According to the International Society for Orthomolecular Medicine (ISOM) website, orthomolecular treatments include "dietary manipulation, nutrition supplementation, herbal remedies, homeopathic treatments, detoxification and safe forms of megavitamin therapy." The megadoses used in "megavitamin" therapy are defined in scientific terms as doses that are 10 times the earlier RDA or more.

The ISOM website contains case studies that the group claims demonstrate the effectiveness of their practices. Andrew W. Saul, PhD, editor-in-chief of the Orthomolecular Medicine News Service, has routinely criticized the media for accepting and promoting all government-sponsored studies showing harmful effects from supplements. In an Internet interview in March 2010, Saul told Nancy Desjardins, of HealthLady.com, that "vitamins save lives. We are a nation of sick, under-nourished, and over-medicated people. Vitamins are not the problem; they are the solution" (Saul, 2010).

The Council for Responsible Nutrition (CRN) likewise claims that vitamins and supplements help prevent disease. This trade association was founded in 1973 and now includes some 70 member companies, including Archer Daniels Midland Company, Bayer Corporation, Shaklee Corporation, and Cargill Health and Food Technologies. The CRN continuously lobbies against any new FDA regulatory controls over vitamins or other supplements. On their website, they rank their ability to maintain and improve consumer confidence in their members' products as a top priority. Recent links focused on the positive effects of vitamin D in lowering cancer risks for older women and on the potential helpful effects of increased vitamin D on lowering blood pressure.

While Pauling focused on establishing orthomolecular medicine, other medical doctors developed their own work with supplements. Dr. Robert C. Atkins, famous for his protein-rich diet, advocated taking 20 vitamins and nutritional supplements a day; he personally took 60 daily. Atkins first appeared on the national stage in 1973 with the publication of his high-protein, low-carbohydrate eating plan. His book, *Dr. Atkins' Diet Revolution* (1972), quickly became a bestseller.

After the success of his book, Atkins opened an alternative healing clinic and continued to publish books. His first book that dealt with alternative healing, *Dr. Atkins' Nutrition Breakthrough: How to Treat Your Medical Condition without Drugs,* was published in 1981. In 1998, he released *Dr. Atkins' Vita-Nutrient Solution: Nature's Answer to Drugs.* Atkins's work with supplements was honored by the National Health Federation (NHF), and he received their National Health Federation Man of the Year Award in 1987. Established in 1955, the NHF is an international consumer-education and health-freedom organization. According to its website, members "work to protect individuals' rights to choose to consume healthy food, take supplements, and use alternative therapies without government restrictions."

It was biochemist Irwin Stone who introduced Linus Pauling to the value of vitamin C in preventing colds. Stone suggested that by treating vitamin C, or ascorbic acid, as a nutrient with a minimum daily requirement instead of a crucial enzyme, people were living in a state of disease he named *Hypoascorbemia.* He believed that people receive only one or two percent of the amount of ascorbic acid they need to be healthy. Stone published his research and findings in 1972, in a book titled *The Healing Factor: Vitamin C against Disease.*

**Vitamins and Disease**   Pauling credited Stone's research for his own developing ideas and wrote the foreword for Stone's book along with Dr. Albert Szent-Gyorgyi, recipient of the 1937 Nobel Prize for his discovery of vitamin C. Szent-Gyorgyi, who originally gave vitamin C the name "ascorbic acid," is also credited as being the first to suggest its use in treating cancer. Szent-Gyorgyi was 80 years old when he founded the National Foundation for Cancer Research (NFCR) in 1973. The NFCR is still active and supports cancer research as well as public education on the prevention, early diagnosis, treatment, and continuing search for a cure for cancer.

The role of B vitamins in improving cardiovascular health was the focus of two studies published on April 12, 2010, in *Stroke: Journal of the American Heart Association*. In those studies, researchers looked at the effects of folate and vitamin B6 on the risk of stroke for women and heart disease for men, respectively. Researchers found that eating more foods rich in folate and B6 reduced the risk of death in women from stroke and heart disease and also reduced death from heart failure in men. A second study, published in that same issue, revealed that eating more folate and vitamin B12 may also lower the risk of stroke in men (Renzhe et al., 2010).

The potential curative effect of vitamins on cancer has been debated for decades by scientists and doctors, including Pauling, Szent-Gyorgyi, and Stone. Researchers in recent years also began to study the reverse, that is, if vitamins promote cancer growth when taken in large doses. Joel Mason, director of the Vitamins and Carcinogenesis Laboratory at the Jean Mayer USDA Human Nutrition Research Center on Aging, at Tufts University, published data showing that colorectal cancer rates rose soon after companies started adding folic acid to foods in the 1990s (Liebman, 2007).

There are theories to explain this early data showing over 15,000 extra cases of colorectal cancer per year. Mason suggested that small doses of folic acid may protect against colorectal cancer, but he cautioned, "we started seeing that an abundant quantity of folic acid might accelerate carcinogenesis in animal studies, and now data from human studies is [sic] starting to emerge" (Liebman, 2007).

Folic acid is necessary for the synthesis of DNA, and cells produce DNA every time they divide. For people who have cancer or precancerous cells, excessive folic acid may increase the body's ability to produce DNA and feed the cancer cells. Whereas foods rich in folate are not a problem because the human body absorbs the folate less efficiently, supplements and fortified foods can quickly bring folate levels to over 800 micrograms of folic acid—double the RDA of 400 micrograms per day.

Another new area of research is whether nutrition can influence the developing and mature brain. Scientists are now looking at the role of vitamins, especially folate, in memory and brain function. Studies are under way to determine if low folate levels play a role in some forms of dementia. including late-onset Alzheimer's disease. Although scientists suggest there may be a connection between a folate deficiency and abnormal mental function, there are not yet sufficient data to make that definitive diagnosis ("Vitamins for the Mind," 2010).

**Buyers Beware?**   Clinical trials compare one group taking a vitamin to another group taking placebos and track those groups to see what conclusions they can draw. Industry officials like to interpret the results in their favor, whereas the government acts to protect consumers. Everyone sees something different in the results. If you are like the majority of Americans, you may take a vitamin of one kind or another. Will vitamins or supplements help those who skip meals, eat out too often, or don't get the recommended amounts of fruits, vegetables, and fiber? Americans think they will, and they assume that vitamins and supplements are safe. But are synthetic vitamins worth it? Several studies have failed to show that vitamins in pill form help prevent chronic disease or prolong life.

Researchers in the Women's Health Initiative study followed eight years of multivitamin use among older women to see if the multivitamins might decrease their risk for heart disease or select cancers. The study results, published in *The Archives of Internal Medicine* concluded there was no benefit (Neuhouser et al., 2009). In January of 2009, an editorial in the *Journal of the National Cancer Institute* noted that most trials had shown little effect in their studies (Parker-Pope, 2009).

The evidence does show that eating a healthy diet and exercising are the best ways to ward off disease, and vitamins are best in their simplest, natural form. Consumers, along with their physicians, should decide whether they need supplements and which ones to take. Services like MedWatch—the FDA Safety Information and Adverse Event Reporting Program—can help keep Americans aware of safety alerts, recalls, withdrawals, and important labeling changes. Whatever the decision, the best advice is still found in the Latin phrase caveat emptor—"let the buyer beware."

*Sharon Zoumbaris*

*See also* Antioxidants; Cancer; Dietary Supplements; Nutritional Diseases.

## References

Alderman, Lesley. "Knowing What's Worth Paying for in Vitamins." *The New York Times,* December 5, 2009: B5.

Atkins, Robert C. *Dr. Atkins' Diet Revolution: The High Calorie Way to Stay Thin Forever.* New York: D. McKay Co., 1972.

Hurley, Dan. *Natural Causes: Death, Lies and Politics in America's Vitamin and Herbal Supplement Industry.* New York: Broadway Books, 2006.

Liebman, Bonnie. "Confusion at the Vitamin Counter: Too Little or Too Much?" *Nutrition Healthletter,* November 2007.

Neuhouser, Marian L., Sylvia Wassertheil-Smoller, Cynthia Thomson, Aaron Aragaki, Garnet L. Anderson, JoAnn E. Manson, Ruth E. Patterson, Thomas E. Rohan, Linda van Horn, James M. Shikany, Asha Thomas, Andrea LaCroix, and Ross L. Prentice. "Multivitamin Use and Risk of Cancer and Cardiovascular Disease in the Women's Health Initiative Cohorts." *Archives of Internal Medicine* 169 (2009): 294–304.

"The NHF Declaration of Health-Freedom Rights." *National Health Federation.* www.thenhf.com/declaration.htm.

"Nutrient Adequacy." *Report of the Dietary Guidelines Advisory Committee on the Dietary Guidelines for Americans, 2010.* October 21, 2011. www.cnpp.usda.gov/DGAs2010-DGACReport.htm.

Parker-Pope, Tara. "Vitamin Pills: A False Hope?" *The New York Times,* February 17, 2009. www.nytimes.com.

Renzhe, Cui, Iso Hiroyasu, D. Chigusa, Kikuchi Shogo, and A. Tamakoshi. "Dietary Folate and Vitamin B6 and B12 Intake in Relation to Mortality from Cardiovascular Diseases." *StrokeAHA.* April 15, 2010. http://stroke.ahajournals.org.

Saul, Andrew W. "Andrew W. Saul, Interviewed by Nancy Desjardins." *HealthLady.com.* March 18, 2010. www.HealthLady.com.

Stampfer, Meir J. The Benefits and Risks of Vitamins and Minerals." *Harvard Special Health Report, Harvard Health Publications,* March 2006.

"Vitamins for the Mind? Evidence Is Growing that Certain Supplements May Be Beneficial for the Brain." *Healthy Years* 7, no. 8 (August 2010): S-2.

Zeratsky, Katherine. "Percent Daily Value: What Does It Mean?" *MayoClinic.com.* May 6, 2010. www.mayoclinic.com/health/food-and-nutrition/AN00284.

# *W*

## WALKING

Walking is a form of exercise that requires no additional equipment. It can be done alone, anywhere, day or evening, and is guaranteed to help take off weight and control blood pressure. Walking can also slow the progression of cognitive illness and, if practiced regularly, may even improve the outcomes for patients with certain forms of cancer. A brisk walk can improve mood, reduce the risk of—or help to manage—Type 2 diabetes, and may even help prevent the onset of Alzheimer's disease. Plus, walking isn't likely to lead to injuries.

Walking simply requires a place to walk, comfortable clothing, and shoes that are comfortable and fit your feet. If jogging is the universal example of aerobic exercise, walking is definitely the best choice for moderate exercise. Unfortunately, statistics show that Americans are far less likely to take a walk then their counterparts in other countries. Australians walk an average of over 9,000 steps per day, Japanese walk over 7,000 steps each day, and the Swiss clock in at 9,000 steps, compared to the average American who takes just over 5,000 steps per day (Bassett, 2010). So why aren't Americans making the most of this easy, simple, effective form of exercise?

While researchers did not answer why, they did note that the comparison of walking between people of various countries does explain at least one reason why obesity rates are higher in the U.S. than in other developed countries.

Walking is routinely suggested by doctors as a form of exercise because it can be combined with many other activities, such as hiking, exercising a dog, sightseeing, or sports like golf. When compared to running or jogging, walking is low impact and does not lead to ankle, knee, and hip injuries that are more often seen in runners. New research now suggests that walking about five miles each week may actually slow down cognitive decline in Alzheimer's patients (Mozes, 2010).

In study results released by the University of Pittsburgh, researchers used data from an ongoing 20-year study. They found weekly walking patterns made a difference among older adults, and those who walked five miles per week had a slower decline in memory loss over time (Mozes, 2010). The study team also noted that the more an individual engaged in physical activity, the larger his or her brain volume remained; larger brain volume is a sign of general brain health.

The researchers did not say that walking was a cure for the disease, but they suggested it may improve resistance to the disease and reduce overall memory loss if practiced regularly. This is important news for the estimated 2 to 5 million Americans who have Alzheimer's disease (Mozes, 2010).

Ways to fit walking into your schedule include choosing a distant parking spot and walking the extra steps to your destination, taking the stairs instead of an elevator, adding a walk break during the day or during lunchtime, and adding extra walks with your pet.

*Sharon Zoumbaris*

*See also* Aerobic Exercise; Alzheimer's Disease; Cancer; Diabetes; Heart Health.

### References

Bardi, Jason. "Brisk Walking May Help Men with Prostate Cancer, UCSF Study Finds." University of California, San Francisco. (May 24, 2011). www.ucsf.edu/news/2011/05/9909/brisk-walking-may-help-men-prostate-cancer-ucsf-study-finds.

Bassett, D. R., Jr., H. R. Wyatt, H. Thompson, J. C. Peters, and J. O. Hill. "Pedometer-measured Physical Activity and Health Behaviors in U.S. Adults." *Medicine & Science in Sports & Exercise* 42, no. 10 (October 2010): 1819–25.

Mozes, Alan. "Regular Walking May Slow Decline of Alzheimer's: Researchers Also Find that Walking 6 Miles a Week Can Help Prevent Onset of Disease." *Consumer Health News.* November 29, 2010. http://consumer.healthday.com/Article.asp?AID=646656.

NIDDK (National Institutes of Health, National Institute of Diabetes & Digestive & Kidney Diseases). *Walking: A Step in the Right Direction.* Bethesda, MD: NIDDK, 2007. NIH Publication No. 07-4155. http://win.niddk.nih.gov/publications/walking.htm.

## WATER

"Water, taken in moderation, cannot hurt anybody."

*—Mark Twain*

Millions of Americans could learn from Mark Twain and could even improve their health if they added more water to their daily diet. In fact, doctors recommend that Americans decrease their consumption of soft drinks, sports drinks, and other fluids and replace it with plain water. Water is the body's principal chemical component and makes up at least 60 percent of our body weight (Mayo Clinic, 2010). Simply put, our bodies need water to function. A human can live for several weeks without food but can survive only for a few days without water.

Water contributes to how well our bodies transport nutrients and oxygen to cells, cushions our joints, and removes wastes through our urine and bowel movements. Water also provides a medium for chemical reactions that take place in

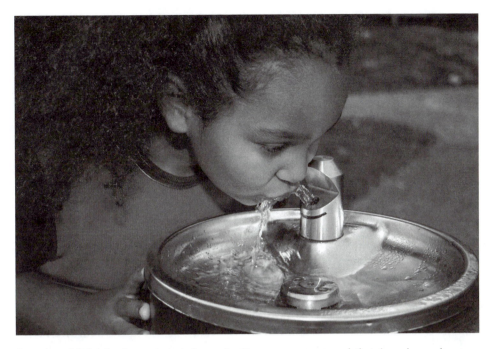

A young girl drinks from a water fountain. Doctors recommend that Americans decrease their intake of soda and sports drinks and increase their consumption of plain water. (Photoeuphoria/Dreamstime.com)

our bodies; keeps the tissues in our mouth, eyes, and nose moist; and helps keep our temperature constant. This basic chemical combination of two molecules of hydrogen and one molecule of oxygen, known as $H_2O$, is found throughout our bodies—in our brains, blood, bones, fat cells, and muscles.

Just how much water does an individual need each day? The answer is not as simple as the question and is based on a formula that involves age and body size, individual fluid intake, normal diet, amount and intensity of physical exercise, climate, and overall health. In general, water intake in a day should range from 8 or 9 cups to as many as 13, depending on those earlier factors. Individuals should routinely consume water from a diet that includes fresh fruits and vegetables and from drinking fluids with each meal and between meals.

In defining good health, doctors suggest that individuals are drinking enough water if they rarely feel thirsty and if their body produces 6 or 7 cups of lightly colored urine each day. One way to measure adequate fluid intake is to check the color of your urine; urine should be pale yellow, so if it is a dark yellow color, more fluids are needed.

One reason it is important to monitor fluid intake and hydration levels is because the human body does not store excess water like it does other key nutrients. It is important to replace lost fluids during the day to keep the body healthy. The sensation of thirst is a key mechanism to remind individuals to maintain the correct fluid balance. When fluid levels are low, the brain stimulates nerves, which in turn create the sensation of thirst, and the feeling of thirst prompts a person to drink. However, doctors recommend individuals not wait until they are exceptionally thirsty to drink water.

Most people are aware that water leaves the body constantly through urine and bowel movements. It also is lost through sweat during exercise. Sports drinks were first created to assist athletes who often sweated out lots of fluids. Sports drinks, like Gatorade, have been around for a long time and were designed to replenish electrolytes for serious athletes who were exercising for long periods of time in hot conditions. They were not originally intended for recreational athletes, children, or spectators. Sports drinks contain sugar, sodium, potassium, and chloride, which are known as "electrolytes." When the human body needs to cool down to remain at a constant temperature, it releases fluid and electrolytes through sweat.

These electrolytes play an important role in most of our body's metabolic activities, such as helping to regulate the levels of oxygen in the blood. Water balance and electrolyte balance are closely intertwined in a healthy body and can be upset by dehydration.

However, health professionals say that fluid lost from exercise that lasts for less than an hour can easily be replaced by water and does not require additional electrolytes. It is only the higher intensity athletes who actually need sports drinks. For the casual athlete or spectator, the same sports drinks add up to excess calories and sugar, which are associated with weight gain, obesity, and dental problems. The American Academy of Pediatrics (AAP) has come out strongly against the routine consumption of sports drinks by children, calling for it to be limited or eliminated (Dotinga, 2011). The exception, according to the AAP, would be for youngsters who are taking part in intense and prolonged exercise.

With the figures for obesity rates for U.S. children continuing to climb, these types of health risks to children are now a growing concern. The Centers for Disease Control and Prevention's (CDC) latest statistics showed that obesity rates for children and teens, ages 2 to 19 years, rose from 5 percent to 17 percent from 1963 to 2008 (CDC, 2010).

Sports drinks were born out of a concern for dehydration, a serious condition caused by the body losing too much water from exercise or from illness and the associated vomiting or diarrhea. Young children and seniors are most at risk for dehydration. Worldwide, dehydration is a very serious health problem for young children. The World Health Organization (WHO) calls dehydration, especially from diarrhea, the second leading cause of child deaths in the world; some 2 million young children each year die from dehydration (WHO, 2006).

Surprisingly it is also possible to take in too much water. This condition is called "overhydration," and it too can lead to serious health problems. Overhydration develops when an individual's intake of water greatly exceeds their output. While drinking large amounts of water does not typically create this problem, overhydration can occur if an individual's kidney's or heart are not functioning correctly. The problem of overhydration is also seen with infants who are most at risk if they are given formula that has been overly diluted with water or just given water to drink. The excess water causes electrolytes to become diluted. In rare cases, this can lead to mental confusion, seizures, or even a coma.

Whether there is too little or too much water, the kidneys are the organ in the human body most responsible for controlling adequate water levels in the body. The kidneys need water to get rid of waste. On the other hand, if there is too much water, the kidneys must also get rid of it. For optimum health, doctors may recommend that those with kidney disease limit the amount of coffee, tea, alcohol, and caffeinated drinks each day, as these beverages act as diuretics, which can increase individual fluid loss. Instead, a well-balanced diet, full of fruits and vegetables as well as water, is important to keep one hydrated and healthy.

Water has played a key role in the dental health of Americans. Cities and other municipalities for decades have used their public water systems as a way to promote and deliver a nationwide fluoride health program. Fluoride was first introduced into U.S. public water systems in the in the 1940s to reduce tooth decay. In 2011, the U.S. Department of Health and Human Services proposed lowering fluoride levels in public drinking water, the first change since 1962 (CDC, 2011). Reasons for the reduction included the fact that Americans have access to more sources of fluoridation than they did decades earlier. Now, toothpastes, dental treatments, and other consumer products include added fluoride and are widely used by a majority of American consumers. The CDC, in recognizing the success and importance of fluoride in dental health, named community water fluoridation as one of the "Ten Great Public Health Interventions of the 20th Century" (CDC, 2011). Americans who worry about the effects of fluoride, especially in young children, have turned to bottled water products that have been distilled or purified. Bottled spring water may not be free of fluoride, because fluoride is naturally present in water, or, in some cases, it has been added to spring water. Also, home water filters do not remove fluoride from tap water.

*Sharon Zoumbaris*

*See also* Caffeine; Centers for Disease Control and Prevention (CDC); Dental Health.

## References

CDC (Centers for Disease Control and Prevention). "Community Water Fluoridation." January 7, 2011. www.cdc.gov/fluoridation/fact_sheets/cwf_qa.htm#.

CDC (Centers for Disease Control and Prevention). "Prevalence of Obesity among Children and Adolescents: United States, Trends 1963–1965 through 2007–2008." June 2010. www.cdc.gov/nchs/data/hestat/obesity_child_07_08/obesity_child_07_08.htm.

Dotinga, Randy. "Pediatricians Group Raps Energy and Sports Drinks for Kids." *Health-Day.* May 31, 2011. www.healthday.com/Article.asp?AID=653354.

Mayo Clinic. "Water: How Much Should You Drink Every Day?" April 17, 2010. www.mayoclinic.com/health/water/NU00283. WHO (World Health Organization). "Improved Formula for Oral Rehydration Salts to Save Children's Lives." March 23, 2006. www.who.int/mediacentre/news/releases/2006/pr14/en/.

"Who Really Benefits from Sports Drinks?" *Harvard Health Commentaries.* July 7, 2007. www.harvardhealthcontent.com/66,COL070607.

## WATERS, ALICE

Alice Waters, the West Coast chef credited with the creation of "California Cuisine" and the transformation of the country's ideas about food through her focus on simple, fresh, seasonal foods is also at the forefront of those fighting childhood obesity in the United States by helping to educate schoolchildren about nutrition in California and across the nation.

The Edible Schoolyard is Water's model garden project started in Berkeley, California, and funded by the Chez Panisse Foundation. Chez Panisse is the restaurant that Waters opened in Berkeley in 1971. The Foundation was developed initially to create financial support for the development of programs that would feature organic gardens in schools with the hope the gardens, food, and nutrition they provided would become part of the school's curriculum and lunch program.

The Chez Panisse Foundation officially began in 1996 in celebration of the 25th anniversary of the restaurant, and it continues working to create partnerships with public schools, to support their efforts to build gardens, and to share with children the lessons of healthy, fresh fruits and vegetables, something Waters has spoken about repeatedly. The Foundation offers lesson plans on its website (www.chezpanissefoundation.org/) that include hands-on experiences for students in the kitchen, garden, and lunchroom, where a nutritious, freshly prepared meal is part of each school day.

Schools with the Edible Schoolyard program include the Martin Luther King Jr. Middle School in Berkeley; the Larchmont Schools in Los Angeles and West Hollywood; the Children's Museum in Greensboro, North Carolina; and the Samuel J. Green Charter School in New Orleans. The Roanoke School District in Virginia began construction on a garden at a middle school and neighboring elementary school in 2010, and a Brooklyn, New York, elementary school opened its garden program in 2010.

Water's also joined forces with a student group at Yale University, where her daughter was enrolled to start the Yale Sustainable Food Project. The project began with a garden on campus, education about food

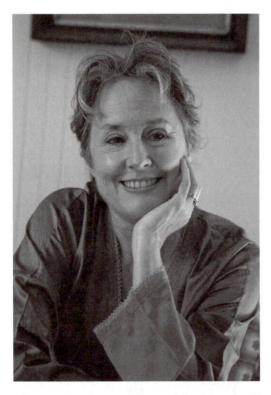

Alice Waters, the grand dame of the "slow food" movement, looks on during an interview in her kitchen in Bolinas, California, Wednesday, August 6, 2008. (AP/Wide World Photos)

and agriculture, and a sustainable-food dining program for one residential dining hall. Due to its popularity with students in 2004, the administration expanded the use of sustainable food in the menus of all the college dining halls, and the students broke ground on an organic garden. The project continues to expand each year, with more staff and interns involved in growing food and sharing information with students and the community.

Waters was born in 1944 in Chatham, New Jersey, the second of four daughters. Her father was a management consultant and her mother was a housewife. Waters left New Jersey for college in California and began her studies at the University of California at Santa Barbara. She later transferred to University of California at Berkeley. Waters majored in French studies and traveled abroad to study at the University of Paris. After she received her undergraduate degree from UC Berkeley in 1967, Waters moved back to Europe where she did postgraduate work at the Montessori School in London, England.

When she returned to the West Coast, she brought with her a European-style delight in food that sees it as something to be enjoyed slowly rather than cheaply and quickly, which at that time was the emerging American model, thanks to the explosion of the U.S. fast food industry. After a brief time teaching at a Montessori school in Berkeley, Waters opened her restaurant, which featured unusual dishes and food items that were unknown at the time, like arugula, goat cheese, and heirloom vegetables. Waters focused on fresh, local, organically grown, seasonal foods that were offered in the European style, with a "fixed price" menu, which gave each diner a minimum of options at a set price. She bought her food largely from local growers and suppliers, a very different business model than other restaurants at that time.

By the end of the decade the restaurant was successful enough for Waters to expand by opening the Chez Panisse Café in the upstairs part of the Shattuck Avenue house. The restaurant became a favorite with the Bay Area's young, urban professional set. Strong supporters of Chez Panisse included *New York Times* food critic Craig Claiborne.

Waters published her first book in 1982, the *Chez Panisse Menu Cookbook,* and other titles have followed. However, she continues to resist joining the ranks of celebrity chefs with television shows. She has not endorsed or offered a line of cookware or foods, and she decided not to open other Chez Panisse restaurants or to franchise her original restaurant. She did receive the cooking world's highest honor in 1992, when she was named the Chef of the Year by the James Beard Foundation. That same year her restaurant was named Restaurant of the Year by the Beard Foundation. Waters was awarded the French Legion of Honor in 2009, joining Julia Child as one of the few chefs to receive that prestigious award.

Called the "Mother of New American Cuisine," Waters is also credited with other food trends, including a growing use by Americans of organic produce and meats, the use of a wide variety of salad greens rather than the traditional iceberg lettuce in salads, and the creation of gourmet pizza. Food legend says the gourmet pizza was invented when a Chez Panisse chef tossed some leftover seafood onto pizza dough and added fresh vegetables.

These honors and accolades have given Waters name recognition that assists in her promotion of her own ideas about the American diet and the importance of nutrition education for U.S. school children. Her Edible Schoolyard project came about after she spoke to a reporter about nutrition education during an interview in the 1990s. During their discussion, she called the lunchroom the most neglected room in the school. Waters told the reporter about a middle school she passed every day on her way to the restaurant and called it an example of the poor food choices children face.

School budget problems had forced the administration to close the cafeteria. Lunch was fast food from plastic containers, which the students ate while sitting on the schoolyard blacktop. After hearing her remarks, the school's principal contacted Waters and invited her to discuss possible solutions. The Edible Schoolyard project was the culmination of their efforts to take the principles of Waters' restaurant into the school's entire lunch program and curriculum. Thanks to donations and fundraising, the school eventually used the blacktop for a garden with fruit trees, berries, and vegetable gardens, and the cafeteria became a kitchen classroom.

Now, the Martin Luther King Jr. Middle School is a model for other schools across the country. The success of this first Edible Schoolyard evolved into Water's School Lunch Initiative project, which offers an entire curriculum based on including a healthy daily lunch and gardening experience into public schools across America. The School Lunch Initiative remains a public–private partnership between the Chez Panisse Foundation, the Berkeley Unified School District, and the Center for Ecoliteracy.

Waters continues to spread her dream of introducing school children to the pleasures of growing, harvesting, and cooking fresh vegetables. She speaks publically about her concern that American children are disconnected from their food. This disconnect, she said during a 2005 interview, was in direct contrast to what she had experienced in France. Water's called mealtime a rich, layered experience (Isenberg, 2005). She talked about important lessons she believes can be learned around the dinner table, including how to curb greed, how to practice patience and generosity through the sharing of food, and how to communicate and pay attention to others through conversation.

It has been suggested that only 15 percent of U.S. children sit down to eat a family meal. Studies have evaluated the relationship between family dinners and the incidence of overweight or obesity in U.S. children. Data revealed that the more frequently children ate dinner with their family, the less likely they were to be overweight. The results of a study published in the March 2010 issue of the journal *Pediatrics* said that preschoolers could reduce their risk of obesity by nearly 40 percent if they followed three basic lifestyle routines, which included more evening family meals, limited TV time, and more sleep. The study was funded by the Food Assistance and Nutrition Research Program within the U.S. Department of Agriculture's Economic Research Service.

Waters praised First Lady Michelle Obama who, in March 2009, assisted by a group of local fifth graders and Secretary of Agriculture Tom Vilsack, broke ground on the south lawn of the White House and planted an organic vegetable garden. It is over 1,000 square feet, and during the summer contained organic herbs, fruits, and vegetables.

Waters is also active in Slow Food International, a nonprofit organization that encourages and promotes local artisanal food. The organization lists over 100,000 members in some 130 countries. Waters has served as Vice President of the organization. Other honors and awards include being a corecipient, with Kofi Annan, of the Global Environmental Citizen Award in 2008. Waters was also inducted into the California Hall of Fame in 2008 and received a Lifetime Achievement Award as having one of *Restaurant* magazine's World's 50 Best Restaurants, in 2007.

The Chez Panisse Foundation named an Ambassador for the Edible Schoolyard program in 2010, Academy Award nominee and actor Jake Gyllenhaal. The actor has agreed to assist the foundation in raising awareness for the program and to encourage schools to include Edible Education.

Waters is not without critics who call her ideas elitist and impractical and say her attempts to prohibit junk food are too far reaching. Some have pointed out that people who are poor cannot afford, or even find, good organic food. Still, she remains a vocal supporter of slow food and sweeping changes in nutrition education, and she continues to gather celebrity endorsements. Members of the Edible Schoolyard Advisory Board include Mikhail Baryshnikov, Frances McDormand, Bette Midler, Chef Jamie Oliver, Robert Redford, and Meryl Streep.

*Sharon Zoumbaris*

*See also* National School Lunch Program (NSLP); Organic Food.

## References

Anderson, Sarah E., and Robert C. Whitaker. "Household Routines and Obesity in U.S. Preschool-Aged Children." *Pediatrics* 125, no. 3 (March 2010): 420–28.

Black, Jane. "Chef Alice Waters Awarded French Legion of Honor." *Washington Post.com.* August 13, 2009. http://voices.washingtonpost.com/all-we-can-eat/chefs-alice-waters-awarded-french-le.html.

Cutright, Courtney. "Middle School Site of Pilot Garden Spot." *Roanoke Times.* November 17, 2010. www.roanoke.com/news/roanoke/wb/267739.

Hendrick, Bill. "Study: Lifestyle Changes Reduce Childhood Obesity Risk by Nearly 40%." *WebMD.* www.webmd.com.

Isenberg, Barbara. "Go Natural: Chef Alice Waters Urges a Switch from Fast Food to a Fresh, Seasonal Cuisine." *Time* 166, no. 19 (November 7, 2005): F12.

Kaiser, Emily. "Reading, Writing & Winnowing Wheat: Thanks to World-Renown Chef Alice Waters, Kids in One California School Went from Eating Fast-Food Lunches on a Crumbling Blacktop to Growing and Preparing Their Own Fresh-Food Feasts." *Diabetes Forecast* 59, no. 7 (July 2006): 52.

"President of Chez Panisse Foundation and Larchmont School Launch Edible Schoolyard." *Pediatrics Week.* (November 28, 2009): 23.

Waters, Alice. "Eating for Credit." *The New York Times,* February 24, 2006: A23.

## WEIGHT TRAINING

Weight training is a form of exercise that uses specialized tools against the force of gravity to build strength and endurance in skeletal muscle. The equipment used in weight training includes dumbbells, kettle bells, heavy plates, weighted bars, weighted balls, and weight machines. Weight training should not be confused with strength training, a broader term that may include weight training but also encompasses the use of non-gravity-based resistance equipment. Examples of equipment not requiring gravity are handheld elastic resistance bands, elastic or spring-loaded resistance machines, and exercise machines that incorporate pneumatic (air) or hydraulic (water) tension to provide resistance.

Milo of Crotona has the honor of being the one of the first recorded weight lifters in history. He was a Greek Olympic champion during the sixth century BCE, who reportedly trained by placing a newborn calf on his shoulders and carrying it for a set distance every day. As the calf grew into a bull, so did Milo's strength, coincidentally providing a good example of the weight training principal called "Gradual Progressive Overload" (GPO). In the second century CE, the Greek physician Claudius Galenus, better known simply as Galen, treated and observed gladiators who were training for the arena. He mentions in his medical texts that these athletes would lift and carry "tabula plumb," which were heavy sheets of rock. They also trained with a pair of "halteres" to build muscular strength and endurance. Halteres were teardrop or C-shaped objects usually made of carved stone and typically weighing from 4 to 20 pounds. They can be seen in the hands of athletes painted on Grecian urns dated to that period, and actual examples of these ancient free weights are on view at the National Archaeological Museum in Athens.

English language texts on weight training first appeared in Europe in the 1500s, during a period of new interest in the science of systematic exercise. In Tudor England, bell ringing became a popular form of exercise, and gentlemen of that time trained their muscles by ringing church-bell apparatus with the sound clappers silenced. For those wondering where the term "dumbbells" may have originated, it is interesting to note this practice was called "the ringing of the dumb [meaning silent] bells." There is no mention of barbells as we know them in English language texts until the year 1828, when a German immigrant to America, physical educator Charles Beck, first described their use. They consisted of bags or hollow spheres filled with various amounts of sand or lead shot attached to each end of a heavy wooden beam.

Not long after, as weight training and calisthenics were promoted as part of the curriculum at men's and women's learning institutions in Europe and America, barbells and dumbbells began to be mass produced and sold to the public. By the beginning of the 20th century, Strongman shows featuring so-called awesome feats of strength were a common sight at traveling circuses. Even today, an old-style drawing of a well-muscled man holding a barbell overhead with one arm comes to mind for many of us when hearing the term "weight training."

With the fitness boom of the 1960s came a renewed interest in looking and feeling healthy. This led to the development of weight machines, which continue as a standard feature in modern day gyms and health clubs. Most weight machines are designed to target individual muscle groups. They help stabilize and isolate specific muscles and work to limit excessive or incorrect range of motion, holding users in the correct body position commonly called "good form." Weight machines are particularly useful for those just starting a weight lifting program.

By contrast, working with free weights requires the ability to align the body properly in relation to the weight to perform the exercises effectively and without injury. There are important advantages for those who master the correct use of free weights. Training with free weights engages the small stabilizer muscles that surround the main muscles being targeted. The result is an improvement in stabilization that helps eliminate muscle imbalances that can cause pain or injury. Free-weight training also calls on the trunk muscles to help control movement, which builds core strength. Additionally, free weight exercises that use multiple muscle groups, commonly referred to as "compound" training, have a higher energy requirement that assists with fat loss. And, free weights have the advantage of being relatively inexpensive and thus available for an individual to purchase and use at home.

Some of the primary principles for any type of fitness training include specificity, overload, progression, and reversibility. The principal of specificity states that the response to training will be specific to the type of training done. In other words, how a person exercises determines exactly what physical ability will change and what will not. One explanation for this is found in the various properties of skeletal muscle. Let us say Exerciser A selects a very heavy weight, so heavy that the individual can only complete five repetitions, or "reps" (lifting and lowering a weight one time is one rep), before total fatigue. Exerciser A will mainly be recruiting large high-threshold motor units in the muscles being worked. These motor units in Type II, or fast-twitch, muscle fibers are activated when great force or power is needed. The result is specific: Exerciser A is training muscles that can lift and hold very heavy loads for short durations.

Conversely, Exerciser B, identical in all other ways to Exerciser A, decides to pick up a moderately heavy weight and perform many reps. Exerciser B's training will mainly recruit the smaller low-threshold motor units in Type I, or slow-twitch, muscle fibers. Slow-twitch fibers have a higher resistance to fatigue and are called into play when the body needs stabilization and endurance. Slow-twitch fibers do not provide great bursts of power, but they do continue to function beyond the point of when fast-twitch fibers have fatigued and reached failure. Again, the results will be specific: Exerciser B is going to be better equipped than Exerciser A to endure a moderate weight load for an extended period of time before the muscles fail.

GPO encompasses both the overload principle and the progression principle. The overload principle states that the human body will not change unless a greater-than-normal stress or load is encountered. Weight training exercisers know overload is occurring when a given exercise becomes difficult or impossible by the last few reps. Hungarian Physician Hans Selye was the first researcher of record to correctly explain the science of biological stress behind the overload principle. In the 1920s, he wrote that all living tissue adapts to stress by increasing cellular activity. That cellular activity in turn forms barriers and strengthens surrounding tissue in order to better handle future stressors. Skeletal muscle being worked to failure develops microscopic tissue tears, leading to inflammation and swelling. The body's immune response then stimulates repairs that lead to muscle fiber growth and greater muscle strength.

The progression principle says the human body will eventually become accustomed to an increased work demand, so the load must be gradually and systematically increased over time to see continued improvement. The act of continuously overloading muscles during long-term training is called "progression" or, more definitively, "gradual progressive overload." Periodization describes exercise programming that will deliver safe and effective progression. Periodization training offers many formats depending on exercise goals, but general guidelines for every periodization-based program call for adequate rest for muscle repair between weight-training sessions, with 48 hours considered an average time for successful recovery, limiting weight increases to 10 percent per week, and periodically alternating those weight increases with other kinds of variations to the workout regimen. Workout variations are considered appropriate and necessary every 5 to 8 weeks, and options include altering the intensity, the movement, the speed, the reps, or the sets (a number of reps done continuously without rest). Well-designed periodization programs can be found in strength training manuals or can be custom designed by certified personal trainers to suit an individual exerciser's starting point and goals.

The principle of reversibility helps us understand the detraining that occurs when an individual completely stops a weight training program. Famed Greek physician Hippocrates, circa 400 BCE, wrote: "that which is used develops, and that which is not used wastes away." Put into modern jargon, we either use it or we lose it. While it is true that muscles must recover between training sessions, even in advanced workouts the rest period needed is seldom more than three or four days. Initial detraining effects begin after just two weeks, and more significant losses are seen as the time of inactivity increases. After five months, nearly complete detraining occurs.

Authors Wilmore and Costill note in their textbook *Physiology of Sport and Exercise* that losses in strength will be measurable after the first four weeks of detraining. However, loss of muscular endurance occurs much faster, typically within just two weeks. On average, after eight weeks of training inactivity about 10 percent of muscular strength is lost, and 30 percent to 40 percent of muscular endurance disappears. Note that the principle of reversibility does not apply to motor skills, like speed and agility, which are defined as sequential movements that combine to produce the smooth, efficient actions used to master tasks. A good example is the ability to ride a bicycle. Such motor skills are stored in long-term memory and remain available when needed.

The U.S. government set a public health goal that 30 percent of American adults would participate in strength-training at least twice weekly by the year 2010. Government figures published in 2007 from the Centers for Disease Control and

Prevention (CDC) show strength training was on an increase between 1998 and 2004. The findings showed a significant increase in Americans who participated in twice weekly strength training sessions, from 17.7 percent in 1998 to 19.6 percent overall by 2004. Still, with less than 20 percent of Americans strength training in 2004, it is unlikely the 2010 goal has been reached. Findings from the same report noted that some racial/ethnic/gender groups had a much lower prevalence of strength training than others. Most notably, strength training was consistently lower among Hispanic male respondents than among non-Hispanic white male respondents. Likewise, strength training was significantly lower among Hispanic women, non-Hispanic black women, and those women classified as "other" when compared to non-Hispanic white women.

Women under age 65 showed twice-weekly workout participation increasing from 14.5 percent in 1998 to 17.5 percent in 2004. By comparison, men under age 65 reported twice-weekly workout sessions at 21.9 percent, but no significant increase in participants over time. Men and women age 65 and older involved in training by 2004 showed the lowest level of overall participants; only 14.1 percent for men and 10.7 percent for women. However, the prevalence of strength training increased significantly between 1998 and 2004 in this group. For older men, participation rose from 11.0 percent in 1998 to 14.1 percent in 2004, and for older women, it rose from 6.8 percent to 10.7 percent.

As we age, a natural loss of muscle mass (*sarcopenia*) and a loss of bone mass (osteoporosis) takes place. The increase in participation noted in older adults is likely a reflection of published results showing these losses could be minimized with strength training. Osteoporosis is an all-too-common disease in women. The leading cause is the gradual loss of estrogen that occurs at menopause. Persons with osteoporosis can become severely disabled due to weakened bones. In particular, hip fractures often lead to the inability to walk independently and are one of the leading causes of admittance to nursing homes. Research showing that osteopenia (low bone mineral density) and osteoporosis (thin bone disease) could be counteracted by weight training reportedly spurred many young adult women to begin a training program.

Some of the common myths that surround weight training include loss of flexibility, the development of bulging muscles in women, and stunted growth in youth. It is true that training incorrectly can lead to a loss of flexibility. Incorporating a full range of motion is important in all resistance work since muscles will strengthen only at the specific joint angle where the work is taking place. Weight training exercises concentrated in only one portion of the muscle instead of using the full range of motion possible, or exercises that favor one muscle group at the expense of the opposing stabilizer muscle group, create short, tight muscles and strength imbalances. Loss of flexibility can be eliminated by following proper training techniques.

Weight training itself does not create hypertrophy (enlargement) of muscle, although specific programs can certainly be designed toward that goal. However, compared to men most women lack the amount of muscle fiber and testosterone (one of the male hormones responsible for hypertrophy) necessary to visually increase muscle size. Because of this, the majority of women who lift weights will increase in strength and endurance without adding bulk. Conversely, weight training promotes a boost to the metabolic system, and women who add weight training to their fitness regimen are likely to see a lithe and toned body as the result.

Weight training has never been shown to stunt growth, but there has been a concern that weight training in children and adolescents might affect the epiphyses (growth plates) in long bones, which are not fully established until adulthood and contain cartilage rather than bone. So while youth are susceptible to epiphyseal fractures, research has shown no greater risk from weight training when using the same safety guidelines of proper form and gradual progression followed by adults. In fact, the most commonly reported injury in young exercisers is low back pain. In a 1996 study of male teenage athletes, 50 percent of reported injuries during weight lifting involved the low back. Attempting to lift very heavy weights, or neglecting to create muscular balance by not including exercises for opposing stabilizer muscle groups, were the reported causes.

Today, weight training is widely considered an important form of exercise that can be used to meet health-related fitness goals. Weight training increases muscle, tendon, and ligament strength, and research shows that weight training provides many corresponding physical benefits. These include a greater physical capacity, a healthy physical appearance, a revved up metabolism, a reduction in injury risk, and good bone health.

*Janice H. Hoffman*

*See also* Back Pain; Exercise; Osteoporosis; Personal Trainer.

### References

CDC (Centers for Disease Control and Prevention). "Trends in Strength Training—United States, 1998–2004." *MMWR Weekly* 55 (28) (July 21, 2006): 769–72.

Delaviere, Frederic, and Michael Gundill. *The Strength Training Anatomy Workout.* Champaign, IL: Human Kinetics, 2011.

Kujala, Urho M., Simo Taimela, Minna Erkintalo, Jouko Salminen, and Jaakko Kaprio. "Low-back Pain in Adolescent Athletes." *Medicine & Science in Sports & Exercise* 28, no. 2 (1996): 165–70.

Maffetone, Philip. *The Big Book of Endurance Training and Racing.* New York: Skyhorse, 2010.

National Strength and Conditioning Association. *Strength Training,* by Lee E. Brown, ed. Champaign, IL: Human Kinetics, 2007.

Rollin, Charles, and Robert Lynam. *The Ancient History of the Egyptians, Carthaginians, Assyrians, Babylonians, Medes and Persians, Grecians and Macedonians.* Vol 3. Philadelphia, PA: Brown and Peters, 1829.

Sandler, David. *Fundamental Weight Training.* Champaign, IL: Human Kinetics, 2010.

Selye, Hans. "A Syndrome Produced by Diverse Nocuous Agents." *Nature* 138 (July 4, 1936): 32.

Todd, Jan. "From Milo to Milo: A History of Barbells, Dumbbells, and Indian Clubs." *Iron Game History* 3, no. 6 (1995): 4–16.

Wilmore, Jack H., David L. Costill, and W. Larry Kenny. *Physiology of Sport and Exercise.* Champaign, IL: Human Kinetics, 2008.

## WEIGHT WATCHERS

Weight Watchers is one of the best-known weight-loss support organizations in the world. It operates through a network of company-owned and franchise operations as well as an online website that offers subscription weight-management products over the Internet. Weight Watchers helps people lose weight at a moderate pace and keep it off with a program that offers a healthy food plan, exercise, and behavior modification in a group support environment.

Weight Watchers sells its products along with publications and programs for individuals and groups interested in weight loss and weight management, both online and in stores and retail shops. The company announced new test sites in the Tampa Bay area and in St. Louis, Missouri, as well as in four other Florida locations. Weight Watcher shops operate during regular business hours, nights, and weekends.

The dieting program now appeals to men in increasing numbers, with male membership up 5 percent in the past decade (Wells, 2010). However, its bread and butter in terms of membership has been and will continue to be women, many of whom are drawn to the organization thanks to famous spokespeople, including singer and actress Jennifer Hudson and Sarah Ferguson, the Duchess of York.

Weight Watchers was started by founder Jean Nidetch in 1961. At the time Nidetch, a 200-plus-pound New Yorker, had met with friends to talk about effective weight loss and provide each other with moral support. With the support of other overweight friends, Nidetch lost 72 pounds, and the organization was formally launched in 1963. Since then, the organization has enrolled millions of members worldwide. In 1978, Weight Watchers was purchased by H.J. Heinz, and 20 years later it was purchased by Luxembourg's Artal Group. In November 2001, the company went public and was listed on the New York Stock Exchange.

New business ventures for Weight Watchers include a spring 2010 deal with McDonald's, New Zealand, to offer meals that will appeal to dieters. The partnership between the two is being called a healthy option for New Zealanders by McDonald's (Clemons, 2010), who say people can now choose from Weight-Watcher-approved items including McDonald's Filet-O-Fish and Chicken McNuggets, which will be teamed with a salad or side salad, water, or a diet drink. The meals will carry a Weight Watchers point value of 6.5.

Weight Watchers offers the Points weight-loss system that includes the Daily Points Range. The Daily Points Range is assigned based on the amount of weight needed to lose. Rather than measure portion size or count calories, points are easier to track and accomplish much the same. Stay within the Daily Points Range and you'll lose weight. For example, a scoop of ice cream is 4 points; a bottle of beer is 3 points, a slice of pizza is 9 points, and a cup of grapes is 1 point. Weight Watchers members are encouraged to eat the daily allowance of food points and are told not to go below the Daily Points Range in an effort to speed up weight loss. People can, however, "earn" extra points by stepping up their physical activity level.

An adult who wants to lose at least 5 pounds can join Weight Watchers. Weight Watchers stresses that it does not market to teens. Members who join can choose to start with a preliminary goal to lose 10 percent of their body weight. For example, a person who weighs 200 pounds and has perhaps been struggling and yo-yo dieting for years to try to reach 150 pounds may quickly find herself or himself disappointed. With the 10 percent goal, the person would reach the first goal at 180 pounds—a weight loss of 20 pounds. That builds up confidence in ability to lose weight. Then he or she can set the next goal.

Weight Watchers is not a quick-fix diet scheme. On its website (www.weight-watchers.com), it states that the organization promotes a "healthy rate of weight loss—up to two pounds per week after the first three weeks." The organization produces a bimonthly magazine and numerous cookbooks and inspirational books for those trying to lose weight and maintain that weight loss. Weekly meetings are key to the concept of Weight Watchers.

The Weight Watchers website states, "preliminary scientific research shows that people who regularly attend Weight Watchers meetings lose more weight than people who try to lose weight on their own. Weight Watchers Leaders, who have all risen through the ranks as Weight Watchers meeting members and learned how to lose and successfully control their weight, lead meetings that follow a weekly curriculum. Their experience, techniques, and suggestions for solving problems can help you do what you're having trouble doing on your own: lose weight."

The organization closely guards its reputation and filed a large lawsuit against rival weight-loss program Jenny Craig in January 2010, when an advertisement implied that Jenny Craig members had lost twice as much weight as an unnamed rival. Weight Watchers took Jenny Craig to federal court over the advertisement. The two weight loss giants battled in court until a federal judge ruled in February of 2010 that the Jenny Craig ad represented false advertising and was unfair and deceptive competition ("Jenny Craig," 2010). The ad had featured actress Valerie Bertinelli, who had claimed that clinical trials showed Jenny Craig users lost twice as much weight as others using other products. Weight Watcher officials had charged that Jenny Craig did not conduct a major clinical trial comparing the two company's products but instead relied on outdated studies to support its claims.

Weight Watchers meeting members are also encouraged to share their weight-loss challenges and to celebrate their weight-loss victories at meetings "knowing that others are facing the same issues you're facing and hearing firsthand how they've solved or are working to solve similar problems can help keep you motivated and inspire you to stay the course."

For those who cannot join weekly meetings, Weight Watchers for years has offered its brand of online support through an Internet-based journal for tracking daily points, an online newsletter, and other support.

Weight Watchers generally receives good ratings from nutritionists because its emphasis is on moderate fat and balanced nutrients. The website contains an FAQ section, success stories, and a search engine that allows a user to find the closest Weight Watchers meetings. Membership charges and special promotions are listed on the local group's contact information.

*Marjolijn Bijlefeld and Sharon Zoumbaris*

*See also* Dieting; Dieting, Online Resources; Yo-Yo Dieting.

## References

Clemons, Rachel. "Marketing Ploy or the Real McCoy? McDonald's Serves up Meals for Waist Watchers." *Choice* (Chippendale, Australia) (May 2010): 7.

Ferguson, Sarah, ed. *Reinventing Yourself with the Duchess of York: Inspiring Stories and Strategies.* New York: Simon and Schuster, 2001.

Ferguson, Sarah, Duchess of York with Weight Watchers. *Energy Breakthrough: Jump-Start Your Weight Loss and Feel Great.* New York: Simon and Schuster, 2002.

Fletcher, Anne M. "Inside America's Hottest Diet Programs." *Prevention,* March 1990, 54.

Frascella, Larry. "An Exclusive Visit with Jean Nidetch." *Weight Watchers Magazine,* January 1988, 37.

Heshka, Stanley, James W. Anderson, Richard L. Atkinson, Frank L. Greenway, and James O. Hill. "Jennifer Hudson Promotes Weight Watcher's Lose for Good Campaign." *Thai Press Reports,* September 20, 2010.

"Jenny Craig, Weight Watchers Settle Suit. *The Recorder,* February 9, 2010.

Miller, Holly G. "Hips, Hips Away!" *Saturday Evening Post,* November 1988, 48.

Neal, Mollie. "Weight Watchers' Winning Marketing Strategy." *Direct Marketing,* August 1993.

Nidetch, Jean. *Story of Weight Watchers.* New York: New American Library, 1979.

"Sales Barb Yields Lawsuit." *Business Insurance* 44, no. 4 (January 25, 2010): 23.

Tisdale, Sallie. "A Weight that Women Carry: The Compulsion to Diet in a Starved Culture." *Harper's Magazine,* March 1993, 49.

"Weight Watchers Shops around New Concept." *The St. Petersburg Times,* September 11, 2010, 10.

Wells, Jeff. "Men Weight In." *Supermarket News* (September 1, 2010). http://supermarket news.com/health_wellness/men-weigh-in-0910.

## WHITE, RYAN

Ryan White was a 13-year-old teenager, living in Indiana in the 1980s. By the time of his death in 1990, he had become the human face of acquired immune deficiency syndrome, or AIDS, a disease at the time thought to affect only gay men and intravenous drug users. White, a hemophiliac, got the virus from infected blood he routinely received as treatment for his disease. When Indiana school officials learned of his illness, he was banned from attending classes in his neighborhood public school.

The fear and anxiety about AIDS in those early days of White's illness was very potent, and people with the disease were forced from their homes, fired from their jobs, and stripped of their health insurance. Personally for White, the diagnosis meant that school administrators, teachers, parents, and some students shunned him, fearful that they would somehow catch the disease through casual contact.

White eventually returned to public school, and his experiences convinced him he could help others through his celebrity. He and his mother turned to activism to improve care for those suffering from the disease, and the teen was quickly embraced as a national spokesperson for AIDS. The White's were eventually successful in their efforts, and in 1990 Congress passed and the President signed the Ryan White Comprehensive AIDS Resource Emergency Care (CARE) Act, a bill that provided health care resources to Americans with AIDS or human immunodeficiency virus (HIV).

The CARE Act is the largest federally funded program created to provide HIV/AIDS-related medical, psychological, and social services, and although it has been amended over the years, it still provides services for those who do not qualify for Medicare, Medicaid, or other insurance coverage for treatment of HIV/AIDS.

The legislation was set to expire in 2006, making it necessary for Congress to pass and for President George W. Bush to sign the Ryan White HIV/AIDS Treatment Modernization Act of 2006 into law. The legislation officially reauthorized the CARE act until 2009. In 2009, Congress passed, and President Barack Obama signed, the Ryan White HIV/AIDS Treatment Extension Act, which now extends the program for an additional four years.

The program is administered by the U.S. Department of Health and Human Services (HHS), Health Resources and Services Administration (HRSA), and the HIV/AIDS Bureau (HAB). Government figures show that an estimated 529,000 people are served each year through the program, with the majority of funds going to support primary medical care and essential support services (HRSA, 2010). A small portion of the over $2 billion budget also goes toward research and clinical training.

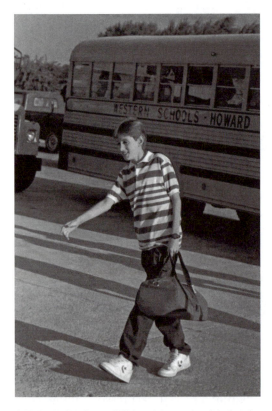

AIDS victim Ryan White, 14, carries his books from the bus on the first day of school at Western High School in Kokomo, Indiana, on August 25, 1986. After his diagnosis, White fought for the right to attend public school. People thought the disease was easily transmitted and they feared their children would catch it from drinking fountains or other casual contact. (AP/Wide World Photos)

However, in the early years of the epidemic, the U.S. government was slow to act, and there was little support for research or treatment. Epidemiologist Donald Francis, working with the Centers for Disease Control and Prevention (CDC) in Atlanta in the early 1980s, lobbied unsuccessfully for $30 million in funding for an AIDS-prevention campaign. He quit the CDC soon after (Jefferson, 2006).

Statistics from the CDC estimate more than 1 million people are living with HIV in the United States. Despite increases in the total number of Americans living with HIV in recent years, the annual number of new infections has remained stable. Still, the CDC's most recent figures estimate some 56,000 people in the United States become infected with HIV each year, and more than 18,000 people with AIDS die each year (CDC, 2008). "AIDS" is the term used to describe the multiple symptoms caused by infection with the human immunodeficiency virus, or HIV.

White was born in December of 1971 and diagnosed with hemophilia as an infant. Hemophilia is an inherited disease and was considered a life-threatening condition until researchers discovered that blood infusions with a clotting compound could control the sometimes uncontrollable bleeding. White received two or three infusions a month, and he and his family were managing his disease when in 1984 he became ill and began to lose weight. Doctors determined he had AIDS, which they suspected he had received from contaminated blood products. At that time, blood and blood products were not being screened for AIDS.

White developed a form of pneumonia common to AIDS patients and was hospitalized until the spring of 1985. During his illness he had kept up with his school work, but he wanted to return to school to be with his friends.

At that point, parents and school administrators joined together, and the teen was banned from returning to school. His mother went to court, and six months later the Whites were successful—Ryan went back to the school. That lasted just one day, as worried parents were again able to have him barred. The court battle continued until a judge ruled White could attend high school if he used a separate bathroom, disposable utensils in the cafeteria, and if he avoided gym class.

Although the legal battle was eventually won by the Whites, the reaction from townspeople left the family ostracized and frightened by threats and harsh treatment. The family decided to move to a nearby small town, and although medical bills had created a difficult financial situation, the proceeds from a television movie about White's battle with the disease helped finance their move. The residents of that town extended a sympathetic welcome, and at the same time White began to respond positively to the experimental drug AZT. AZT, or azidothymidine, is a drug used to delay development of AIDS in patients infected with HIV, and in 1987 it was the first drug approved by the Food and Drug Administration (FDA) for treatment of AIDS patients.

At age 16, White was invited to testify before the President's Commission on AIDS. He described his experiences with people who feared catching the disease from him, and he also shared information about his family's financial problems, caused by his illness. White told the hearing he hoped others would not have to suffer as he had, even if they had the same deadly disease.

White continued to live a normal life until his senior year, when he developed several serious health problems related to his AIDS. The 18-year-old White died from complications on April 8, 1990, and over 1,500 people attended his funeral in Indianapolis. In his autobiography, *Ryan White: My Own Story,* he described his desire to live a normal life rather than be a permanent invalid. White inspired celebrities like singer Elton John and Indiana native Michael Jackson with his courage and determination, and they in turn supported his work as an AIDS activist. At White's funeral, Elton John led the congregation in singing a hymn and then performed a song he wrote in White's honor.

*Sharon Zoumbaris*

*See also* Acquired Immune Deficiency Syndrome (AIDS); Health Insurance; Human Immunodeficiency Virus (HIV); U.S. Department of Health and Human Services (HHS).

### References

CDC (Centers for Disease Control and Prevention). "HIV in the United States." *MMWR* 57 no. 39 (2008): 1073–76.

CDC (Centers for Disease Control and Prevention). "HIV Prevention in the United States at a Critical Crossroads." 2009. www.cdc.gov/hiv/resources/reports/hiv_prev_us.htm.

HRSA (Health Resources and Services Administration). "Ryan White HIV/AIDS Program Overview." August 2010. http://hab.hrsa.gov/aboutthab/aboutprogram.html.

Huber, Joseph H. "Pediatric AIDS: A New Professional Challenge." *Palaestra* (Spring 1991): 64. www.palaestra.com.

Jefferson, David. "How AIDS Changed America; The Plague Years: It Brought out the Worst in Us at First, but Ultimately it Brought out the Best, and Transformed the Nation. The Story of a Disease that Left an Indelible Mark on Our History, Our Culture and Our Souls." *Newsweek,* May 15, 2006, 36.

Johnson, Dirk. "Ryan White Dies of AIDS at 18; His Struggle Helped Pierce Myths." *The New York Times* (April 9, 1990). www.nytimes.com/1990/04/09/obituaries/ryan-white-dies-of-aids-at-18-his-struggle-helped-pierce-myths.html?pagewarted=all&src=pm.

Sidewater, Nancy. "The Boy Next Door: Ten Years ago, Ryan White Succumbed to AIDS after a Lengthy Struggle that Moved the Nation." *Entertainment Weekly* (April 14, 2000): 80. www.ew.com/ew/article/0,,275882,00.html.

## WOMEN'S HEALTH INITIATIVE (WHI)

The Women's Health Initiative (WHI) is considered the premier national health study examining some specific diseases in older women as well as their causes and cures. The results have given women and their doctor's new information about hormone therapy, diet and its relationship to disease, vitamin supplementation, and the effects of some specific lifestyle choices on women's health.

Launched in 1991, this 15-year project sponsored by the National Institutes of Health (NIH) along with the National Heart, Lung and Blood Institute (NHLBI) has involved over 100,000 women and millions of dollars as researchers studied strategies for preventing breast and colorectal cancer, heart disease, and fractures due to osteoporosis in postmenopausal women. According to the government, these diseases account for the majority of death, disability, and poor quality of life in U.S. women of all ethnicities.

There are three parts to the WHI, a randomized clinical trial (CT), an observational study (OS), and a community prevention study (CPS). Women enrolled in the WHI study had the option of enrolling in one, two, or all three parts as well as choosing one, two, or all three of the major clinical trials. Those three main trials were hormone therapy trial (HT), dietary modification trial (DM), and calcium/ vitamin D trial (CaD).

The first trial, HT, looked at the effects of combined hormones, or estrogen, alone on the prevention of heart disease and osteoporotic fractures along with any associated risk for breast cancer. Participants in this trial were given hormone pills or a placebo, but this study was halted in 2002 when researchers noticed increased risks of heart disease and breast cancer in the women taking the study pills compared with those taking the placebo pills. After the trial was halted, researchers continued to gather data from the women and then used that information to evaluate the effects of stopping hormone therapy.

The second trial, DM, evaluated the effect of a low-fat and high vegetable, fruit, and grain diet and any role it might have in the prevention of colorectal and breast cancer or coronary heart disease. Study participants were asked to follow their usual diet or a specific low-fat diet.

The third trial, CaD, looked at the effect of calcium and vitamin D supplements on the possible prevention of fractures in women with osteoporosis or the prevention of colorectal cancer. The women in this trial were given a placebo or took calcium and vitamin D pills.

The second portion of the WHI, the observational study, or OS, was designed to evaluate the relationship between health, lifestyle, risk factors, and how that would or would not change disease outcomes. Researchers followed the medical history and health habits of over 93,000 women for up to a dozen years to gather that data. The last component, the community prevention study (CPS), was a cooperative effort with the Centers for Disease Control and Prevention (CDC) that lasted for five years, with the goal of putting in place community-based public health intervention models that would assist women over age 40 incorporate healthful behaviors into their lifestyles.

In its efforts to add to the body of research on women's health issues, the WHI research is now posted on the WHI website (www.whi.org). The site connects users directly to the results of the studies, with links to the journals where the findings were published. For example, there is the link to the Estrogen Plus Progestin and Breast Cancer study, as well as a link to *The New England Journal of Medicine,* where it was published. Those results revealed that women who stopped taking estrogen plus progestin hormones showed a decreased risk of breast cancer. Dietary study findings include "Low-Fat Dietary Pattern and Risk of Treated Diabetes Mellitus in Postmenopausal Women." The calcium and vitamin D results include "Calcium/Vitamin D Supplementation in the Prevention of Weight Gain in Postmenopausal Women."

*Sharon Zoumbaris*

*See also* Cancer; National Institutes of Health (NIH); Osteoporosis.

### References

Hawkins, Joellen Watson, and Lois A. Haggerty. *Diversity in Health Care Research: Strategies for Multisite, Multidisciplinary, and Multicultural Projects.* New York: Springer Publishing, 2003.

"Highlights of NIH Women's Health and Sex Differences Research: 1990–2010." *National Institutes of Health (NIH).* Bethesda, MD: Office of Research on Women's Health; NIH Coordinating Committee on Research on Women's Health, 2010.

Minikin, Mary Jane, and Carol V. Wright. *A Woman's Guide to Menopause & Perimenopause.* New Haven, CT: Yale University Press, 2005.

Women's Health Initiative. "Participant Website." n.d. www.whi.org.

Women's Health Initiative. "WHI Background and Overview." n.d. www.nhlbi.nih.gov/whi/background.htm.

## WORKPLACE WELLNESS

Wellness has moved up in the world. Stock in wellness is rising, fueled by concerns about rising health costs and the realization by companies that having a healthy workforce not only benefits their workers but also their bottom lines.

There's been a shift from viewing wellness as a soft benefit, a feel-good benefit, to recognizing it as part of the organization's overall health care strategy. Savvy organizations have come to realize that, effectively managed, a healthy workforce is a competitive advantage in a tough market. They've also come to realize that the payoff for their investment won't be years down the road but more immediately, because a healthier workforce is a more productive one.

It's certainly no secret that for the past two decades spending on health insurance has significantly outpaced both workers' earnings and the rate of inflation. In 2009, companies were expected to spend, on average, $9,660 per employee for health benefits, an increase of 6 percent from 2008 (Perrin, 2008). If food prices had risen at the same rates as medical inflation since the 1930s, we would be paying $80.20 for a dozen eggs and $107.90 for a dozen oranges (Powell, 2002).

Everyone is concerned about health care costs, employee and employer alike. The Congressional Budget Office (CBO) has gone so far as to call the rising costs of health care and health insurance "a serious threat to the future fiscal condition" of the United States (CBO, 2008).

**Absenteeism and Presenteeism** In addition to ever-higher medical costs, employers must cope with the high cost of absent workers. Absenteeism is linked to as much as 36 percent of payroll, or more than twice the cost of health care (Mercer and Kronos Incorporated, 2008). The 300 largest employers in the United States estimated that unscheduled absenteeism costs their businesses, on average, more than $760,000 per year in direct payroll costs (CCH, Inc., 2007).

The cost of absence can be far greater than only wage replacement payments for lost time. Dr. Thomas Parry, president of Integrated Benefits Institute in San Francisco, notes that a company also bears "the opportunity costs associated with how it manages those absences—additional staff to have workers in reserve, the use of overtime or temporary help; the impact on the work performance of other team members or revenue lost through production shortfalls."

Smart employers have learned to measure not just the cost of absenteeism but also the productivity cost of *presenteeism*—which occurs when an underperforming worker is present but distracted, for example, by physical or mental illness. Presenteeism accounts for 61 percent of an employee's total lost productivity and medical costs (Goetzel et al., 2004).

But there is hope. The health care costs of people with chronic diseases such as diabetes and cardiovascular disease accounts for more than 75 percent of the medical care costs in the United States (Aldana et al., 2006). That means that there's much that individuals, with the help of their employers, can do to bring these costs down by making healthy lifestyle changes.

**Hard Numbers** Organizations are searching for proof that wellness programs can reduce health-related costs and help improve the bottom line. Academics, company wellness professionals, and consultants have compiled a wealth of proof.

Watson Wyatt's 2007 "Staying @ Work Report" has some impressive numbers to offer: employers with the most effective health management programs achieved 20 percent more revenue per employee, had 16.1 percent higher market value, and delivered 57 percent higher shareholder returns (Towers Watson, 2008).

Dr. D. W. Edington, director of the University of Michigan Health Management Research Center, has done extensive research on the effect of risk factors such as high cholesterol, obesity, and tobacco use on health costs. He finds that costs increase as the number of dangerous risk combinations increases. "However, wellness interventions designed to shift a high-risk individual into a lower-risk category can save as much as $4,078 in annual costs," notes Edington. The earlier people engage in changing their health status, the sooner risks are minimized and health-care costs are reduced, according to Edington. His research also shows that employee productivity decreases as health risks increase (Edington, 2001).

Larry Chapman, senior vice president of WebMD Health Services, and a trustee of the National Wellness Institute, has conducted an evaluation of 56 peer-reviewed journal articles on worksite health-promotion programs. Chapman found such programs produced an average 26.1 percent reduction in health costs, an average 26.8 percent reduction in sick-leave absenteeism, and an average 32 percent reduction in workers' compensation and disability management claims costs. He also measured an average $5.81 savings for every dollar invested.

Return on investment (ROI) is a key measure in the business world. In the wellness world, ROI is usually measured by determining the ratio of medical expenses not incurred to the total costs of wellness, including incentives paid to employees to participate. One commonly cited ROI range is 1.5:1 to 3:1 after three to five years, meaning that for every dollar invested in wellness, employers saved or can expect to save between $1.50 and $3 (Wells, 2008).

Experts warn against dazzling ROI claims that purport to show many dollars saved in a short period of time, but they say a well-designed, well-implemented program can positively affect health care and health-related costs. One analyst says that while in the first year you should expect a net investment rather than a return, it's possible to start seeing a return on your investment in the second year and more likely in three to five years.

A 3-to-1 return specifically on health care costs is the rule of thumb, but that doesn't look at other productivity factors that are estimated to be 3 to 10 times the direct medical costs. Even taking the conservative estimate, it's a significant return, according to one prominent analyst, David Anderson, senior vice president and chief health officer of StayWell Health Management, St. Paul, Minnesota.

The Health Project, a private–public organization formed to bring about behavioral changes in the American health care system, carefully tracks the success of its C. Everett Koop Award winners:

- For every dollar Motorola invested in wellness benefits, the company saved $3.93. In 2000, that meant a $6,479,673 savings in the United States. The company and employees saved approximately $6.5 million a year for lifestyle-related diagnoses such as obesity, hypertension, and stress.
- The Pepsi Bottling Group reported a return on investment of $1.70 for every dollar spent. Annual medical savings were estimated as averaging $264 per participant.
- USAA reported that workplace absences have decreased, with an estimated three-year savings of more than $105 million.
- The UAW-GM LifeSteps Health Promotion Program reported medical savings of $97 per participant per year and a disability/absence savings of $240 per participant per year.

**ROI Models**  It's often difficult to measure the ROI of a wellness program, but several nonprofit organizations are offering models to help you get started. Wellness Council of America (WELCOA) offers a free ROI calculator at Wellsteps.com. To use WELCOA's calculator, you'll need your company's total health care costs over the past year, the total number of employees receiving benefits, and the percentage change in health care costs per year for the past five years.

The calculator can show the cost of doing nothing—what will happen to your health care costs over the next few years if you make no changes, based on health care cost increases continuing as they have. Second, the calculator can project about how much money you could save if you decreased the percentage of workers who smoke or who are obese. Finally, the calculator can project what you would save on employee costs after implementing a low-, medium-, or high-intensity wellness program, according to WELCOA (Adams, 2008).

The Alliance for Wellness ROI Inc., which is working to standardize wellness programs so that return on investment can be objectively measured, is launching an ROI valuation modeler that will be able to calculate an estimated ROI for your company's wellness program, including individual components as well as aggregate program costs, compared to other companies.

The Corporate Executive Board also offers tools to estimate the returns you can expect from wellness, according to Michal Kisilevitz, who leads The Corporate Executive Board's benefits roundtable. "You used to be able to get away with 'Trust me. It will have an impact,'" she says. "But now a lot of our members feel that pressure to demonstrate returns. They hear, 'Make the case and convince me.'" It's initially difficult to show the value of wellness, she adds, because "if you do it well you are avoiding cost, not reducing costs. But over time you will see a reduction in cost because you won't have as many people sick."

Mary Liz Murphy, head of LifeForce Solutions Inc., sees a shift from measuring ROI to measuring "value on investment." It's a more meaningful measurement, according to Murphy, who is also project leader for the Conference Board's research working group "The Wellness Advantage." "Value on investment looks not only at financial indicators but also at participation indicators, screening indicators such as getting mammograms, health-risk indicators, clinical indicators, and utilization indicators," she says.

It's more challenging to add productivity indicators and shareholder value indicators, Murphy says, but researchers are in the frontier stages of research in those areas. With all of these indicators, you can better assess if what you're doing is working or not, she says, and if you are meeting the expectations of the different stakeholders—the CEO, the COO, shareholders, employees.

**The Bottom Line**   Health care insurance isn't likely to get cheaper. Productivity isn't going to become any less important in this competitive climate. But the experience of workplace experts and a review of literature that examines the business rationale for worksite health promotion shows that when properly designed, a wellness program can increase employees' health and productivity (Goetzel & Ozminkowski, 2009).

Now is the time to look at the numbers, to look at the potential payoff, and to implement a well-thought-out wellness strategy that truly benefits the bottom line. To execute that successful wellness strategy, you'll need a champion at the top. Profile: Union Pacific Tracks Wellness Results (www.up.com).

Union Pacific Corporation sees a substantial payoff for its wellness initiative because it identifies its workers' most serious health risks, designs effective programs to reduce those risks, and tracks the results of its efforts. Barb Schaefer, senior vice president, human resources, is adamant that "healthier employees who make good, informed decisions about their medical care help hold down rising health care costs" (Union Pacific, 2005).

Her motto is "An ounce of prevention is worth a pound of cure," because working on the railroad can be physically demanding for the mostly older workforce, some of whom are on call 24 hours a day. Fatigue is a chronic hazard. The prevention has plenty of time to pay off—the average employee stays more than 30 years with the company.

Union Pacific has had plenty of time to hone its wellness initiative; it started the program back in 1987. Today, the "HealthTrack" program has four main components: employee assessment, analysis of the assessment results, targeted interventions, and periodic follow-ups. After evaluating the data, the Union Pacific health-promotion program seeks to raise awareness and control 10 targeted risk factors: alcohol consumption, blood glucose, blood pressure, cholesterol, nutrition, fitness, mental health, tobacco use, stress, and weight.

Over the years, Union Pacific has earned many honors for its efforts, including the WELCOA Well Workplace Platinum Award. WELCOA praises Union Pacific for "the most sophisticated approach available for supporting employee behavior change and affecting positive health and productivity outcomes. Instead of shooting from the hip, blindly hoping to help their population, UP uses assessment to develop the specific goals for Health Track. After gathering and evaluating this information, they are poised to implement targeted interventions designed to effectively reduce risk factors" (WELCOA, 2001).

The results, according to WELCOA, include the following:

- Blood pressure interventions have yielded a ratio of $4.29 saved for every $1 spent.
- Cholesterol interventions have yielded a ratio of $5.25 to $1.
- Smoking cessation interventions have yielded a ratio of $2.24 to $1.

The net effect of these interventions has been a cost ratio of $3.24 to every $1 invested, WELCOA notes, which is "highly significant when you consider that prior claims analyses have revealed that unhealthy behaviors cost approximately 40 million dollars per year during the 1990s" (Union Pacific, 2000).

**Linking Safety and Health**   Union Pacific coordinates safety, productivity, and health care costs, says Jackie Austad, general director of health promotion and wellness, because "studies correlate health risks with safety. If you can improve health risks, the probability of injury goes down."

These studies show that stress, depression, fatigue, obesity, diabetes, and high blood pressure "significantly increase the likelihood of injury," she says. "We're trying to decrease the number of health risks, so we're confident we will get a corresponding decrease in costs. The goal is to make people healthier, to get that improvement to the bottom line."

The biggest challenge at Union Pacific now is weight, according to Austad. "It's the biggest health risk, and it impacts so many other health risks, such as cholesterol, blood pressure and diabetes. If we can improve weight, we can improve health in general."

To win the battle against the bulge, the company has given employees free access to more than 525 fitness centers system-wide, as well as a fitness facility at headquarters in Omaha, Nebraska. The Union Pacific Center also houses a dining room that features healthy cuisine. The company is proud to point out that

25 percent of sales are generated through the salad bar offerings. Even the vending machines offer healthy snack alternatives.

As the largest railroad in North America, Union Pacific has a lot of ground to cover to make sure its health message is communicated to its 50,000 employees in 23 states. A network of on-site regional health coordinators and occupational health nurses conduct health screenings and health fairs.

The unions are committed to improving employee health, says Austad. So is senior management. Union Pacific declared health and welfare one of its eight "Big Financial Deals" for the years 2001–2006, putting health on the same level as fuel costs and business in Mexico. Everyone wants "employees going home in as good or better shape than they came to work," she says.

*Stephenie Overman*

*See also* Blood Pressure; Fatigue; Health Insurance; Obesity; Stress.

## References

Adams, Troy. "The ROI Calculator." *WELCOA's Absolute Advantage* 7 no. 5 (2008): 28–33.

Aldana, Steven G., Roger L. Greenlaw, Audrey Salberg, Hans A. Diehl, Ray M. Merrill, Camille Thomas, and Seiga Ohmine. "The Behavioral and Clinical Effects of Therapeutic Lifestyle Change on Middle-aged Adults." *Centers for Disease Control and Prevention* 3, no. 1 (2006): A05.

CBO (Congressional Budget Office). *Key Issues in Analyzing Major Health Insurance Proposals.* Summary. December 2008.

CCH Inc. *Unscheduled Absence Survey.* 2007. www.cch.com/press/news/2007/20071010h.asp.

Edington, D.W. "Emerging Research: A View from One Research Center." *American Journal of Health Promotion* 15, no. 5 (2001): 341–49.

Goetzel, Ron Z., and Ronald J. Ozminkowski. *Annual Review of Public Health* 29 (April 2009): 303–23.

Goetzel, Ron Z., Stacey R. Long, Ronald J. Ozminkowski, Kevin Hawkins, Shaohung Wang, and Wendy Lynch. "Health, Absence, Disability, and Presenteeism Cost Estimates of Certain Physical and Mental Health Conditions Affecting U.S. Employers." *Journal of Occupational & Environmental Medicine* 46, no. 4 (April 2004): 398–412.

Mercer and Kronos Incorporated. *The Total Financial Impact of Employee Absences.* Survey. October 2008. www.fmlainsights.com/mercer-survey-highlights%5B1%5D.pdf.

Perrin, Towers. *Health Care Cost Survey,* 2008. www.towersperrin.com/tp/getwebcachedoc?webc=HRS/USA/2008/200801/hccs_2008.pdf.

Powell, Don R. "How to Achieve an R.O.I. on Your Health Care Dollars." *Employee Benefits Journal* 27, no. 1 (2002): 24–7.

Towers Watson. "Few Employers Addressing Workplace Stress, Watson Wyatt Surveys Find." Press Release. February 14, 2008. www.watsonwyatt.com/render.asp?catid=1&id=18643.

Union Pacific. "Raising Heart and Overall Health Awareness: Union Pacific Links Wellness Programs with Business and Medical Initiatives." Press Release. February 11, 2005. www.uprr.com/newsinfo/releases/human_resources/2005/0211_hearthealth.shtml.

Union Pacific. "WELCOA Well Workplace Platinum Award: Executive Summary, 2000." www.welcoa.org/wellworkplace/platinum/apps/unionpacaific.pdf.

WELCOA. "Union Pacific . . . On the Right Track." WELCOA website, Platinum Award 2001.

Wells, Susan J. "Finding Wellness's Return on Investment." *HR Magazine* (June 2008): 74–84.

## WORLD HEALTH ORGANIZATION (WHO)

Neither diseases nor the organisms that cause them recognize the political boundaries that separate human populations into nations. The natural boundaries that long isolated islands and continents—and their unique biological populations—have been crossed with increasing frequency and effectiveness. Today, we live in a truly global society, sharing pathogens with the world. Never has international cooperation in monitoring, planning for, and confronting infectious diseases been more important.

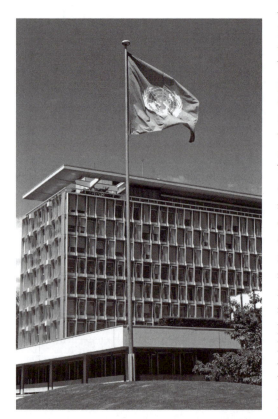

The headquarters of the World Health Organization (WHO) is located in Geneva, Switzerland. The WHO is a specialized agency of the United Nations that began operation in 1948. (WHO/ P. Virot)

The World Health Organization (WHO) is an international body that works to safeguard public health. Nearly 8,000 people from more than 150 countries work for the WHO in their capacity as doctors, public health specialists, researchers, and epidemiologists along with administrative staff and experts in the fields of health statistics, economics, and emergency relief. The WHO objectives include several core functions: providing leadership on public health matters and engaging in partnerships with countries where joint action is needed; working to shape the research agenda and in the dissemination of health information; setting norms and standards and promoting and monitoring implementation of those standards around the world. It also provides technical support and monitors health situations and assesses health trends as they change. These functions were established for the 10-year period from 2006 to 2015 under the 11th General Programme of Work titled "Engaging for Health."

**Early Attempts at Public Health**   The idea of an international response to disease and public health crisis began back in Medieval Europe. The plague prompted Italian city-states to surveil their neighbors for signs of an outbreak and to recognize each other's health passes, guaranteeing a traveler's lack of disease. Early modern maritime nations at least tacitly recognized each others' quarantine and isolation procedures, and *cordons sanitaires* along national borders were generally respected because no one had an interest in spreading pestilential disease. Yet the earliest multistate effort to confront epidemic disease began only in the mid-19th century as cholera raged across European countries and their colonies.

By the 1850s, Europe was rapidly undergoing industrialization and urbanization and was beginning to experience the closer ties created by such innovations as steamships, railroads, and the telegraph. Imperialism linked a lengthening list of European states to far-flung colonies, many of which served as reservoirs for infectious tropical diseases. At the same time, the medical profession in Europe was gaining increasing popular respect, raising the prospect that diseases might soon be understood and conquered. In 1830, an outbreak of epidemic cholera prompted the Ottoman Empire to initiate a program of international monitoring of sea and land routes between Asia and Western nations, directed by the Conseil Supérieur de Santé de Constantinople (Istanbul). Two decades later, in the midst of another cholera pandemic, diplomats, physicians, and scientists from 12 nations participated in the First Sanitary Conference, which opened on July 23, 1851. A lack of consensus on causation led to a lack of consensus on action, but the first step had been taken. In 1859, the Second Conference convened again in Paris, but with only the diplomats present. Even so, no agreement on measures to combat cholera was ratified. The medical men rejoined the diplomats for the Third Conference in Istanbul in 1866, and yellow fever was added to the agenda, but no real headway resulted. Though the agendas broadened somewhat, the same must be said for the Fourth Conference (Vienna, 1874), the Fifth (Washington, DC, 1881; with a greater emphasis on yellow fever), and the Sixth (Rome, 1885).

During this period, other developments reinforced international collaboration on matters of health and disease. The International Statistical Congresses, beginning in 1853, helped disseminate the emerging ideas and tools of the new science of epidemiology; the International Congress of Medicine held 11 sessions between 1867 and 1900; and the U.S. Surgeon-General began publication of the *Index Medicus,* an up-to-date international catalogue of books and articles of medical relevance. The German Robert Koch and Frenchman Louis Pasteur made their respective microbiological discoveries that confirmed modern germ theory of disease, while Rudolf Virchow in Germany and John Snow and William Farr in England paved the way for modern epidemiology.

The Seventh International Sanitary Conference, held in Rome in 1892, was a breakthrough, as it unanimously ratified the First International Sanitary Convention (agreement). Though limited to establishing quarantine protocols for ships passing into the Mediterranean through the new Suez Canal, it opened the door to a series of conventions drafted and approved by the subsequent conferences. The Eighth Conference met in Dresden, Germany, in 1893 and agreed on certain prophylactic measures and required notification during future cholera outbreaks.

In 1894, the Ninth Conference convened in Paris and established guidelines for reducing the spread of cholera during the annual Islamic pilgrimage to Mecca. By 1897, bubonic plague had reemerged in the form of the Third Plague Pandemic and was appropriately the focus of the Tenth Conference, held in Venice. The Fourth Convention dealt with international notification and quarantining to contain the spread of plague. Six years later, the Eleventh Conference met in Paris. Delegates agreed to work toward controlling rat populations, which had only recently been linked to the plague; toward codifying the quarantine and other procedures established at previous conferences; and toward establishing a new organization, the Office International d'Hygiène Publique (International Office of Public Hygiene [OHIP]), which would have a largely European scope. The OHIP was founded by 12 countries—including the United States and Brazil—and met for the first time in Paris in 1908. It tackled the issue of monitoring leprosy, tuberculosis, typhoid, sexually transmitted diseases, and water quality (for cholera). Only three more conferences of this series would be held, the last in Paris in 1938.

**The WHO Is Established**   Following World War II, the United Nations Conference on International Organization established a new World Health Organization (WHO) that would absorb earlier organizations including the League of Nations Health Organization (LNHO), OHIP, Pan American Sanitary Bureau (PASB), and UNRRA. The Allied-sponsored United Nations Relief and Rehabilitation Administration (UNRRA) had emerged in 1943 amid fears of pandemics like those that followed World War I.

World War I (1914–1918) not only killed millions of combatants and countless civilians in Europe but also spawned terrible outbreaks of cholera and typhus in its wake. More deadly than the war itself was the worldwide influenza pandemic of 1918–1919. The failures of international diplomacy that sparked the war led to the founding of the League of Nations (1919), and the medical emergencies to the LNHO, in 1923. Because the United States was not a member of the League, it could not participate in LNHO activities, so the OHIP and ISB (now the Pan American Sanitary Bureau) remained independent and active as monitors and quarantine supervisors that worked with the LNHO.

Based in Washington, DC, the ISB was directed by the U.S. Surgeon-General and often collaborated with the Rockefeller Foundation's International Health Division and the U.S. Institute for Inter-American Affairs. As with the OHIP, the chief function of the ISB was to monitor and report on levels or outbreaks of infectious disease in the Western Hemisphere and to supervise its quarantine procedures.

Complementarily, the LNHO took a much more proactive role in supporting practical measures to prevent the outbreak and spread of disease. Aided by Rockefeller Foundation funds, the Organization disseminated the latest information, strategies, and techniques, and published a monthly report on medical situations worldwide. Unlike earlier international efforts, the LNHO covered East Asia, from an office in Singapore. It collaborated with the International Red Cross and the International Labor Office in providing public education, sending experts to trouble spots, and sponsoring committees and conferences. It sponsored research and development of treatments, public hygiene, and worldwide standardization of epidemiological matters from cause of death reporting to medical products.

On April 7, 1948, the required 26 nations ratified the WHO constitution, and it assembled for the first time in June. The International Sanitary Conventions evolved into the World Health Organization's International Health Regulations (IHR), adopted in 1969. Updated in 2005, the new IHR was implemented in 2007; 192 countries are currently party to the regulations. These require cooperating governments to inform the WHO of any reportable diseases in a timely way but do not require further action.

Since 1948, the WHO has been in the forefront as an organizer of international efforts to maintain high levels of general health, prevent the emergence or spread of disease, treat victims, and, in some cases, eradicate diseases. Controlling and eventually eradicating infectious diseases are among the highest of WHO's priorities, and success with smallpox eradication in 1977 set the tone for current efforts against measles, tuberculosis, malaria, and polio.

The United Nations and WHO consider good health to be a fundamental human right and a positive goal for their activities. The WHO is thus proactive and not merely reactive to dangerous outbreaks of disease. Though headquartered in Geneva, Switzerland, WHO has six regional offices through which many of its efforts are directed. In the Western Hemisphere it is the Pan American Health Organization (Washington, DC; formerly the PASB). WHO also maintains offices in countries that have needs being met by the organization. Collaboration with host countries is of utmost importance, as is collaboration with nongovernmental organizations, especially those that can provide technical expertise or funding. The Bill and Melinda Gates Foundation is a good example of the latter. WHO also works with other international organizations—such as the Food and Agriculture Organization (FAO), UNICEF, and UNESCO—in areas such as nutrition, health and personal hygiene education, prenatal care, children's diseases, and vaccinations.

*Joseph P. Byrne*

*See also* Immunizations; Pandemics; Pasteur, Louis.

## References

Baldwin, Peter. *Contagion and the State in Europe, 1830–1930.* New York: Cambridge University Press, 1999.

Harvard University Library. *Contagion: Sanitary Conferences.* n.d. http://ocp.hul.harvard.edu/contagion/sanitaryconferences.html.

Howard-Jones, Norman. *The Pan American Health Organization.* Geneva: World Health Organization, 1981.

Huber, Valeska. "The Unification of the Globe by Disease? The International Sanitary Conventions on Cholera, 1851–1894." *The Historical Journal* 49 (2006): 453–76.

Merson, Michael. *International Public Health: Diseases, Programs, Systems and Policies.* Boston: Jones & Bartlett, 2006.

Pan-American Health Organization. n.d. www.paho.org/.

Siddiqi, Javed. *World Health and World Politics: The World Health Organization and the U.N. System.* Columbia: University of South Carolina Press, 1995.

Stern, Alexandra Minna, and Howard Merkel. "International Efforts to Control Infectious Diseases, 1851 to the Present." *Journal of the American Medical Association* 292 (2004): 1474–79.

UNICEF. n.d. www.unicef.org/.

Weindling, Paul, ed. *International Health Organizations and Movements, 1918–1939.* New York: Cambridge University Press, 1995.

World Health Organization. October 2011. www.who.int/en/.

# Y

## YOGA

Yoga means different things to different people, in part because it involves a variety of ways to create wellness through strength and flexibility. The different styles of yoga are rich and varied, but they share a common lineage. Yoga began as an ancient school of Indian philosophy that originated some 6,000 years ago. Unlike other schools of philosophy, yoga is also considered a science and a discipline that can govern many areas of life. Within the umbrella of yoga there is *karma* yoga, the yoga of action; *bhakti* yoga, the yoga of devotion; *jnana* yoga, the yoga of knowledge; and *hatha* yoga, the physical practice of yoga. While hatha yoga is indeed grounded in physical movement, for many yogis it is first and foremost a mental exercise. One swami describes hatha yoga as such: "The postures of hatha yoga are a form of physical action, yet they lead to detachment from physical action. Outer movements are taking place, of course—the physical body is becoming stronger and more supple. Yet the whole purpose of hatha yoga is to draw the attention inward" (Chidvilasananda, 1996).

The yoga asanas (postures) known today were created as a way to prepare the body for meditation by calming the mind, body, and spirit. Each yoga style has a different emphasis, but overall, hatha yoga remains at its core the practice of calming and strengthening the body while drawing individual attention inward.

There are many styles of hatha yoga; some of the most common hatha yoga styles are as follows:

- Ananda Yoga: A classical style of hatha yoga that uses asanas (postures) and pranayama (breath control) to awaken the body to sensations and control subtle energies within oneself. Ananda is typically gentle, and not athletic or aerobic. Students are encouraged to use silent affirmations in the poses to coax themselves into a deeper practice.
- Anasura Yoga: A newer style of hatha yoga that is heart oriented and spiritual in nature. Each student's abilities and limitations are deeply respected.

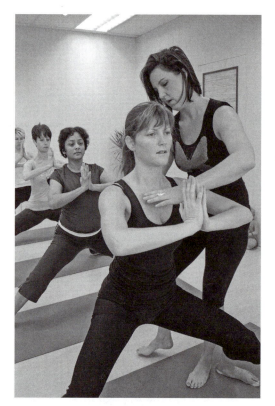

A yoga instructor adjusts a student during class. Classes featuring different forms of yoga have been gaining in popularity. (Hongqi Zhang/ Dreamstime.com)

- Ashtang Yoga: Modern yoga classes in this style are often called "power yoga." Ashtang is aerobic and physically demanding; this practice is intended to build strength and stamina. Practitioners often jump from one posture to another.
- Bikram Yoga: Modern yoga classes in this style are often called "hot yoga" because the room is heated to ensure that practitioners sweat out toxins. Bikram was designed to warm and stretch muscles and even harder-to-reach ligaments and tendons. Bikram classes utilize a set routine of asanas (postures) each time.
- Integral Yoga: A yoga style that has a focus on pranayama (breath control), meditation, and that incorporates chanting. This style was used by Dr. Dean Ornish as part of his work to reverse heart disease in patients.
- Iyengar Yoga: This style is known for great attention to and precise alignment of postures, and it utilizes props such as blocks and belts. Iyengar teachers must complete a rigorous 2 to 5 year training program for certification.
- Kali Ray TriYoga: TriYoga combines flowing and sustained postures that allow individuals to move intuitively at their own pace. Synchronizing breath with movement is very important to achieve the best results. Students of all levels can practice Kali Ray at their own pace and level.
- Kripalu Yoga: Kripalu is called "the yoga of consciousness"; students learn to focus on their emotions caused by various postures. There are three stages in Kripalu: Stage one is about learning the postures; stage two involves holding the postures for an extended period of time with greater awareness; stage three is like a meditation, while one moves from posture to posture unconsciously and spontaneously.
- Kundalini Yoga: One of the more spiritual types of yoga, it goes beyond the physical postures with its emphasis on breathing, meditation, and chanting. Kundalini yoga is great for those who want both a mental and physical challenge.

- Sivananda Yoga: Sivananda is one of the world's largest schools of yoga. Sivananda yoga follows a set routine of postures that includes pranayama (breath control), asanas (postures), and relaxation. The founder of Sivananda wrote one of the contemporary yoga classics, *The Complete Illustrated Book of Yoga,* in 1960.
- Svaroopa Yoga: Svaroopa focuses on spinal articulation and therefore changes the experience of doing familiar poses. It is a relatively gentle form of yoga and emphasizes inner experience as the focus of each practice.
- Viniyoga: Viniyoga a methodology for developing practices for individual conditions and purposes. Key characteristic of the asana practice are the careful integration of the flow of breath with movement of the spine, with sequencing, adaptations and intensity dependent upon the ability of the student. Many Viniyoga classes are taught privately because of the personal adaptation necessary for many students coping with physical limitations.

While each style differs in its approach, there are many common elements to be found. For example, when beginning any yoga practice, it is important to include warm-up movements and stretches. Yogis say warm-ups bring awareness to the body and help ease the transition from daily life to focusing on the inner self. Warm-ups increase oxygen flow to muscles while lubricating joints to facilitate easy movements. A complete warm-up session should include the six movements of the spine; backward/forward, lateral, and spinal twists to each side. The movements can be done sitting, kneeling, or standing.

Almost every yoga style includes some type of pranayama (breath control) and a complete diaphragmatic breath. The purpose of breathing from the diaphragm is to fill the lungs completely with oxygen and force out trapped carbon dioxide in the lungs, as yogis suggest trapped, stale air causes fatigue and nervousness. A full diaphragmatic breath starts in the belly, progresses to the rib cage, and completely fills the upper chest. Other common pranayama exercises include *kapalabhati,* a rapid, forceful exhale from the belly that stirs creative energy; *ujjayi,* a throat constricting, audible breath that helps individuals concentrate; and *nadi sodhana,* alternate nostril breathing that aims to balance and relax the mind and body. Pranayama is helpful to detect subtle changes in mental peace and clarity, the ultimate goal of pranayama is to release stress from the mind and body.

Stress has many insidious effects on the body, so limiting daily stressors and dealing with the response to stress is an important component of well-being. Many health benefits achieved by a regular yoga practice can be attributed to learning effective stress management techniques. Most modern stress reduction techniques originated from ancient yoga practices, including pranayama (breathing exercises), progressive relaxation techniques, and meditation. A regular yoga practice can help individuals master these skills and enjoy an improved state of health as a result.

In fact, in a recent study conducted by the Boston University School of Medicine, yoga was shown to increase the level of gamma-aminobutyric acid (GABA), a chemical in the brain that helps regulate nerve activity ("Yoga's Ability to Improve

Mood," 2010). GABA activity is reduced in people with mood and anxiety disorders, so finding how to stimulate the body to produce GABA naturally is at the center of finding a safe, nondrug treatment for depression. The calming effects of yoga are just beginning to be studied by the medical world, but yogis have described these benefits for ages. The forward bend group of asanas has long been cited as an excellent treatment for relieving anxiety and anxiety-based depression. Backward bending asanas are also thought to help some forms of depression by releasing pent-up emotions.

Scientists are not only considering yoga as a potential treatment for those suffering from anxiety and depression, they are also studying the effects of yoga on people with fibromyalgia, a chronic pain syndrome. Fibromyalgia is characterized by multiple tender points on the body, fatigue, insomnia, anxiety, depression, and memory and concentration problems (Goodwin, 2010). After an eight-week hatha yoga class, the patients reported improvements in both physical and psychological aspects of fibromyalgia, including decreased pain, fatigue, tenderness, anxiety, and better sleep and mood (Goodwin, 2010). An important part of the yoga treatment was the focus on meditation and breathing exercises to help sufferers with chronic pain reduce stress and cope with pain.

Cancer survivors are another group that may benefit from a gentle, inward-focusing yoga class. A study conducted by the University of Rochester monitored the effects of a yoga regime on recent cancer survivors. Researchers found an increase of 22 percent in sleep quality after the yoga classes and a 21 percent drop in the use of sleep medication ("Yoga Benefits Cancer Survivors," 2010). Yogis have traditionally taught that many inversion asanas aid sleep and soothe the nervous system, so it is not surprising that medical findings demonstrated those substantial benefits. The study concluded that participation in a twice-weekly hatha yoga class led to an increase in the quality of life of cancer survivors.

Yoga has great potential as a nondrug treatment for anxiety, depression, fibromyalgia, and for those in cancer remission. Its effectiveness at treating real medical issues can be attributed to the mind–body link that many medical professionals are beginning to recognize. Yogis have long touted the connection between the physical self and inner spirit. They developed many styles of yoga as a way to teach others how to cultivate awareness and grow mentally and physically strong. Yoga does not have to be a spiritual practice; it is incredibly useful as exercise alone, but individuals can gain even greater benefits by using their yoga practice as a time to look inward.

*Leslie Shafer*

*See also* Cancer; Depression; Fibromyalgia; Meditation; Ornish, Dean; Stress.

## References

Chidvilasananda, Gurumayi. *The Yoga of Discipline.* South Fallsburgh, NY: SYDA Foundation, 1996.

Goodwin, Jenifer. "Yoga May Combat Fibromyalgia Symptoms: Less Pain, Fatigue, Anxiety Reported by Study Participants after 8 Weeks Researchers Say." *Consumer Health News,* October 14, 2010.

Haupt, Angela. "Benefits of Yoga: How Different Types Affect Health." *U.S. News & World Report,* September 24, 2010. http://health.usnews.com/health-news/diet-fitness/fitness/articles/2010/09/24/benefits-of-yoga-how-different-types-affect-health.

Park, Alice. "Yoga Improves Quality of Life After Cancer." *Time,* May 19, 2010. www.time.com/time/health/article/0,8599,1990540,00.html.

"Study: Yoga May Ease Fibromyalgia Pain." *UPI NewsTrack.* October 15, 2010. www.upi.com/Health_News/2010/10/15/Study-Yoga-may-ease-fibromyalgia-pain/UPI-49381287122330/.

"Yoga Benefits Cancer Survivors." *Health News* 16, no. 8 (August 2010): 7.

"Yoga Styles." www.yogasite.com. "Yoga's Ability to Improve Mood and Lessen Anxiety Is Linked to Increased Levels of a Critical Brain Chemical." *Biotech Week,* December 1, 2009. www.newsrx.com/health-articles/2269860.html.

## YO-YO DIETING

Yo-yo dieting, also known as weight cycling, occurs when a person experiences cycles of weight loss and weight gain resembling the up and down of a yo-yo. The pattern begins with rapid weight loss normally associated with the use of fad diets or diet pills. Celebrities including Oprah Winfrey, Russell Crowe, Kirstie Alley and Janet Jackson have all been featured in the tabloids over their weight losses and gains.

Doctors say once yo-yo dieters reach a goal weight they often return to their original eating habits. This causes the lost pounds to return, followed by extra weight gain. Each time yo-yo dieters lose weight through the use of pills, liquid diet drinks or fads like a high-protein, high-fat, and low-carbohydrate diets, they lose mostly lean muscle and water but only a small amount of fat. Those pounds return and statistics show that more than 80 percent of people who lose weight this way regain all of it, or more, after two years. In fact, researchers at the University of California at Los Angeles released the results of a long-term diet survey that showed about two-thirds of dieters regained even more weight than they initially lost in just four or five years time (Voss, 2010).

One of Oprah's most memorable televised weight loss moments was in 1988 when she lost 67 pounds using the Optifast liquid protein diet and appeared on stage pulling a wagon loaded with 67 pounds of fat. But after one year she was almost 20 pounds heavier and eventually went on to regain that weight and more. In 2009, she once again announced a serious weight loss attempt after years of putting on more pounds.

The sad news for many dieters is that when those pounds return, it is in the form of fat with very little muscle regained. The psychological effects of yo-yo dieting include depression and the erosion of confidence and self-esteem. That emotional loss is intensified by the physical effects of the extra weight and researchers are now suggesting the gain-lose-gain cycle may cause other problems as well including high blood pressure, high cholesterol and heart disease.

That's not all. Researchers at the Fred Hutchinson Cancer Research Center announced findings that suggest weight cycling or yo-yo dieting may also have a negative impact on immune health (Shade, 2004). The report noted that immune function, measured by natural-killer-cell activity, was higher for women who had kept a stable weight for several years. Natural-killer cells, also known as NK cells, are an important aspect of the human immune system. They are a type of white blood cell that kills cells infected by viruses or other abnormal body cells such as cancer cells. The higher the natural-killer cell levels the better. Low NK activity has been associated with increased susceptibility to colds and infections and the possibility of a link to increased incidence of cancer is being researched. In the plus column, results showed that exercise appeared to counteract the negative effects of weight loss on immune function according to researchers (Shade, 2004). The study, funded by the National Cancer Institute, interviewed overweight but otherwise healthy older women about their weight-loss history during the previous 20 years.

While research shows weight cycling may not benefit individuals who have only small amounts of weight to lose, doctor's caution that severely obese individuals should not allow concerns about the hazards of weight cycling to deter them from efforts to control their body weight. Instead, individuals who undertake a weight loss program should consult a doctor first. They should also expect to make life-long changes in their eating, behavior, and physical activity. Studies show that, for obese individuals, keeping off just 5 to 15 pounds permanently can have a positive impact on overall health (Douketis, 2005).

A simple way to increase exercise is to be more active during the day. For example, take the stairs instead of the elevator, park farther away and walk to your destination. If possible do errands on foot or on a bicycle instead of driving everywhere. Walking is also an easy and affordable exercise. For anyone looking for a more organized exercise program, the ideal choice is to include a combination of strength training, anaerobic exercise and aerobic exercise.

If a yo-yo dieter decides to make a permanent lifestyle change rather than "go on a diet" there are several other key behavioral choices that will improve chances for long-term weight loss and maintenance. Along with the number one suggestion to increase daily physical activity, the next best tip is to eat only when hungry. Loneliness, boredom or anxiety can cause people to eat when they are not hungry.

Weight loss experts also suggest when snacking, remove a portion based on the package label rather than eating from the container. Then put the container away so you only eat one serving. Another simple and effective suggestion is to get plenty of sleep. Studies have shown that lack of sleep increases hormone levels and can promote fat storage. Research presented at a Canadian conference showed that lack of sleep lead to chemical changes which triggered weight gain (Europe, 2005). Sleep deprivation has been shown to cause leptin levels to drop and levels of ghrelin to rise. Ghrelin is a hormone produced in the stomach which contributes to a feeling of hunger.

Eating breakfast is considered important because it helps control hunger and can prevent binge eating later in the day. Maintaining consistent eating patterns rather than dieting and then taking days off was also a key to success as was making careful food selections instead of restricting whole categories of foods, such as carbohydrates.

There is good news for yo-yo dieters who do make lasting behavioral changes. In a report published in the American Journal of Clinical Nutrition, researchers analyzed people who had successfully maintained weight loss and discovered the basic simple changes mentioned above were the key to their success. Researchers looked at the National Weight Control Registry (NWCR), a collections of people who have maintained an average weight loss of 73 pounds for approximately 6 years. Although individual weight loss techniques varied among group members, those basic tips were commonly shared by the successful registrants.

More good news for many women who had feared years of yo-yo dieting may have permanently lowered their body's metabolism. A study published in the *Journal of the American Dietetic Association* says the effect is only short term. The results tracked overweight women for 18 years and found that their slowed metabolism, a byproduct of severe calorie restriction, was only temporary (Sass, 2008). Once the women raised their food intake levels to a healthy number their ability to burn calories also returned to normal.

*Marjolijn Bijlefeld and Sharon Zoumbaris*

*See also* Diets, Fad; Exercise; Ghrelin.

## References

Douketis, J.D., Macie, C., Thabane, L., Williamson, D.F. "Systematic Review of Long-Term Weight Loss Studies in Obese Adults: Clinical Significance and Applicability to Clinical Practice." *International Journal of Obesity* 29 (2005): 1153–1167.

Freed, Ellen. "Oprah Needs to Change Her Lifestyle to Remain Healthy." *Nursing Standard* 23, no. 23 (February 11, 2009): 32.

"Healthiest Way to Weight Loss: A Healthy Diet and Exercise Regimen Will Subtract Pounds and Add Years to Your Life." *Healthy Years* 6, no. 5 (May 2009): 1.

Lofshult, Diane. "Should Teens Weigh Themselves?" *IDEA Fitness Journal* 4, no. 5 (May 2007): 75.

"Long-Term Weight Loss: Six Keys to Keeping It Off." *Tufts University Health & Nutrition Letter* 24, no. 5 (July 2006): 4.

Sass, Cynthia A., RD. "Eat to speed metabolism." *Prevention*. 60.5 (May 2008): 076.

Shade, E.D., Ulrich, C.M.; Wener, M.H., Wood, B., Yasui, Y., Lacroix, K., Potter, J.D., McTiernan, A. *Journal of the American Dietetic Association* 104 (June 1, 2004): 892.

"Studies Show Good Night's Sleep Could Help Weight Loss." *Europe Intelligence Wire* (October 20, 2005).

Voss, Gretchen. "When fat comes back." *Women's Health* 7, no. 3 (April 2010): 104.

# Glossary

**addiction:**  Physical or emotional dependence on a substance, most often alcohol or another drug.

**ADHD:**  "Attention deficit hyperactivity disorder," a condition usually diagnosed in children that is marked by inattention, hyperactivity, and impulsiveness. Sometimes referred to as ADD (attention deficit disorder), especially if there is no hyperactivity component.

**adrenaline:**  A naturally occurring hormone that increases heart rate and blood pressure and affects other body functions.

**AED:**  "Automated External Defibrillator" is a portable electronic device that automatically diagnoses serious heart problems such as arrhythmias and treats them using defibrillation, an electronic therapy that allows the heart to reestablish its normal rhythm.

**aerobic activity:**  When the human body's large muscles move in a rhythmic manner for a sustained period of time, which increases heart rate and respiration bringing more oxygen to muscles. Examples include walking, running, swimming, or bicycling.

**AIDS:**  "Acquired immune deficiency syndrome," a disease due to infection with the human immunodeficiency virus (HIV). Also referred to as "acquired immune deficiency disease."

**allergen:**  A substance that triggers an allergy. Common triggers include molds, pollens, ragweed, animal dander, feathers, cosmetics, and dust mites.

**allergic reaction:**  An exaggerated immune system response to an allergen. Signs and symptoms include rashes, nasal congestion, asthma, and, occasionally, shock.

**amino acids:**  Organic compounds composed of carbon, hydrogen, oxygen, nitrogen, and, in some cases, sulfur, which are bonded in formations. Eight amino acids cannot be manufactured by the body and must be obtained from the diet.

**anaerobic exercise:**  Exercise that improves the efficiency of the anaerobic (without oxygen) energy-producing systems and increases muscular strength.

**anaphylaxis:**  An immediate and severe allergic response to a substance that can result in severe breathing difficulties, severe drop in blood pressure, or loss of consciousness. This allergic reaction can be fatal if not treated promptly.

**anesthesiologist:** Decides which type of anesthesia should be used and administers it during surgery, then monitors its effects after surgery.

**anorexia nervosa:** An eating disorder characterized by markedly reduced appetite or total aversion to food. Anorexia is a serious psychological disorder.

**antibiotic:** A drug used to treat infections caused by bacteria and other microorganisms.

**antibodies:** Immune-system proteins that counteract or eliminate foreign substances known as "antigens."

**antidepressant:** Anything, especially a drug, used to prevent or treat depression.

**antigens:** Substances foreign to the body that cause antibodies to form.

**antioxidants:** Substances that protect cells against the actions of free radicals.

**anxiety:** A feeling of apprehension and fear characterized by physical symptoms such as palpitations, sweating, and feelings of stress. Anxiety disorders are serious medical illnesses that affect approximately 19 million American adults.

**asthma:** A chronic disease in which the bronchial airways become narrow and swollen, making it difficult for an individual to breathe.

**bacteria:** The plural for "bacterium," a single-cell microorganism without nuclei. Some bacteria cause infections.

**balance:** A component of physical fitness that involves maintenance of equilibrium, whether standing or moving.

**bariatric surgery:** Surgery on the stomach and/or intestines to assist with weight loss in cases of extreme obesity.

**benefit period:** In health insurance, the number of days for which benefits are paid to the insured and his or her dependents.

**beriberi:** A disease caused by a deficiency of thiamine and characterized by nerve and gastrointestinal disorders.

**beta carotene:** A nutrient that the body converts to vitamin A, found in orange and yellow fruits and vegetables such as cantaloupe and carrots as well as in green leafy vegetables such as broccoli and spinach.

**biofeedback:** A behavior-training program that teaches a person how to control autonomic reactions such as heart rate, blood pressure, skin temperature, and muscular tension.

**bipolar disorder:** A mood disorder sometimes called "manic-depressive illness," or "manic-depression," that characteristically involves cycles of depression and elation or mania.

**blood:** A tissue with red blood cells, white blood cells, platelets, and other substances suspended in fluid called "plasma." Blood takes oxygen and nutrients to the tissues and carries away waste products.

**blood count:** The calculated number of white or red blood cells in a cubic millimeter of blood.

**blood pressure:** The force placed on the inner walls of the arteries.

**blood vessel:** A tube through which the blood circulates through the body, and which includes a network of arteries, arterioles, capillaries, venules and veins to transport the blood.

**BMI:** "Body mass index" is the measure of body fat based on height and weight.

**booster:** Administration of an additional vaccination to help increase or speed the immune response to a previous vaccination.

**bulimia:** Also called "bulimia nervosa," an eating disorder characterized by episodes of secretive excessive eating (binge eating) followed by inappropriate methods of weight control, such as self-induced vomiting (purging), abuse of laxatives and diuretics, or excessive exercise.

**calcium:** A mineral found throughout the body, needed for healthy bones and teeth as well as for blood clotting and nerve function.

**calorie:** A unit of energy in food used by the body to breathe, circulate blood, digest food, and be physically active.

**cancer:** A term for diseases in which abnormal cells divide without control and that can invade nearby tissues and spread to other parts of the body through the blood or lymph systems.

**carbohydrate:** A compound consisting of carbon, hydrogen, and oxygen, found in plants and used as food by humans and other animals.

**carcinogen:** Any substance that causes cancer.

**cardiologist:** One who specializes in diagnosing and treating heart disease and other heart conditions.

**carotenoids:** Any of the more than 600 yellow-orange pigments found in fruits and vegetables like apricots, sweet potatoes, carrots, tomatoes, and winter squash. Many are thought to protect against heart disease and certain types of cancer.

**cataract:** The clouding of the natural lens of the eye, located behind the iris and pupil.

**cavity:** A small hole in a tooth caused by tooth decay.

**cell:** The basic structural and functional unit in people and all living things. Each cell is a small container of chemicals and water wrapped in a membrane.

**chi:** The vital energy in Traditional Chinese Medicine, believed to circulate around the body in currents.

**cholesterol:** A fat-like substance that is made by the body and found naturally in animal foods such as meat, fish, poultry, eggs, and dairy products. If cholesterol levels are too high, some of the cholesterol is deposited on the walls of the blood vessels and can build up over time, causing decreased blood flow.

**chromosome:** One of the 46 rod-shaped structures in the nucleus of each cell that carries hereditary information.

**chronic:** Relating to a disease or condition lasting over a period of time, or a recurrent medical condition.

**COBRA:** "Consolidated Omnibus Budget Reconciliation Act," a federal law in effect since 1986 that permits individuals and their dependents to continue in an employer's group health-insurance plan after their job ends, which generally lasts 18 months, or 36 months for dependents in certain circumstances.

**cocaine:** The most potent stimulant of natural origin, a bitter, addictive anesthetic (pain blocker) that is extracted from the leaves of the coca shrub (*Erythroxylon coca*), indigenous to the Andean highlands of South America.

**complete protein:**  A protein that includes all eight essential amino acids.

**contagious:**  Describing a disease with the potential to spread from one person to another.

**coronary artery disease:**  A disease that causes narrowing of the heart arteries.

**CPR:**  "Cardiopulmonary resuscitation" is a combination of rescue breathing and chest compressions given to people thought to be in cardiac arrest. It supports a small amount of blood flow to the heart and brain until normal heart function is restored.

**cross-training:**  Changing a regular fitness routine to incorporate new and different activities to reduce repetitive stress injuries and to improve fitness by providing the body with new challenges.

**crown:**  The portion of the tooth outside the gum.

**CT scan:**  "Computerized tomography scan." Pictures of structures within the body created by a computer that takes the data from multiple X-ray images and turns them into pictures on a screen.

**deficiency diseases:**  Diseases caused by poor nutrition and inadequate amounts of vitamins and minerals in the diet.

**dehydration:**  Excessive loss of body water. Diseases of the gastrointestinal tract that cause vomiting or diarrhea may, for example, lead to dehydration. There are a number of other causes of dehydration, including heat exposure, prolonged vigorous exercise (e.g., as in a marathon), kidney disease, and medications (diuretics).

**dementia:**  Mental deterioration due to organic causes.

**dentin:**  The tissue of a tooth found beneath the enamel that encloses the pulp cavity.

**depression:**  An illness that involves the body, mood, and thoughts that affects the way one eats and sleeps, the way one feels about oneself, and the way one thinks about things.

**detoxification:**  The process of cleansing the body of a drug or toxin, such as alcohol.

**diabetes:**  A disorder characterized by high levels of sugar or glucose in the blood caused by a failure of the pancreas to produce sufficient insulin or by resistance of the body to the action of insulin.

**diastolic pressure:**  The lowest blood pressure reached during the relaxation of the heart. It is recorded as the second number in the measurement of blood pressure.

**diet:**  What a person eats and drinks; a type of eating plan.

**Dietary Guidelines for Americans (DGA):**  Nutritional advice for Americans ages two years and older issued by the U.S. Department of Agriculture and the Department of Health and Human Services, updated every five years to serve as the cornerstone of the federal nutrition policy and nutrition education activities.

**disinfectant:**  A chemical agent applied to inanimate surfaces to destroy germs.

**diuretic:**  A substance that increases fluid output through urination. Caffeine, alcohol, and other medications act as diuretics.

**DNA:**  "Deoxyribonucleic acid," a double-helix shaped molecule inside cells that carries genetic information.

**dopamine:**  An important neurotransmitter (messenger) in the brain.

**duration:**  The length of time in which an activity or exercise is performed and which is generally expressed in minutes.

**ECG:** "Electrocardiogram," a test to record the electrical processes from within the heart to diagnose heart problems. Electrodes are attached to the check, neck, arms, and legs, and the electrical activity is recorded.

**EEG:** "Electroencephalogram," a technique for studying the electrical current within the brain. Electrodes are attached to the scalp. Wires attach these electrodes to a machine that records the electrical impulses.

**electrolytes:** Minerals in the blood and other body fluids that carry an electric charge. They are lost through perspiration and replaced by drinking fluids.

**emergency department:** The department of a hospital that is responsible for the provision of medical and surgical care to patients in need of immediate care.

**endorphins:** Chemical substances produced by the central nervous system and other organs that suppress pain.

**enrollment period:** The time during which employees and their dependents can sign up for health-insurance coverage under an employer group health plan.

**enzymes:** Proteins produced by the cells that are involved in every chemical reaction in the body.

**epidemic:** An outbreak of a disease that spreads at an extremely rapid rate in a specific region and/or country.

**essential fatty acids:** Fatty acids that the body cannot produce and must be obtained from food.

**exercise:** A physical activity that is planned, repetitive, and that is performed in an effort to maintain one or more components of physical fitness.

**Family and Medical Leave Act (FMLA):** A federal law that guarantees up to 12 weeks of job-protected leave for certain employees when they need to take time off due to serious illness, to have or adopt a child, or to care for another family member. Those who qualify for leave under FMLA can continue health-insurance coverage under their group health plan during the leave.

**fat-soluble vitamins:** Vitamins A, D, E, and K, which are soluble in the fatty parts of plants and animals.

**fats:** Organic compounds composed of fatty acids that are either saturated or unsaturated.

**fatty acids:** Acids produced when fats are broken down; may be saturated, polyunsaturated, or monounsaturated.

**fertilizer:** Natural or synthetic materials spread on soil to increase its capacity to support plant growth.

**fiber:** A food substance that resists chemical digestion and passes through the system essentially unchanged.

**flavonoids:** Also known as "bioflavonoids," flavonoids are polyphenol antioxidants found in plants.

**fluoride:** A chemical solution or gel put on the teeth that hardens the teeth and prevents tooth decay. Is often added to municipal water as a preventative treatment.

**food additive:** A substance added to foods to improve nutrition, taste, appearance, or shelf-life. In some instances, additives such as dyes or antibiotics have created food safety issues.

**food poisoning:** The common term for any illness caused by eating contaminated food or water. Food safety experts use the term "food-borne illness."

**food safety:** A system to ensure that illness or harm will not result from eating food. Everyone in the process—from food production and processing to transportation, retail, or use in the home has an important role in keeping food safe.

**Food Safety and Inspection Service (FSIS):** The public health agency in the U.S. Department of Agriculture responsible for ensuring that the nation's commercial meat, poultry, and egg products are safe, wholesome, and correctly labeled and packaged as required by the Federal Meat Inspection Act, the Poultry Products Inspection Act, and the Egg Products Inspection Act.

**Food-borne illness:** Also known as "food poisoning," an infection caused by the transfer of microbial contaminants from food or drinking water. In most cases the contaminants are bacteria, parasites, or viruses.

**fortified foods:** Foods with added nutrients that were not originally present or were present in insignificant amounts, such as iron-fortified cereal.

**free radicals:** Highly reactive oxygen molecules that are a by-product of normal metabolism and that can damage cells, proteins, and DNA by altering their chemical structure.

**frequency:** The number of times an exercise or activity is performed and is generally expressed in sessions, episodes, or times per week.

**gene:** The basic biological unit of heredity. A segment of deoxyribonucleic acid (DNA) that carries instructions for a particular inherited feature, such as hair color or height.

**generic drug:** An identical copy of a brand-name drug that usually costs considerably less than the brand-name drug.

**genetically modified organism (GMO):** An organism with new genetic material added to create desirable traits. This form of genetic engineering was made possible by the discovery of DNA and other scientific advances.

**geneticist:** One who specializes in diagnosing and predicting inherited disorders such as cystic fibrosis, hemophilia, and other metabolic disorders.

**genome:** All the genetic information possessed by an organism. Genomics is the study of this genetic information.

**gingivitis:** The inflammation of gums caused by improper brushing and the first sign of periodontal or gum disease.

**gluten:** Plant proteins found in grains such as wheat, oats, rye, and barley.

**group health plan:** Health insurance that covers at least two employees and is sponsored by an employer, union, or professional association.

**gums:** The pink area around the teeth.

**health care directive:** A document giving someone else the power to make medical decisions for you or directing what kind of care you are willing to accept if incapacitated and unable to make medical decisions.

**health savings account:** A plan that allows an individual to contribute pretax money to be used for qualified medical expenses.

**heart:** The muscle that pumps blood received from veins into arteries throughout the body. It is positioned in the chest behind the sternum (breastbone); in front of the trachea, esophagus, and aorta; and above the diaphragm muscle that separates the chest and abdominal cavities.

**herbal:** Refers to herbs, as in an herbal tea or botanical or medicinal aspects of herbs.

**herbicide:** A chemical substance used to kill weeds or undesirable plants.

**high blood pressure:** The force of blood pushing against the walls of the arteries, measured in two numbers: the systolic measures the pressure when the heart beats and pumps blood into the arteries and the diastolic measure when the heart is at rest between beats. A measurement of 140/90 mmHg (millimeters of mercury) or higher is considered hypertension, or high blood pressure.

**high-density lipoprotein (HDL):** Commonly called "good cholesterol," this form of cholesterol circulates in the blood and lowers the risk of heart disease.

**high-glycemic foods or high glycemic index foods:** Foods that release energy quickly and result in fluctuations in blood glucose and insulin levels.

**HIPAA:** The "Health Insurance Portability and Accountability Act," also known as Kassebaum-Kennedy, for the two senators who spearheaded the bill. The law was passed in 1996 to help individuals buy and keep health insurance, even when they have a serious preexisting health condition.

**HIV:** Acronym for the "human immunodeficiency virus," the cause of AIDS (acquired immunodeficiency syndrome). HIV has also been called the human lymphotropic virus type III, the lymphadenopathy-associated virus, and the lymphadenopathy virus.

**HMO:** "Health maintenance organization," a type of health insurance plan that limits coverage to care from doctors who work for or contract with the HMO.

**hormone:** A chemical substance produced in the body that controls and regulates the activity of certain cells or organs.

**hydrogenation:** A chemical process to turn liquid fat or oil into solid fat, creating a new type of fat called "trans fatty acids." Eating a large amount of trans fatty acids may raise heart disease risk.

**hygiene:** The practice of cleanliness or grooming of skin, hair, or nails that promotes health and prevents disease.

**hyperglycemia:** High concentrations of glucose in the blood, usually associated with diabetes.

**hypoglycemia:** An abnormally low level of glucose in the blood.

**hypertension:** Another term for high blood pressure.

**immune system:** The system that protects the body against disease, infection, and foreign substances.

**immunity:** The condition of being immune or protected against infection, disease, and foreign substances.

**immunodeficiency:** Inability to mount a normal immune response. Immunodeficiency can be due to a genetic disease or acquired, as in AIDS due to HIV.

**immunoglobulin E (IgE):** The primary antibody associated with an allergic response.

**incisors:** The eight front teeth, four in the upper jaw and four in the lower jaw.

**infection:** An invasion and multiplication of germs in the body that can occur in any part of the body and can spread through the body.

**inoculation:** The introduction of a vaccine or other material into the body to create immunity.

**insomnia:** Poor-quality sleep because of difficulty falling asleep, waking up frequently during the night with difficulty returning to sleep, waking up too early in the morning, or restless sleep.

**insulin:** A hormone secreted by the islet cells in the pancreas in response to an increase in blood sugar, which facilitates the absorption of glucose.

**insulin resistance:** A condition in which the body cannot process glucose well because cells are not using the insulin effectively.

**insulin sensitivity:** The human body's ability to use glucose, a sugar.

**irradiation:** A process in which ionizing energy is used to kill pathogens and other harmful organisms in food by causing breaks in the DNA of the organisms' cells.

**isoflavones:** A type of phytoestrogen (plant estrogen) found primarily in soybeans.

**isometric exercise:** A form of exercise in which muscles contract without moving a joint and the muscle does not lengthen or shorten.

**isotonic exercise:** A form of active exercise in which the muscle contracts and causes movement.

**kidney:** One of a pair of organs located in the right and left side of the abdomen which clean "poisons" from the blood, regulate acid concentration, and maintain water balance in the body by excreting urine.

**lactose:** The sugar found in milk, composed of glucose and galactose.

**legumes:** The protein powerhouses of the plant kingdom, these plants have their seeds arranged in pods and include black, garbanzo, great northern, kidney, lima, mung, navy, pinto, and soy beans as well as lentils and peas.

**lipids:** Fats or fat-like substances in the blood, such as cholesterol.

**liposuction:** The process that removes fat deposits from beneath the skin by using a suction device.

**live vaccine:** A vaccine that contains a living, yet weakened, organism or virus.

**liver:** An organ in the upper abdomen that aids in digestion and removes waste products and worn-out cells from the blood. The liver is the largest solid organ in the body.

**living will:** A legal document describing what type of medical care and intervention a person authorizes in the event of a terminal illness or incapacity of that person.

**long-term care insurance:** Private insurance that pays for nursing home care.

**low-density lipoprotein (LDL):** Commonly known as "bad cholesterol," this form of cholesterol circulates in the blood and increases the risk of heart disease.

**low-glycemic foods:** Foods that release energy slowly.

**lumbar:** Referring to the five lumbar vertebrae that are situated below the thoracic vertebrae and above the sacral vertebrae in the spinal column. The five lumbar vertebrae are represented by the symbols L1 through L5. There are correspondingly five lumbar nerves.

**lymphatic system:** The system of the body that is responsible for the immune response. A tiered system of defense that uses physical barriers, such as the skin, and general defense mechanisms, such as the white blood cells, as well as specialized cells called "lymphocytes" that detect specific invaders (such as fungi, bacteria, and viruses) and eliminate them from the body.

**macrobiotics:** A dietary program in which foods are classified according to the principles of yin and yang and consist mainly of whole grains and vegetables.

**magnesium:** A mineral needed for healthy muscles, nerves, and bones. It also helps maintain normal blood sugar levels and blood pressure.

**malnourished:** Lacking adequate nutrients in the diet.

**malnutrition:** The chronic lack of sufficient nutrients to maintain health.

**mania:** A mental disorder characterized by an intense feeling of elation and excitability, often accompanied by increased activity.

**meditation:** Contemplation of spiritual matters or reflection, as a religious practice or as a form of relaxation and stress relief.

**mental illness:** Any disease of the mind or the state of mind of someone who has emotional or behavioral problems serious enough to require psychiatric intervention.

**metabolism:** All the processes that occur in the human body that turn food into energy the body can use.

**microorganism:** A microscopic life form that cannot be seen with the naked eye. Types of microorganisms include bacteria, viruses, protozoa, fungi, yeasts, and some parasites and algae.

**migraine:** Strong headaches on one or both sides of the head that may be accompanied by nausea, vomiting, increased sensitivity of the eyes to light (photophobia), increased sensitivity to sound (phonophobia), dizziness, blurred vision, cognitive disturbances, and other symptoms.

**minerals:** Inorganic substances that serve a function similar to vitamins. They include chemical elements such as calcium or iron as well as some compounds.

**molars:** The 12 grinding or chewing teeth, located at the back of the upper and lower jaws.

**monosaccharide:** A sugar that may no longer be broken down into simpler sugars by hydrolysis.

**monounsaturated fat:** The fat found in canola oil, olive oil, nuts, and seeds that may help lower cholesterol and reduce the risk of heart disease.

**nausea:** The urge to vomit, brought on by many causes, including systemic illnesses such as influenza, medications, pain, and inner-ear disease.

**neurotransmitters:** Chemicals in the brain and other nervous-system tissues that aid in the transmission of nerve impulses.

**nicotine:** A chemical found in tobacco that is addictive and poisonous. When it enters the human body it causes an increased heart rate and a sense of well-being and relaxation.

**nutrients:** Materials essential to the survival of an organism, including proteins, carbohydrates, lipids or fats, vitamins, and minerals.

**nutrition:** The study of nutrients, their consumption, and how they are processed by the human body.

**Nutrition Facts Label:** The labeling required by the FDA that offers specific nutrition information for that packaged product. Food packaged in bulk is exempt from the labeling requirement, but manufactures may voluntarily include such labeling.

**nutrition standards:** A collective term for the nutrition goals that school meals must meet when averaged over a school week for students, based on Reference Daily Intake or Recommended Daily Intake (RDI) levels for specific nutrients.

**obese:** Having a body mass index (BMI) greater than 30.

**OCD:** "Obsessive-compulsive disorder" is an anxiety disorder characterized by uneasiness, apprehension, fear, or worry with symptoms that include repetitive behaviors or nervous habits used to reduce anxiety.

**omega-3 fatty acids:** A group of polyunsaturated fatty acids found in fish oil and seeds, such as linseed oil, which are thought to reduce blood clotting and may reduce the risk of heart attack or stroke.

**oncologist:** One who diagnoses and recommends treatment for cancer.

**organic farming:** A method of farming that does not use chemicals to kill weeds or pests.

**osteoporosis:** A disease in which bones become more fragile and brittle and are at increased risk of breaking.

**out-of-pocket limit:** A predetermined amount of money that an individual must pay before insurance will pay 100% of an individual's health care expenses.

**outbreak:** Spread of disease, which occurs in a short period of time and in a limited geographic location, such as a neighborhood, community, school, or hospital.

**outpatient:** A patient who is not an inpatient (not hospitalized) but instead is cared for elsewhere—as in a doctor's office, clinic, or day surgery center.

**over-the-counter:** A designation for a drug that can be sold without a prescription. Common examples include cold medicines, pain relievers, and laxatives.

**overweight:** Being too heavy for one's height, defined as a body mass index (BMI) of 25 to 30.

**pain:** An unpleasant sensation that can range from mild, localized discomfort to agony. Pain has both physical and emotional components. The physical part of pain results from nerve stimulation. Pain may be contained to a single area, as in an injury, or it can be more diffuse, as in disorders like fibromyalgia.

**pandemic:** An outbreak of disease that spread throughout the world.

**paranoia:** A mental disorder characterized by suspicion, delusions of persecution, or jealousy.

**pasteurization:** The process of destroying disease-causing microorganisms by heating food to a high enough temperature to kill the bacteria. The process was named for scientist Louis Pasteur.

**pathogen:** Any microorganism that is infectious or toxigenic and causes disease, including parasites, viruses, and some yeast and bacteria.

**periodontitis:** A serious gum infection that kills soft tissue and bones that support teeth.

**perspiration:** Sweat or salty fluid excreted from the sweat glands of the skin, usually through exercise or some form of physical exertion.

**pesticide:** A chemical used to kill plants or pests, such as crop-damaging insects.

**physical activity:** Any form of exercise or movement that may include planned activities such as walking, running, or other sports or daily activities such as yard work or house cleaning.

**phytochemicals:** Plant compounds found in dark fruits and vegetables, which are believed to have health-protecting qualities.

**phytoestrogens:** Naturally occurring plant compounds that are thought to have a number of different health benefits.

**plaque:** A film or deposit of bacteria and other material on the surface of a tooth that may lead to tooth decay or periodontal disease.

**point-of-service plan:** Health insurance policy that allows the employee to choose between in-network or out-of-network care each time medical treatment is needed.

**polysaccharide:** A carbohydrate that may be broken down by hydrolysis into two or more molecules of monosaccharides.

**polyunsaturated fat:** An unsaturated fat that is liquid at room temperature. These fats are found in the greatest amounts in corn, soybean, and safflower oils.

**polyunsaturated fatty acids:** Fats consisting of a large percentage of unsaturated fatty acids that include corn, safflower, and sesame oils. They are believed to lower LDL cholesterol, reducing the amount of artery-clogging cholesterol in the bloodstream.

**PPO:** "Preferred provider organization," a health care organization composed of doctors, hospitals, or other providers to offer health care services at a reduced price.

**preexisting condition:** Any physical illness, mental illness, or chronic disease for which medical advice, diagnosis, care, or treatment was recommended or received within the six-month time immediately before enrollment in a health plan. Pregnancy cannot be counted as a preexisting condition.

**prescription:** A physician's order for the preparation and administration of a drug or device for a patient. A prescription has several parts, including the superscription or heading, with the symbol "R" or "Rx," which stands for the word "recipe" (meaning, in Latin, "to take"); the inscription, which contains the names and quantities of the ingredients; the subscription, or directions, for compounding the drug; and the signature, which is often preceded by the sign "s," standing for signa (Latin for mark), giving the directions to be marked on the container.

**prognosis:** A prediction of the course or outcome of a disease.

**proteins:** Large molecules that are essential to the structure and functioning of all living cells.

**psychiatric:** Pertaining to or within the purview of psychiatry, the medical specialty concerned with the prevention, diagnosis, and treatment of mental illness.

**psychiatrist:** A physician or medical doctor (MD) who specializes in the prevention, diagnosis, and treatment of mental illness. Psychiatrists must receive additional training and serve a supervised residency in their specialty.

**psychosis:** A mental disorder of serious magnitude where an individual loses touch with reality and may suffer from delusions and hallucinations.

**pterostilbene:** A naturally occurring antioxidant in blueberries.

**qualified high-deductible health plan:** A health plan with lower premiums that covers health care expenses after the insured has paid a yearly large amount out of pocket.

**quarantine:** To isolate an individual who has or is suspected of having a disease, in order to prevent the spread of that disease to others. Quarantine can be voluntary or can be ordered by public health officials during a state of emergency.

**radiologist:** One who administers technology such as X-rays and ultra sounds to diagnose medical problems.

**recall:** The voluntary action of removing a product from retail or distribution. The action is conducted by a manufacturer or distributor to protect the public from products that may cause serious health problems or possible death.

**RDAs:** "Recommended Dietary Allowances," or the estimated amount of nutrients needed daily for good health.

**recombinant bovine growth hormone:** A synthetic hormone marketed to dairy farmers to increase milk production in cows. Its use, while allowed in the United States, has been banned in the European Union and Canada since 1999.

**reflexology:** An alternative medicine or treatment that involves the application of pressure to the feet and hands through a system of zones and reflex areas.

**refrigeration:** The process of chilling food for preservation.

**registered dietitian (RD):** A health professional who is a food and nutrition expert and who has completed an American Dietetic Association (ADA) approved program of study and passed an exam.

**reiki:** A Japanese technique for stress reduction and relaxation that promotes healing and is administered by laying on hands.

**relapse:** The return of a disease or symptoms of a disease after an apparent recovery.

**REM sleep:** "Rapid eye movement sleep," when dreaming occurs and the eyes move even though they are closed.

**resting metabolic rate (RMR):** The total amount of energy the human body uses in a given period of time when at rest. Factors that influence RMR include body size, composition, activity level, and diet.

**rhinovirus:** A large subgroup of viruses that is responsible for a large percentage of cases of the common cold.

**root canal:** The space in the root of a tooth that contains nerves.

**roughage:** Indigestible fiber of fruits, vegetables, and cereals that assist in the elimination of waste for the digestive system.

**Salmonella:** A group of bacteria that is one of the most common causes of food poisoning and that is a frequent contaminator of foods.

**saturated fat:** A fat that is solid at room temperature and found in high-fat dairy products, meats, palm oil. and coconut oil. Eating a diet high in saturated fat may raise cholesterol and increase the risk of heart disease.

**sciatic nerve:** The largest nerve in the body, formed by the motor and sensory nerves to and from the legs and feet. It begins at the base of the spinal cord and passes through the pelvis and down the back of each thigh to the heel.

**scurvy:** A disease caused by a deficiency of vitamin C. Symptoms include a weakening of connective tissue in bone and muscle.

**sedentary:** Describing a person or lifestyle characterized by inactivity that can contribute to obesity and associated health problems.

**serotonin:** A hormone, also called "5-hydroxytryptamine," that acts both as a chemical messenger that transmits nerve signals between nerve cells and that causes blood vessels to narrow.

**sexually transmitted disease:** Any disease transmitted by sexual contact; caused by microorganisms that survive on the skin or mucus membranes of the genital area; or transmitted via semen, vaginal secretions, or blood during intercourse. They include AIDS, chlamydia, genital herpes, genital warts, gonorrhea, syphilis, yeast infections, and some forms of hepatitis. Also known as a *morbus venereus,* or venereal disease.

**sleep:** The body's rest cycle.

**sterile:** Clean and free of bacteria and/or microorganisms.

**strength training:** Increases the strength of muscles, bones, ligaments, and tendons and also builds muscle mass through the use of resistance via the body's weight, such as in push-ups or with equipment that includes free weights, bands, tubes, or weighted medicine balls.

**stress:** Forces from the outside world impinging on the individual.

**stroke:** The loss of blood flow to any part of the brain, which then damages brain tissue. The risk for stroke is increased by conditions including high blood pressure, smoking, diabetes, high cholesterol, or heart disease.

**substance abuse:** The excessive use of a substance, especially alcohol or a drug.

**Supplemental Security Income (SSI):** A program providing cash benefits to certain low-income, disabled, or elderly individuals. Those who qualify for SSI generally also qualify for Medicaid.

**surgeon:** A physician who treats disease, injury, or deformity by operative or manual methods. A medical doctor specialized in the removal of organs, masses, and tumors and in doing other procedures using a knife (scalpel).

**sustainable agriculture:** A method of farming designed to preserve the environment of the land, livestock, and surrounding area while ensuring profitability.

**systolic pressure:** The highest blood pressure produced by the contraction of the heart. It is recorded as the first number in a blood pressure measurement.

**target heart rate:** The level at which the human heart is beating with moderate to high intensity and is 50 percent to 85 percent of the maximum heart rate of 220 minus your age.

**tartar:** Plaque deposits on the teeth.

**tincture:** A medication made up of an alcoholic solution of a vegetable or animal extract or a chemical substance.

**tobacco:** A plant with leaves that have high levels of the addictive chemical nicotine. The leaves may be smoked, applied to the gums, or inhaled. The scientific name is *Nicotiana tabacum.*

**tocopherol:** A class of compounds, many of which have vitamin E activity.

**topical:** Designed to have an effect on a limited area of the body, a description of creams and lotions that are applied to the skin, eyes, ears, hair, or mucous membranes for maximum effectiveness.

**toxic:** Having to do with poison or a substance that is harmful to the human body and that can cause unwanted side effects.

**trans fatty acid:** A fat that is produced when liquid fat or oil is turned into solid fat through a chemical process called "hydrogenation." Eating trans fat is considered more of a health risk than eating saturated fat.

**triglyceride:** A form of fat that the body makes from sugar, alcohol, or excess calories.

**tryptophan:** An amino acid well-known to foster drowsiness.

**unsaturated fat:** A fat that is liquid at room temperature and includes polyunsaturated fats and monounsaturated fats. It includes most nuts, olives, avocados, and fatty fish.

**urine:** Fluid containing water and waste products that is made by the kidneys, stored in the bladder, and exits the body through the urethra.

**vaccination:** Injection of a weakened or dead microorganism such as a bacterium or virus, given to prevent or treat infectious diseases.

**vaccine:** The weakened or dead microorganisms or viruses of a disease that are introduced through vaccination into the body to stimulate immunity.

**vegan:** A vegetarian who does not consume any animal products and does not use products derived from animals, such as leather or fur.

**vegetarian:** A person who excludes all meat, poultry, and fish from his or her diet and instead eats plant foods. Some vegetarians include dairy products and eggs in their diets and are known as "lacto-ovo-vegetarians"; others who exclude all animal foods are known as "vegans."

**vertebra:** Any one of the 33 bones that make up the human spine.

**virus:** A microorganism, smaller than bacteria, that cannot grow or reproduce apart from a living cell. A virus invades living cells and uses their chemical machinery to keep itself alive and to replicate itself.

**vitamins:** Organic substances essential to the nutrition of humans, animals, and some plants. Vitamins are needed in differing quantities. They work with enzymes in regulating metabolic processes.

**X-ray:** A diagnostic imaging technique that shows a two-dimensional image and is used to analyze various bones or some diseases of soft tissue.

**waiting period:** The time period required to work for an employer before an individual is eligible for health benefits as part of that employers' group health plan. If an employer requires a waiting period, a preexisting condition exclusion period begins on the first day of the waiting period.

**water-soluble vitamins:** Vitamins, such as vitamin C and the B-complex vitamins, that are soluble in the watery parts of plant and animal tissues.

**weight control:** Achieving and maintaining a healthy weight by eating well and getting regular physical activity.

**weight cycle:** Losing and gaining weight over and over again, also known as "yo-yo dieting."

**yang:** A principle in Chinese philosophy that is positive, active, dry, hot, and masculine in nature and balances the other fundamental principle of yin.

**yin:** A principle in Chinese philosophy that is negative, dark, passive, cold, wet, and feminine in nature and balances the principle of yang.

**yoga:** Derived from the Sanskrit word for "yoke" or "join together," it means "union." It is the science of uniting the individual with the cosmic spirit through physical postures and meditation.

**yo-yo dieting:** Constant weight loss and gain over and over again due to fad dieting or other short-term diet plans.

# Internet Resources

The following resource list offers online sites of nonprofit, government, and private organizations that provide information on numerous aspects of wellness and health. While there are many different facets of wellness covered in this encyclopedia and in this list, there are many organizations not listed here that could also be useful. If you do not find the information you seek, we suggest using these websites to follow the numerous links they offer. The organizations are listed alphabetically under broad topics.

## GENERAL RESOURCES

American Association for the Advancement of Science
1200 New York Avenue NW
Washington, DC 20005
www.aaas.org

The AAAS is a nonprofit, professional association made up of scientists, engineers, and science educators. Their mission is to educate the general public about science and technology.

American Council on Science and Health
1995 Broadway, 2nd Floor
New York, NY 10023-5860
www.acsh.org

The ACSH is a consumer-education consortium of physicians, scientists, and policy advisors that works to provide education to consumers.

American Dental Association
211 E. Chicago Avenue
Chicago, IL 60611
312-440-2500
www.ada.org

The ADA labels itself the country's leading advocate for oral health and offers professional resources for members as well as information for the public on all aspects of dental health and related research.

American Medical Association
515 N. State Street
Chicago, IL 60654
800-621-8335
www.ama-assn.org

The AMA provides resources for physicians with additional information aimed at the general consumer. The site offers a members-only portion and related links to various health issues.

American Red Cross
2025 E. Street NW
Washington, DC 20006
202-303-5000
www.redcross.org

The website for this world-renowned emergency response organization features information about volunteering, classes, assistance, and news.

Centers for Disease Control and Prevention (CDC)
1600 Clifton Road
Atlanta, GA 30333
www.cdc.gov

This government agency is part of the Department of Health and Human Services, and its website offers information to consumers on all aspects of health and disease.

Consumer Information Center
Pueblo, CO 81009
www.usa.gov/topics/consumer.shtml

The CIC is a government agency included under the General Services Administration (GSA) that maintains a large catalog of consumer publications on a variety of health, food, and nutrition issues.

Consumers Union
101 Truman Avenue
Yonkers, NY 10703-1057
www.consumersunion.org

This independent, nonprofit testing organization publishes the popular *Consumer Reports Magazine.* The website offers consumers links to information and to various government agencies that handle consumer complaints.

Family Doctor.Org
American Academy of Family Physicians

11400 Tomahawk Creek Parkway
Leawood, KS 66211-2680
http://familydoctor.org/online/famdocen/home.html

Easy to read and understand, FamilyDoctor.org is operated by the American Academy of Family Physicians (AAFP), a national medical organization of family physicians, family practice residents, and medical students. Information on the website is written and reviewed by physicians and patient education professionals at the AAFP. Topics range from diseases and conditions to health insurance.

Health Resources and Services Administration
5600 Fishers Lane
Rockville, MD 20857
301-443-3376
www.hrsa.gov

This U.S. Department of Health and Human Services website links to a great deal of government health information, including information about transplants, HIV and AIDS, and the National Health Service Corps as well as public health links.

Healthfinder/U.S. Department of Health and Human Services
PO Box 1133
Washington, DC 20013-1133
www.healthfinder.gov

This government agency website, from the Department of Health and Human Services, covers everything from breast-feeding to nutrition information from federal and state agencies. The site also includes information about support and self-help groups.

Healthy People 2020
200 Independence Avenue SW
Washington, DC 20201
http://www.health.gov/healthypeople/default.htm

This website offers details about the U.S. Department of Health and Human Services Healthy People 2020 Initiative, with progress reports, updated statistics and information.

Mayo Clinic
200 First Street SW
Rochester, MN 55905
904-953-2000
www.mayoclinic.org

The Mayo Clinic, a nonprofit, worldwide leader in medical care, research, and education developed this website to further provide information to medical professionals, patients, and their families in the form of past articles, current research, as well as providing a question-and-answer format.

Medical Library Association
65 East Wacker Place, Suite 1900
Chicago, IL 60601-7246
312-419-9094
www.mlanet.org

This nonprofit, educational organization of health sciences information professionals supports research and works to promote the importance of quality information for improved health in the community. Their resources section includes
recommended, authoritative sites for consumers and for the conditions or cancer,
diabetes, and heart disease: http://www.mlanet.org/resources/userguide.html.

Medline Plus
8600 Rockville Pike
Bethesda, MD 20894
www.nlm.nih.gov/medlineplus

A service of the U.S. National Library of Medicine through the National Institutes of Health, this online resource connects consumers with the latest research
in health topics, drugs, supplements, and other health facts.

National Health Information Center
PO Box 1133
Washington, DC 20013-1133
800-336-4797
www.health.gov

Sponsored by the U.S. Department of Health and Human Services, this health
referral service answers questions for professionals and consumers on all kinds of
health issues. It also provides support through the Healthfinder website, another
government resource for consumer health information.

National Institutes of Health (NIH)
9000 Rockville Pike
Bethesda, Maryland 20892
301-496-4000
http://health.nih.gov

This government website provides a comprehensive list of resources on health
issues from ADHD to stress or viruses. The NIH is under the U.S. Department of
Health and Human Services.

National Library of Medicine
8600 Rockville Pike
Bethesda, MD 20894
888-346-3656
www.nlm.nih.gov

Located on the campus of the National Institutes of Health, this is the world's
largest medical library with a collection of material that is available for research in

all areas of medicine and health care. The various reading rooms are open during the week for research or for those interested in learning more about diseases, drugs, clinical trials, and other medical resources.

Physicians Committee for Responsible Medicine
5100 Wisconsin Avenue NW, Suite 400
Washington, DC 20016
www.pcrm.org

The PCRM promotes nutrition and preventive medicine and supports research programs for diabetes, cancer, and other issues. This website offers restaurant reviews, physician referrals, and other resources for students and educators.

## ALTERNATIVE HEALTH CARE AND COMPLEMENTARY MEDICINE

American Academy of Medical Acupuncture
5820 Wilshire Boulevard, Suite 500
Los Angeles, CA 90036
800-521-2262
www.medicalacupuncture.org

This medical-physician-only professional organization works to promote the integration of acupuncture with Western medical training. The organization is open only to physician acupuncturists.

American Association of Acupuncture and Oriental Medicine
PO Box 162340
Sacramento, CA 95816
866-455-7999
www.aaom.org

Formed in 1981, the AAAOM is a national association promoting the professional standards in the practice of acupuncture and oriental medicine in the United States, with the goal of promoting excellence and integrity in the profession.

American Association of Naturopathic Physicians
4435 Wisconsin Avenue NW, Suite 403
Washington, DC 20016
866-538-2267
www.naturopathic.org

This website provides consumer information and the ability to search for a naturopathic doctor by zip code. There is also a database of members and information concerning professional education for members.

American Botanical Council
PO Box 144345

Austin, TX 78714-4345
512-926-4900
www.herbalgram.org

This nonprofit research and information organization is dedicated to providing accurate and reliable information for consumers about the use of herbs and medicinal plants.

American College for Advancement in Medicine
24411 Ridge Route, Suite 115
Laguna Hills, CA 92653
949-309-3520
www.acamnet.org

This not-for-profit corporation is dedicated to the education of physicians and other health care professionals in complementary, alternative, and integrative medicine. The website offers a public connection to physicians who use integrative medicine and information on integrative treatment options.

American Holistic Medical Association
PO Box 2016
Edmonds, WA 98020
425-967-0737
www.holisticmedicine.org

This organization serves it members and provides advocacy about the use of holistic and integrative medicine by licensed health care providers. It also provides links to those patients interested in choosing a holistic provider.

American Meditation Institute
PO Box 430
Averill Park, NY 12018
518-674-8714
www.americanmeditation.org

The AMI is a nonprofit education organization working to improve training and education in mind-body medicine by offering information as well as a speaker's bureau and links to other organizations.

American Yoga Association
PO Box 19986
Sarasota, FL 34276
912-927-4977
www.americanyogaassociation.org

This website offers information about yoga, its history, types, and how to choose a qualified teacher.

Association of Accredited Naturopathic Medical Colleges
4435 Wisconsin Avenue NW, Suite 403
Washington, DC 20016

202.237.8150
www.aanmc.org

This website provides information about naturopathy and naturopathic medicine, including a list of schools offering the program, admission and application information, career information, and open house and campus tour details.

Ayurvedic Institute
PO Box 23445
Albuquerque, NM 87192
www.ayurveda.com

This nonprofit organization features a school and spa plus links to information about the practice of ayurvedic medicine, along with education, membership information, an events calendar, and other online resources.

Center for Mind-Body Medicine
5225 Connecticut Avenue NW, Suite 414
Washington, DC 20015
202-966-7338
www.cmbm.org

This nonprofit educational organization offers facts about resources, research, a list of CMBM certified practitioners, and a job and internship list.

National Ayurvedic Medical Association
620 Cabrillo Avenue
Santa Cruz, CA 95065
800-669-8914
www.ayurveda-nama.org

This website links Ayurvedic medical professionals from across the country and works to promote the science and practice of Ayurveda.

National Center for Complementary and Alternative Medicine
NCCAM Clearinghouse
9000 Rockville Pike
Bethesda, MD 20892
888-644-6226
http://nccam.nih.gov

The NCCAM is the U.S. government's lead agency for scientific research on unconventional or complementary medical practices, research, and products. The website offers information as well as links to research, grants, training, and legislative updates.

National Commission for Certification of Acupuncture and Oriental Medicine
76 South Laura Street, Suite 1290
Jacksonville, FL 32202
904-598-1005
www.nccaom.org

This nonprofit organization evaluates entry-level programs and competency in the practice of acupuncture and oriental medicine through its program of professional certification.

## DISEASES AND DISORDERS

AIDSinfo: National Institutes of Health (NIH)
PO Box 6303
Rockville, MD 20849-6303
http://aidsinfo.nih.gov

This government website is provided by the U.S. Department of Health and Human Services to offer information about HIV/AIDS treatment, prevention, research, and related health topics and offers a link to clinical trials.

AllergyKids
PO Box 20236
Boulder, CO 80308
www.allergykids.com

This organization is working to provide information about additives used in food. It is run entirely by volunteers, and donations are contributed toward research on the role of food in the health of children.

Alliance for Lupus Research
28 West 44th Street, Suite 501
New York, NY 10036
212-218-2840 or 800-867-1743
www.lupusresearch.org

The ALR is a national health organization founded in 1999 by Robert Wood Johnson IV. Its focus is to discover better treatments and to ultimately prevent and cure systemic lupus erythematosus (SLE).

Alzheimer's Association
225 N. Michigan Avenue, Floor 17
Chicago, IL 60601-7633
800-272-3900
www.alz.org

This nonprofit association seeks to improve care for Alzheimer's sufferers on a national and international level. The website offers links to support groups, a 24-hour helpline, and links to information on clinical trials.

Alzheimer's Disease Education and Referral Center
PO Box 8250
Silver Spring, MD 20907-8250
800-438-4380
www.nia.nih.gov/alzhemers/alzheimersInformation/generalinfo

This government site, under the U.S. National Institutes of Health National Institute on Aging, offers research-based information on Alzheimer's disease via publications, clinical trials, and research and news.

American Academy of Allergy, Asthma & Immunology
555 East Wells Street, Suite 1100
Milwaukee, WI 53202-3823
800-822-2762
www.aaaai.org

The AAAI is a professional medical specialty organization that represents allergists, physicians, clinical immunologists, and health professionals, and their online site offers consumers a referral directory and resource center along with information.

American Autoimmune Related Diseases Association
22100 Gratiot Avenue East
Detroit, MI 48021
800-598-4668
www.aarda.org

The AARDA is a national, nonprofit health agency dedicated to eradication of autoimmune diseases through education, public awareness, research, and patient services.

American Cancer Society
250 Williams Street
Atlanta, GA 30303
800-227-2345
www.cancer.org

The ACS is a national voluntary health organization whose goal is to assist those with cancer by providing information and by supporting research.

The American College of Allergy, Asthma, and Immunology
85 West Algonquin Road, Suite 550
Arlington Heights, IL 60005
847-427-1200
www.acaai.org

This professional organization of allergists, immunologists, and allied health professionals works to promote excellence in the practice of allergy and immunology and provides members with continuing education, publications, and other resources.

American Diabetes Association
1701 North Beauregard Street
Alexandria, VA 22311
www.diabetes.org

This association works to prevent and cure diabetes through funding for research and by providing information for diabetics and others interested in the disease.

American Gastroenterological Association
4930 Del Ray Avenue
Bethesda, MD 20814
301-654-5920
www.gastro.org

This professional site focuses on serving its members and their information needs and supports both researchers and clinicians through education, job openings, and by offering resources to members to support their efforts to provide clinical care.

American Heart Association
7272 Greenville Avenue
Dallas, TX 75231
www.americanheart.org

This association provides clear, concise information on heart disease as well as on nutrition, exercise, and stroke-related illness for a general audience.

American Institute for Cancer Research
1759 R Street, NW
Washington, DC 20009
www.aicr.org

This is a national charity offering information on cancer along with legislative and news updates. The site also offers a resource to answer questions for newly diagnosed cancer patients and their families.

American Lung Association
1301 Pennsylvania Avenue NW, Suite 800
Washington, DC 20004
www.lungusa.org

This organization has been in operation for over 100 years, according to its website, and continues to improve lung health and prevent lung disease by supporting education and research.

Arthritis Foundation
1330 West Peachtree Street
Atlanta, GA 30309
800-283-7800 or 404-872-7100
www.arthritis.org

This organization is dedicated to improving the lives of people with arthritis through information, access to health care, advocacy, and supporting research.

Asthma and Allergy Foundation of America
1233 20th Street NW, Suite 402
Washington, DC 20036
800-727-8462
www.aafa.org

This organization and its website is geared toward allergy suffers and provides information about clinics, support groups, and health professionals with links to regional chapters around the United States.

Autism Society of America
7910 Woodmont Avenue, Suite 300
Bethesda, MD 20814-3067
800-AUTISM
www.autism-society.org

The website for this grassroots organization features its quarterly journal, publications, and programs while it continues to advocate for the rights of all people with autism.

Celiac Disease Foundation
13251 Ventura Boulevard, Suite 1
Studio City, CA 91604
818-990-2354
www.celiac.org

This website is designed to provide resources, information, diet and lifestyle suggestions, and treatment information for those suffering from celiac disease.

CFIDS Association of America
PO Box 220398
Charlotte, NC 28222-0398
704-365-2343
www.cfids.org

The CFIDS Association is a charitable organization dedicated to conquering chronic fatigue and immune dysfunction syndrome, and its website offers links to research, free brochures, a youth home page, along with patient support and advocacy.

Christopher & Dana Reeve Foundation
636 Morris Turnpike, Suite 3A
Short Hills, NJ 07078
800-225-0292
www.christopherreeve.org

This international website, which can be accessed in eight different languages, is designed to provide information for those dealing with spinal cord injury as well as resources for those working with spinal injury patients. There is additional research, including a link to the Quality of Life grants program and the Paralysis Resource Center.

Crohn's and Colitis Foundation of America
386 Park Avenue South, 17th Floor
New York, NY 10016
800-932-2423
www.ccfa.org

This website provides information about the nonprofit organization and its resources aimed at assisting those living with Crohn's disease and ulcerative colitis. There are links to research, disease management choices, and even a youth and teen page.

Gluten Intolerance Group of North America
31214 124th Avenue, SE
Auburn, WA 98092
253-833-6655
www.gluten.net

The website for this nonprofit organization provides medical information, a recipe database, links to gluten-free restaurants and a list of local branches across the United States for those suffering from gluten intolerance.

HIV-UCSF Center for HIV Information
4150 Clement Street, Box 111V
San Francisco, CA 94121
http:// hivinsite.ucsf.edu

This program from the University of California San Francisco school of Medicine has partnered with government agencies, international organizations, and charitable foundations to advance the prevention and care of HIV infection and its related illnesses. The site has an international focus along with a list of projects that target services for specific HIV populations.

Immune Deficiency Foundation
40 W. Chesapeake Avenue, Suite 308
Towson, MD 21204
800-296-4433
www.primaryimmune.org

Although immunodeficiency diseases are considered relatively rare, this organization provides accurate information on research, treatment, and patient needs to an international audience.

International Association for Chronic Fatigue Syndrome CFS/ME
27 N. Wacker Drive, Suite 416
Chicago, IL 60606
847-258-7248
www.iacfsme.org

This not-for-profit organization, started in 1992, works to support those with CFS by providing information for researchers, clinicians, health care workers, and support groups. Membership is also available internationally for those interested in the organization.

International Foundation for Functional Gastrointestinal Disorders (IFFGD)
PO Box 170864
Milwaukee, WI 53217
414-964-1799
www.iffgd.org

This nonprofit organization is focused on education and research dedicated to assisting people with gastrointestinal disorders. Information is available for patients, their families, and medical professionals.

Juvenile Diabetes Research Foundation International
120 Wall Street
New York, NY 10005-4001
800-533-2873
www.jdrf.org

This international organization works with other groups around the world to provide information, research, and assistance in developing new and better treatments for patients with juvenile diabetes. The website features research, publications, and information about advocacy.

Learning Disabilities Association of America
4156 Library Road
Pittsburgh, PA 15234-1349
412-341-8077
www.ldanatl.org

This nonprofit organization, started in the 1960s, now serves tens of thousands of members with learning disabilities as well as their families and the professionals who assist them. The website offers resources for teachers, parents, adults, and professionals as well as links to a bookstore, resources, state chapters of the organization, and legislative updates.

Leukemia & Lymphoma Society
1311 Mamaroneck Avenue
White Plains, NY 10605
800-955-4572
www.leukemia-lymphoma.org

This organization supports fund researchers who are working to find a cure for leukemia, lymphoma, Hodgkin's disease, and melanoma and offers information that links individuals with clinical trials and to services they need as they manage their disease.

Lupus Foundation of America
800-558-0121
www.lupus.org

This interactive website offers basic information about lupus, connects individuals to local chapters of this national nonprofit health organization and support groups, and sponsors a Walk for Lupus fund-raiser.

March of Dimes Foundation
1275 Mamaroneck Avenue
White Plains, NY 10605
888-663-4637
www.marchofdimes.com

This organization was started by President Franklin D. Roosevelt to help fight the disease of polio. Over the years, the mission of the organization has shifted to support research in finding and curing the causes of premature birth and birth defects.

MRSA Survivors Network
PO Box 241
Hinsdale, IL 60522
630-325-4354
www.mrsasurvivors.org

This network was founded in early 2003 to inform consumers and health providers about the serious health issues association with MRSA. The organization lobbies for change in national policy concerning MRSA and public health.

National Cancer Institute
NCI Public Inquiries Office
6116 Executive Boulevard, Suite 300
Bethesda, MD 20892-8322
800-422-6237
www.cancer.gov

This government website offers information on cancer-related questions along with medical research related to cancer and has a list of clinical trials. It also links to the National Institute of Health for additional cancer and health issues.

National Center for Learning Disabilities
381 Park Avenue South, Suite 1401
New York, NY 10016
212-545-7510
www.ncld.org

This organization advocates for U.S. children, adolescents, and adults with learning disabilities, and its site offers a resource locator, age-related content, a blog to connect members, and a newsletter.

National Center on Sleep Disorders Research
6701 Rockledge Drive
Bethesda, MD 20892
301-435-0199
www.nhlbi.nih.gov/about/ncsdr

This branch of the National Institutes of Health offers sufferers of sleep disorders links to research, patient information, and training for health professionals.

National Eye Institute
31 Center Drive
Bethesda, MD 20892-3655
301-496-5248
www.nei.nih.gov

Established in 1968 by President Lyndon B. Johnson, this government organization is dedicated to promoting research and finding a cure for human eye diseases and disorders. The website links to jobs, training, resources, research, news, and health information.

National Institute of Allergy and Infectious Diseases
6610 Rockledge Drive, MSC 6612
Bethesda, MD 20892
866-284-4107
www.niaid.nih.gov

Sponsored by the Department of Health and Human Services and its National Institutes of Health, this organization is designed to improve research, understanding, treatment, and responses to immunologic, infectious, and allergic diseases. There are links to scientific resources, funding sources, research, and news and legislative updates.

National Osteoporosis Foundation
1232 22nd Street NW
Washington, DC 20037-1292
800-231-4222
www.nof.org

This national organization is dedicated to the prevention of osteoporosis and works to promote education, legislation, and research to improve treatment and diagnosis of this disease.

Obsessive-Compulsive Foundation
337 Notch Hill Road
North Bramford, CT 06471
203-315-2190
www.ocfoundation.org

This international not-for-profit organization was founded in 1986 and works to link individuals with obsessive compulsive disorder or related disorders with health care professionals and information to assist them in their treatment. The website lists resources, programs, research, and legislative updates for interested individuals.

PCOSupport
PO Box 3403
Englewood, CO 80155-3403
www.pcosupport.org

This site, sponsored by the Polycystic Ovarian Syndrome Association, Inc., is dedicated to serving women who have been diagnosed with PCOS. The website offers information on medical treatments and supplements and also offers a message board for women who need support and a newsletter with links to recent research in PCOS and its treatment.

## ENVIRONMENTAL HEALTH

American Association of Poison Control Centers
515 King Street, Suite 510
Alexandria, VA 22314
800-222-1222
www.aapcc.org

The AAPCC is a private association that represents the poison control centers and their staff in the United States. The website provides tools to find poison control centers around the country.

EarthSave International
20555 Devonshire St., Suite 105,
Chatsworth, CA 91311
www.earthsave.org

The organization is funded by memberships and contributions, and the site offers information on how a vegetarian diet helps the planet.

National Institute of Environmental Health Sciences (NIH)
111 T.W. Alexander Drive
Research Triangle Park, NC 27709
www.niehs.nih.gov

This environmental organization promotes the health of the community and supports research under the umbrella of the National Institutes of Health. The website offers information on a large variety of issues ranging from carcinogens, like formaldehyde and aristolochic acids, to cell phone health concerns, environmental diseases, and a follow-up to the environmental impact of the Gulf Oil Spill.

Union of Concerned Scientists
161 First Street, Fourth Floor
Cambridge, MA 02142
www.ucsusa.org

Calling itself the leading science-based nonprofit working for a healthy environment, this organization offers scientific research, encourages citizen action through legislative updates, and offers individuals an opportunity to donate in support of various environmental issues.

U.S. Environmental Protection Agency (EPA)
1200 Pennsylvania Avenue, NW
Washington, DC 20460
www.epa.gov

This highly interactive website, provided by the U.S. government, offers an A to Z index of issues facing Americans, including acid rain, mold, radon, and climate change. The website includes news and announcements as well as a map of the United States that offers a breakdown of environmental issues unique to each state, additional research, and contact information.

## EXERCISE AND WEIGHT CONTROL

Aerobic and Fitness Association of America (AFAA)
15250 Ventura Boulevard, Suite 200
Sherman Oaks, CA 91430
www.afaa.com

The AFAA website offers fitness education for professionals and upholds the Basic Exercise Standards and Guidelines for safe fitness practice.

American Anorexia/Bulimia Association
165 West 46th Street, Suite 1108
New York, NY 10036
212-575-6200
www.aabainc.org

The AABA is a nonprofit organization for those dedicated to the treatment of eating disorders, and the information on this site is geared for the general public.

American College of Rheumatology
2200 Lake Boulevard NE
Atlanta, GA 30319
404-633-3777
www.rheumatology.org

The organization is overseen by a foundation established in 1985, with the goal of advancing research and training to improve the treatment and understanding of rheumatology.

American College of Sports Medicine (ACSM)
PO Box 1440
Indianapolis, IN 46206
317-637-9200
www.acsm.org

This professional organization provides access to research, education, and advocacy for certified professionals, graduate students, and undergraduate students in the field of applied exercise science and clinical sports medicine.

American Council on Exercise (ACE)
4851 Paramount Drive
San Diego, CA 92123
800-825-3636
www.acefitness.org

This nonprofit organization is a resource for fitness professionals and consumers, provides research on fitness products and programs, and offers certification and continuing education standards for fitness professionals.

American Society of Bariatric Physicians
5600 South Quebec Street, Suite 109A
Englewood, CO 80111
303-770-2526
www.asbp.org

While there is a members-only section for doctors, there is also information for the general public about obesity and related surgical treatments.

President's Council on Physical Fitness and Sports
1101 Wootton Parkway, Suite 560
Rockville, MD 20852
www.fitness.gov

This government site is part of the U.S. Department of Health and Human Services and provides information about the history of the President's Council along with exercise and nutrition tips.

Shape Up America!
6707 Democracy Boulevard, Suite 306
Bethesda, MD 20817-1129
www.shapeup.org

This website features information about the national initiative to promote healthy weight, called "Shape Up America!" There is advice from fitness and nutrition experts as well as practical tips and support, plus a tool to determine body mass index (BMI).

## GOVERNMENT, LEGISLATION, AND PUBLIC POLICY

Administration on Aging
One Massachusetts Avenue NW
Washington, DC 20001
800-677-1116
www.aoa.gov
Eldercare locator (www.eldercare.gov)

The AoA is a government agency created to develop a comprehensive, coordinated, and cost-effective system of home and community-based services. The website offers information to help elderly individuals maintain their health and independence in their homes and communities.

American Association of Retired Persons (AARP)
601 E Street NW
Washington, DC 20049
800-424-3410
www.aarp.org

This organization is a nonprofit, nonpartisan group that works to assist people age 50 and over with issues by providing information, advocacy, and service.

Centers for Medicare and Medicaid
7500 Security Boulevard
Baltimore, MD 21244-1850
800-MEDICARE
www.medicare.gov

This government website, through the U.S. Department of Health and Human Services, is packed with information about both programs, along with legislative highlights, regulations, research, and statistics.

Department of Veterans Affairs (VA)
810 Vermont Avenue NW
Washington, DC 20420
800-827-1000
www.va.gov

Sponsored by the U.S. Department of Veterans Affairs, this website features everything from information about health and wellness to links for burial and memorial information, benefits, and news.

National Institute for Occupational Safety and Health
1600 Clifton Road
Atlanta, GA 30333
800-232-4636
www.cdc.gov/niosh

Established under the Centers for Disease Control and Prevention (CDC), the NIOSH works to prevent workplace illness and injuries. The website offers safety and health topics for workers and industry owners as well as emergency information, acts on hazards related to chemical exposure, and diseases and common workplace injuries.

Office of the Surgeon General
5600 Fishers Lane, Room 18-66
Rockville, MD 20857
www.surgeongeneral.gov

This website links to the surgeon General of the United States and the 6,500 member Commissioned Corps of the U.S. Public Health Service. Information on the site ranges from scholarship, internship and employment links to the history of the office, facts and research on health topics including childhood obesity, as well as links to other government sponsored websites.

U.S. Department of Agriculture (USDA)
14th and Independence Avenue, SW
Washington, DC 20250
www.usda.gov

This website has a great deal of information, beginning with the history of American agriculture. There is a link to the Code of Federal Regulations and to the USDA Fraud Hotline.

U.S. Department of Health and Human Services (HHS)
200 Independence Avenue, SW
Washington, DC 20201
www.hhs.gov

The HHS is the government's chief agency overseeing all aspects of health, covering everything from Medicare and Medicaid to drug safety. It includes the Food and Drug Administration (FDA), which is listed under "Nutritional Health," below.

World Health Organization (WHO)
525 23rd Street NW
Washington, DC 20037
202-974-3000
www.who.int

This website emphasizes international health issues and offers reports, research, and information on issues from eradicating polio to advances in medications. There is a great deal of information for those interested, but it is not geared for the casual browser.

## INSURANCE AND HEALTH CARE COSTS

HeathCare.gov
200 Independence Avenue, SW
Washington, DC 20201
www.healthcare.gov

A federal government website, managed by the U.S. Department of Health & Human Services, that provides information on types of health insurance available by state, how to find health insurance, and how to understand information on government laws related to health insurance.

## MENTAL, SOCIAL HEALTH, AND ADDICTION

Alcoholics Anonymous
475 Riverside Drive, 11th floor
New York, NY 10115
www.aa.org

Alcoholics Anonymous is an organization for individuals who are working to achieve sobriety from alcohol. The site offers information, how to find an AA meeting, as well as information for family members. The organization was founded in the 1950s and is self-supporting through contributions. There are no dues or fees for membership.

American Anorexia/Bulimia Association
165 West 46th Street, Suite 1108
New York, NY 10036
212-575-6200
www.aabainc.org

The AABA is a nonprofit organization for those dedicated to the treatment of eating disorders, and the information on this site is geared for the general public.

Anxiety Disorders Association of America
8730 Georgia Avenue, Suite 600
Silver Spring, MD 20910
240-485-1001
www.adaa.org

Along with resources for professionals, this website offers information about anxiety, self-help publications, finding a therapist, and explanations of treatment options.

Attention Deficit Disorder Association
PO Box 7557
Wilmington, DE 19803
800-233-4050
http://www.add.org

The ADDA website offers information, resources, and networking opportunities for adults with ADHD, including facts, articles, research, support group information, and links to other helpful resources.

Depression and Bipolar Support Alliance
730 N. Franklin Street, Suite 501
Chicago, IL 60654-7225
800-826-3632
www.dbsalliance.org

The website for this national organization, serving patients with mental illness, offers support, information about mood disorders, links to research and clinical trials, as well as a calendar of educational programs and events.

Dressing Room Project
PO Box 834
Black Mountain, NC 28711
828-318-4438
www.thedressingroomproject.org

This website supports the promotion of a positive body image for girls and women and was developed through the Emerging Women Projects (EWP), a nonprofit organization that works to empower teen girls. The project offers girls and women opportunities to create positive body image cards and place them in public places.

Hospice Foundation of America
1621 Connecticut Avenue, NW, Suite 300
Washington, DC 20009
800-854-3402
www.hospicefoundation.org

This organization conducts professional development for hospice providers and offers research, publications, and assists individuals who are coping with caregiving, terminal illness, and grief through links on its website.

National Alliance on Mental Illness
2107 Wilson Boulevard, Suite 300
Arlington, VA 22201-3042
800-950-6264
www.nami.org

This advocacy organization works to improve treatment and quality of life for individuals suffering from mental illness. Founded in 1979, the organization supports research and awareness of mental illness, offering resources to patients and their families. There is also a link to legislative information, a magazine, a blog, and a ranking of states and the quality of their mental health services.

National Association of Anorexia Nervosa and Associated Disorders
PO Box 640
Naperville, IL 60566
www.anad.org

The ANAD, among the country's oldest nonprofit organizations, offers access to a wealth of resources for eating-disorder victims and their families.

National Attention Deficit Disorder Association
1788 Second Street, Suite 200
Highland Park, IL 60035
847-432-ADDA
www.add.org

This national organization works to support adults with ADHD through sharing information, resources, and advocacy about issues relating to ADHD.

National Institute of Mental Health (NIMH)
Science Writing, Press, and Dissemination Branch
6001 Executive Boulevard, Room 8184, MSC 9663
Bethesda, MD 20892-9663
301-443-4513
www.nimh.nih.gov

This organization, under the U.S. National Institutes of Health, supports basic and clinical research to prevent and cure mental illness. The website offers links to research and funding, news and legislative updates, as well as basic mental health information.

National Mental Health Association
2001 North Beauregard Street, 12th Floor
Alexandria, VA 22311
800-969-6642
www.nmha.org

This nonprofit organization addresses all aspect of mental health and illness and supports reform and education to improve treatment and conditions for Americans with mental illness.

## NUTRITIONAL HEALTH

American Culinary Federation
180 Center Place Way
St. Augustine, FL 32095
www.acfchefs.org

The ACF is a not-for-profit, professional organization developed to support professional chefs through education, directories of accredited culinary programs, and information on certification.

American Dietetic Association
120 South Riverside Plaza, Suite 2000
Chicago, IL 60606-6995
800-877-1600
www.eatright.org

This user-friendly site offers a tool to help find a dietitian along with links to other nutrition-related sites, medical and health professionals, and dietetic associations.

Center for Food Safety & Applied Nutrition, Food and Drug Administration
666 Pennsylvania Avenue, SE, Suite 302
Washington, DC 20003
www.centerforfoodsafety.org

This public interest, environmental advocacy organization addresses the impact of issues and their effects on food. The website also contains an interactive tool for consumers to submit comments to government agencies and members of Congress.

Center for Foodborne Illness Research and Prevention (CFI)
PO Box 206
Grove City, PA 16127
www.foodborneillness.org

This national nonprofit organization is dedicated to preventing foodborne illness through research, education, and advocacy. The website features a speaker's bureau, brochures, and research.

Center for Nutrition Policy and Promotion, USDA
3101 Park Center Drive, 10th Floor
Alexandria, VA 22302-1594
703-305-7600
www.cnpp.usda.gov

This website links consumers with the USDA Center for Nutrition Policy and Promotion, which features the MyPlate materials as well as a link to The Dietary Guidelines for Americans, a food planning tool and other USDA resources.

Center for Science in the Public Interest (CSPI)
1875 Connecticut Avenue, NW, Suite 300
Washington, DC 20009
202-332-9110
www.cspinet.org

The CSPI is a nonprofit education and advocacy organization that offers information on the safety and nutritional quality of food. The website links to jobs, nutrition information, food safety outbreaks, and legislation.

Edible Schoolyard
Martin Luther King Jr. Middle School
1781 Rose Street
Berkeley, CA 94703
510-558-1335
www.edibleschoolyard.org

This website links the program of kitchen classrooms to the Chez Panisse Foundation, which began the program. The site offers a look at gardens created by different participating schools, a list of events, and links to resources.

Five-a-Day
5301 Limestone Road, Suite 101
Wilmington, DE 19808-1249
www.fruitsandveggiesmatter.gov

This site was created by the National Cancer Institute and the Centers for Disease Control and Prevention (CDC) to provide information about the basics of eating five or more servings of fruits and vegetables per day.

The Food Allergy Initiative (FAI)
515 Madison Avenue, Suite 1912
New York, NY 10022
212-207-1974
www.faiusa.org

The website for this nonprofit organization, founded to fund food allergy research, links to news stories, upcoming events, a research library, a resource directory, and support groups.

Food Allergy Network
11781 Lee Jackson Highway, Suite 160
Fairfax, VA 22033-3309
www.foodallergy.org

This website offers facts on food allergies as well as the latest research on allergies and product alerts.

Food and Drug Administration (FDA)
U.S. Department of Health and Human Services
10903 New Hampshire Avenue
Silver Spring, MD 20993
www.fda.gov

This government agency is part of the U.S. Department of Health and Human Services and provides information on a wide range of topics as well as links to other government resources.

Food and Nutrition Service
3101 Park Center Drive
Alexandria, VA 22302
800-221-5689
www.fns.usda.gov

This website, sponsored by the U.S. Department of Agriculture and its Food and Nutrition Information Center, links to a huge variety of government-sponsored nutrition information as well as nutrition assistance programs.

Food First: Institute for Food & Development Policy
398 60th Street
Oakland, CA 94618
www.foodfirst.org

The organization's mission statement of eliminating the injustices that cause hunger is supported by the website, which offers links to publications, programs, issues, a blog, as well as the opportunity to volunteer or participate in an internship.

International Food Information Council (IFIC)
1100 Connecticut Avenue, NW, Suite 430

Washington, DC 20036
www.ific.org

The IFIC collects and disseminates scientific information about nutritional health and food safety to government officials, consumers, and educators. The site for the nonprofit organization is filled with facts as well as a glossary.

Linus Pauling Institute
Oregon State University
571 Weniger Hall
Corvallis, OR 97331
541-737-5075
http://lpi.oregonstate.edu

Located on the campus of Oregon State University, this institute, cofounded by Dr. Linus Pauling, investigates the role vitamins and minerals play in overall health. The organization and website support the research in a variety of health-related areas, including how diet and dietary supplements affect human health.

McDonald's Corporation
2111 McDonald's Drive
Oak Brook, IL 60523
www.McDonalds.com

This website offers nutritional information on menu choices from fat grams to calories. This corporation's site also features promotional products from McDonalds.

Meals for You (My Menus)/Point of Choice
PO Box 2309
Fairfield, IA 52556
www.MealsForYou.com

This website, sponsored by a small, independent company, provides menus and recipes arranged by type, ingredients, or nutrient content and also by categories such as diabetic, vegetarian, and diet.

National Academy of Science; Institute of Medicine/Food Nutrition Board
500 Fifth Street, NW
Washington, DC 20001
www.nas.edu
www.iom.edu

The NAS is a private, nonprofit corporation of biomedical scientists who provide independent advice on issues to government. The information offered here is geared for the professional rather than a general audience. The IOM, an independent, nonprofit organization, works outside of the government to provide information about health and health care and to provide information to government and the private sector.

Nourish America
PO Box 567
Ojai, CA 93024
866-487-1484
www.nourishamerica.org

Nourish America is a charity developed to help low-income families and homeless individuals and families get the nutritional support they need to be healthy. Programs available through Nourish America include Children First, Healthy Moms & Babies, Teen Support, and Senior Support. The program receives donations to support distribution of high-nutrient food and supplements to identified programs and individuals.

Office of Dietary Supplements, National Institutes of Health
6100 Executive Boulevard, Room 3B01, MSC 7517
Bethesda, MD 20892
301-435-2920
www.ods.od.nih.gov

This government website offers an analysis of dietary supplements, the laws that govern them, research and information about the ODS, and its role in dietary supplements in the United States.

Oldways Preservation and Exchange Trust
266 Beacon Street
Boston, MA 02116
www.oldwayspt.org

This nonprofit, education organization features information on traditional cuisines from other countries along with an assortment of articles about nutrition, educational programs, and a bookstore.

Organic Consumers Association (OCA)
6771 South Silver Hill Drive, Finland, MN 55603
www.organicconsumers.org

This nonprofit public interest organization works to promote health and sustainable farming practices in the United States and around the world. They provide consumers information on issues such as food safety, genetic engineering, fair trade, and other key topics.

President's Council on Food Safety
200 Independence Avenue, SW
Washington, DC 20201
www.foodsafety.gov

This government website provides a gateway to government food safety information and is sponsored by the Department of Commerce, the Environmental Protection Agency, the Department of Health and Human Services, and the USDA and is maintained by the FDA's Center for Food Safety and Applied Nutrition.

Rodale Institute
611 Siegfriedale Road
Kutztown, PA 19530-9320
www.rodaleinstitute.org

The Rodale Institute is a nonprofit organization dedicated to organic farming, research, and the spread of information about best farming practices. Founded in 1947 by J. I. Rodale, the institute continues Rodale's goal of preserving and improving soil fertility through organic means.

Safe Tables Our Priority (STOP)
3759 N. Ravenswood, Suite 224
Chicago, IL 60613
www.safetables.org

This national nonprofit public health organization works to prevent foodborne illness through advocacy as well as changes in public policy. The website provides information and awareness for business, nutrition, and health care providers and features the personal stories of victims of foodborne illness.

School Nutrition Association
120 Waterfront Street, Suite 300
National Harbor, MD 20745
301-686-3100
www.schoolnutrition.org

This nonprofit professional organization represents more than 55,000 members across the country employed in some aspect of school nutrition. The organization and website offer opportunities for education and training, legislative and industry information about school nutrition, links to a resource center, publications and current legislative updates.

Snack Food Association
1600 Wilson Boulevard, Suite 650
Arlington, VA 22209
www.sfa.org

The association, founded in 1937 supports the snack food industry through information aimed at consumers. There are also regional recipes using every conceivable snack food.

Vegetarian Resource Group (VRG)
PO Box 1463,
Baltimore, MD 21203
www.vrg.org

This nonprofit group works to educate the public on vegetarian and related health issues. There is information about world hunger and nutrition along with recipes and a list of nutrition-related links.

Wheat Foods Council
51D Red Fox Lane
Ridgway, CO 81432
970-626-9828
www.wheatfoods.org

Wheat producers created this organization to improve understanding of wheat and other grain foods to American consumers. This nonprofit organization works to provide information and increase awareness of the health values of wheat and grain consumption.

## PHYSICAL HEALTH

American Society on Aging
833 Market Street, Suite 512
San Francisco, CA 94103
415-882-2910
www.asaging.org

This website is geared toward the researchers, educators, health practitioners and others who work with older adults.

MedicAlert Foundation
2323 Colorado Avenue
Turlock, CA 95382
888-633-4298
www.medicalert.org

Founded in 1956, this organization calls itself the only nonprofit emergency medical information service in the world, with over 4 million members. They provide MedicAlert jewelry designed to be recognized by emergency responders along with basic information on health topics for consumers.

National Clearinghouse on Families & Youth
PO Box 13505
Silver Spring, MD 20910
888-650-9127
www.canceradvocacy.org

This information resource through the U.S. Department of Health and Human Services seeks to assist individuals and organizations that work with at-risk youth and families.

National Council on Aging
1901 L Street NW, 4th Floor
Washington, DC 20036
202-479-1200
www.ncoa.org

The NCOA is a nonprofit service and advocacy organization that works to serve older Americans through their community organizations by bringing together other nonprofits, businesses, and government to improve the lives of older adults.

## PROFESSIONAL ORGANIZATIONS

American Academy of Family Physicians
11400 Tomahawk Creek Parkway
Leawood, KS 66211-2680
800-274-2237
www.aafp.org

This national medical association represents family physicians and medical students interested in the science of family medicine.

American Academy of Pediatrics
141 Northwest Point Boulevard
Elk Grove Village, IL 60007-1098
847-228-5005
www.aap.org

This doctor-sponsored organization provides health resources, publications, and information about health issues affecting children.

American Academy of Sleep Medicine
2510 North Frontage Road
Darien, IL 60561
630-737-9700
www.aasmnet.org

Membership in this organization is open to clinicians, students, and research professionals specializing in sleep medicine. The website offers links to journals, information on legislation, and an online learning center for members.

American College of Obstetricians and Gynecologists (ACOG)
PO Box 96920
Washington, DC 20090-6920
202-638-5577
www.acog.org

This organization offers membership to doctors and medical students and provides everything from information and updates on technology to advocacy, publications, and a host of other services. The website provides links to a physician's directory of its members.

American Pharmaceutical Association
2215 Constitution Avenue NW
Washington, DC 20037-2985

202-628-4410
http://parmacyandyou.org

This website offers a variety of information choices, including myths about pharmacists, information about specific medicines, health news, along with links to information about pharmacist education.

American Psychiatric Association
1000 Wilson Boulevard, Suite 1825
Arlington, VA 22209
888-357-7924
www.psych.org

This website for members includes news, information about research, changes in public policy, a schedule of events for professional members, and a job bank.

American Public Health Association
800 I Street, NW
Washington, DC 20001-3710
202-777-2742
www.apha.org

The APHA is among the oldest organizations supporting public health professionals in the world. The website offers publications, membership information, career assistance, and links to other information.

Homeopathic Academy of Naturopathic Physicians
PO Box 126
Redmond, WA 998073
www.hanp.net

Affiliated with the American Association of Naturopathic Physicians, the HANP encourages development of curriculum for naturopathic colleges, publishes a journal, and offers continuing education seminars for its membership.

International Society for Orthomolecular Medicine (ISOM)
16 Florence Avenue
Toronto, Ontario, Canada M2N 1E9
www.orthomed.org

This organization, started by Dr. Linus Pauling and others, works to raise awareness of orthomolecular medicine, and the website provides links to other international orthomolecular organizations.

North American Society of Homeopaths
PO Box 450039
Sunrise FL 33345-0039
206-720-7000
www.homeopathy.org

This organization, started in the 1990s, was founded to set standards and certification programs for those interested in classical homeopathy. Besides certification for practitioners, it offers links to resources, research, and how to find a homeopathic practitioner in various geographic areas.

Wellness Council of America (WELCOA)
9802 Nicholas Street, Suite 315
Omaha, NE 68114
www.welcoa.org

This not-for-profit organization was founded in the 1980s with the goal of improving workplace wellness by providing business leaders, public health professionals, and health care practitioners with information, research, and resources.

## WOMEN'S HEALTH

La Leche League International
957 N. Plum Grove Road
Schaumburg, IL 60173
www.lalecheleague.org

This organization offers information on all aspects of breast-feeding and provides links to support groups and volunteer counselors.

National Women's Health Information Center
8270 Willow Oaks Corporate Drive
Fairfax, VA 22031
800-994-9662
www.womenshealth.gov

This federal government source for information on women's health is sponsored by the U.S. Department of Health and Human Services and its Office on Women's Health. The office was established in 1991 to improve the health and well-being of U.S. women and girls by sponsoring programs that focus on health, educate physicians and researchers, and by providing information to the public.

National Women's Health Network
1413 K Street, NW 4th Floor
Washington, DC 20005
202-682-2646
www.womenshealthnetwork.org

This membership-based organization was founded in 1975 and works to influence health policy by promoting women's health issues. It monitors the actions of the federal government and funding agencies as well as industry and health professionals, and supports grassroots action to improve health care outcomes for women.

# *About the Editor and Contributors*

## THE EDITOR

**Sharon Zoumbaris** is a professional librarian, freelance writer, editor, and author of *Nutrition: Health & Medical Issues Today* (ABC-Clio, 2009), coauthor of *Teen Guide to Personal Financial Management* (Greenwood, 2000), *Food and You: A Guide to Healthy Habits for Teens* (Greenwood, 2001), and *Encyclopedia of Diet Fads* (Greenwood, 2003).

## THE CONTRIBUTORS

**Antoine Al-Achi** is associate professor of pharmaceutical sciences, Campbell University, Buies Creek, North Carolina. He is the author of *An Introduction to Botanical Medicine: History, Science, Uses and Dangers* (Praeger, 2008). His research interests include protein delivery systems and complementary and alternative medicine.

**Linda Wasmer Andrews** is a journalist and author with a master's degree in psychology. She is the author of *The Encyclopedia of Depression* (2010) and specializes in writing about health, psychology, and the mind/body connection.

**Devon Atchison** is an assistant professor at Grossmont College in San Diego, California. She teaches early and modern American history and American women's history. She is also the archivist for the Women's History Museum & Educational Center.

**Anja Becker** is a postdoctoral fellow at Vanderbilt University, funded by the German Academic Exchange Service (DAAD). Her current research is on higher education in the American South and West between the Civil War and World War II.

**Jennifer Berg** is the director of graduate food studies at New York University. Her research focuses on New York's new immigration.

**Marjolijn Bijlefeld** is a medical reporter and editor from Fredericksburg, Virginia. She has authored and coauthored numerous books, including *The Encyclopedia of Diet Fads* (2003) and *It Came from Outer Space: Everyday Products and Ideas from the Space Program* (2003), both published by Greenwood.

**Joseph P. Byrne,** PhD, MUP, is a cultural and social historian of medieval and early modern Europe and professor of honors humanities at Belmont University in Nashville, Tennessee. He has written extensively for a wide variety of historical reference works and journals and is the editor of and contributor to *Encyclopedia of Pestilence, Pandemics, and Plagues* (2008); *Encyclopedia of the Black Death* (2012); and *Daily Life during the Black Death* (2006), all from Greenwood Press.

**Stephanie Jane Carter** is administrative director of the Southern Food and Beverage Museum in New Orleans as well as a writer, speaker, and food historian.

**David Chen** is an MD-MPH Candidate (2015) at the University of Virginia, Charlottesville.

**Robert William Collin** is the senior research scholar at Willamette University Center for Sustainable Communities in Salem, Oregon. His published works include *Battleground: Environment; The EPA: Cleaning Up America's Act;* and, with Robin Morris Collin, *The Encyclopedia of Sustainability,* all published by Greenwood Press.

**Jacob Cunningham,** MA, teaches history at Hebrew Union College–Jewish Institute of Religion, Los Angeles, California. He studied at the University of California, Santa Cruz, and did his graduate work at the University of California, Los Angeles. He is the coauthor, with Howard Padwa, of *Addiction: A Reference Encyclopedia* (ABC-CLIO, 2010).

**Don E. Davis** is an assistant professor at Georgia State University. His research interests include religion/spirituality, forgiveness, humility, and multicultural issues.

**Margo DeMello** received her PhD in cultural anthropology from University of California at Davis and currently lectures at Central New Mexico Community College, teaching sociology, cultural studies, and anthropology. Her books include *Bodies of Inscription: A Cultural History of the Modern Tattoo Community* (2000), *Feet and Footwear: A Cultural Encyclopedia* (Greenwood, 2009), and *Faces Around the World* (2011).

**Roni K. Devlin,** MD, practices infectious disease medicine, internal medicine, and pediatrics in Muskegon, Michigan. Dr. Devlin graduated from the University of Colorado School of Medicine and completed her residency at Spectrum Health in Grand Rapids, Michigan. She is the author of *Influenza* (Greenwood, 2008).

**Megan Moore Duncan** coauthored *Autism Spectrum Disorders: A Handbook for Parents and Professionals* (Praeger, 2007).

**Kevin J. Eames** is associate professor of psychology at Covenant College in Lookout Mountain, Georgia. Recent book chapters include "Evil in Mind: Psychopathy and Anomalous Cognitive Function," in *Explaining Evil,* J.H. Ellens, ed., Praeger, 2011, and "Traits, Factors, and Faith: A Review of the Relationship between Personality Traits and Religiosity," in *The Healing Power of Spirituality,* J.H. Ellens, ed., Praeger, 2010.

**Reverend Dr. J. Harold Ellens** is professor emeritus of Philosophy, Wayne State University, Farmington Hills, Michigan. A former research scholar at the University of Michigan, Department of Near Eastern Studies, he has also been a psychotherapist in private practice (now retired) and a U.S. Army colonel. Currently, he is an independent scholar, published in 201 volumes and 167 journal articles.

**Ruth C. Engs,** RN, EdD, is professor emeritus, applied health science, Indiana University, Bloomington. She has published numerous articles and over 11 books, including *The Eugenics Movement* (2005) and *Clean Living Movements: American Cycles of Health Reform* (2000).

**Abena Foreman-Trice** is a communications professional at the University of Virginia who writes about business and health topics. She has received numerous awards for her journalistic work in the medical field, including an editorial bronze award from Parenting Publications of America for coverage of Sudden Infant Death Syndrome.

**Myron D. Fottler,** PhD, is Director of Programs in Health Services Administration in the College of Health and Public Affairs at the University of Central Florida in Orlando, where he teachers courses in human resources management and is the author of 18 books, including *The Retail Revolution in Healthcare* (Praeger, 2010). He has an MBA from Boston University and a PhD in business from Columbia University.

**Cheryl Fracasso,** MS, is a doctoral candidate at Saybrook University, San Francisco. She is a research assistant at Saybrook with Stanley Krippner and a faculty member at the University of Phoenix. She serves on the editorial/advisory board of *NeuroQuantology Journal* and as associate managing editor with the *International Journal of Transpersonal Studies.*

**Harris Friedman** was research professor of psychology (now retired), at the University of Florida, Gainesville. He has published more than 100 scholarly works and is senior editor of *International Journal of Transpersonal Studies.* He is currently a clinical-consulting psychologist and independent scholar.

**Mark A. Goldstein,** MD, is chief of the division of adolescent and young adult medicine at Massachusetts General Hospital, and assistant professor of pediatrics at Harvard Medical School. His published works with Myrna Chandler Goldstein include *Healthy Foods: Fact versus Fiction* (Greenwood, 2010), *Food and Nutrition Controversies Today: A Reference Guide* (Greenwood, 2009), and, with Myrna Chandler Goldstein and Larry Credit, *Your Best Medicine: From Conventional and Complementary Medicine* (2008).

**Myrna Chandler Goldstein** is a writer, independent scholar, and author of numerous books with Mark A. Goldstein, MD, including *Food and Nutrition Controversies Today* (Greenwood, 2009), *Healthy Foods: Fact versus Fiction* (Greenwood, 2010), and *Controversies in the Practice of Medicine* (Greenwood, 2001). Her website is Doing Good, While Doing Business: Support Socially Responsible Companies (www.changethemold.com).

**Gina Graci,** PhD, CBSM, is a licensed clinical psychologist and certified behavioral sleep medicine specialist and is employed as a private practitioner specializing in both sleep disorders and psychosocial oncology. She is the coauthor, with Kathy Sexton-Radek, of *Combating Sleep Disorders* (Praeger, 2008).

**Janice Gronvold** is the founder and director of Spectrec and has over 25 years of experience in business development in the hospitality, resort, spa, and health industries. She graduated from the Stuart Graduate School of Business at the Illinois Institute of Technology and the eBusiness Strategy Program at the University of Chicago. Her book projects include a chapter contribution to *Whole Person Healthcare* (Praeger, 2007), and she contributed to *Bust the Silos: Opening Your Organization for Growth* (2010).

**Joan H. Hageman,** PhD, is an international research scientist, chair of research at PSYmore Research Institute, Inc., and associate professor for dissertation committees at Northcentral University. She has been published in books and journal articles, and her recent publications include *Cross Cultural Boundaries: Psychophysiological Responses, Absorption, and Dissociation Comparison between Brazilian Spiritists and Advanced Meditators* (2011), *The Neurobiology of Trance and Mediumship in Brazil* (2009), and "Not All Meditation is the Same: A Brief Overview of Perspectives, Techniques, and Outcomes" (2008).

**Victoria A. Harden** retired in 2006 as director of the Office of NIH History and the Stetten Museum at the National Institutes of Health, an office she created during the 1986–1987 observance of the NIH centennial. She has written and edited several books, including *Rocky Mountain Spotted Fever: History of a Twentieth-Century Disease* and *AIDS and the Public Debate: Historical and Contemporary Perspectives,* and she oversaw an oral history project on the 1960s eradication of smallpox in West Africa.

**Janice H. Hoffman** is a clinical exercise specialist and fibromyalgia and chronic pain conditions research studies coordinator at Oregon Health and Science University, Portland. She is a board member on the Fibromyalgia Information Foundation in Portland, Oregon. She is coauthor, with Kim Dupree Jones, of *Fibromyalgia* (Greenwood, 2009).

**Jeanne Holcomb** is completing her PhD in sociology at the University of Florida. Her project is focused on women's experiences with breast-feeding and, more specifically, challenges women might face as they breast-feed over time. Her interests include work and family issues, sociology of childhood, and social change. She lives with her husband, Greg, and their daughter and son.

**Kathryn H. Hollen** is a freelance science writer and editor who works with her husband, a technical illustrator, out of her rural home west of Washington, DC. She writes for the National Cancer Institute and other organizations engaged in biomedical reporting and research. She is the editor of *The Encyclopedia of Addictions* (Greenwood, 2008).

**Jeanne Holverstott,** MS, is an autism spectrum specialist with Responsive Centers for Psychology and Learning, Overland Park, Kansas, and coauthored *Autism Spectrum Disorders: A Handbook for Parents and Professionals* (Praeger, 2007).

**Joshua Hook** is assistant professor of psychology, University of North Texas, Denton. His research interests include positive psychology, religion/spirituality, and treatments for alcohol dependence and hypersexuality.

**Jonelle Husain** is a doctoral student in sociology at Mississippi State University. Her research interests focus on the diversity and negotiation that characterize pro-life activism, the turning points that propel activists into public activism, the multivalent ways pro-life activists construct abortion as a moral problem, and the ways activists create and use action strategies to disseminate their worldviews and to stop abortion.

**Barbara Froling Immroth,** PhD, is a professor in the School of Information at the University of Texas at Austin. She received her degree from the University of Pittsburgh and is the author of *Health Information in a Changing World: Practical Approaches for Teachers, Schools and School Librarians* (2010).

**Leonard Jason,** PhD, is professor of psychology at DePaul University in Chicago, where he heads the Center for Community Research. He has published extensively on preventive school-based interventions; the prevention of alcohol, tobacco, and drug abuse; media interventions; and program evaluation. His own experience with chronic fatigue syndrome has been a motivating factor in his efforts to promote the healing effects of community on chronic illness and other conditions described in *Havens: Stories of True Community Healing* (2004).

**Elizabeth Jones,** MDiv, CADC, is a coordinator and instructor in the program in religion, spirituality, and mental health in the department of psychiatry at the University of Illinois at Chicago.

**Kim D. Jones,** RN, FNP, PhD, is associate professor of nursing and assistant professor of medicine at Oregon Health and Science University in Portland, Oregon. She is coauthor, with Janice H. Hoffman, of *Fibromyalgia* (Greenwood, 2009). She has been the principal investigator on five major research studies funded by National Institutes of Health, Industry, and Foundations and a coinvestigator on over 25 fibromyalgia research studies, mostly in collaboration with colleagues on the Oregon Fibromyalgia Research and Treatment Team.

**Stanley Krippner,** PhD, is Alan Watts Professor of Psychology and Humanistic Studies at Saybrook University, San Francisco, California. He is coauthor of *Haunted by Combat: Understanding PTSD in War Veterans* and co-editor of *Debating Psychic Experience: Human Potential or Human Illusion?* He has received lifetime achievement awards from the Parapsychological Association and the International Association for the Study of Dreams.

**Shobha S. Krishnan,** MD, is a board certified family physician and gynecologist at Barnard College, Columbia University, New York. Prior to joining Barnard, she was in private practice for 10 years and worked as a surveillance physician for the Centers for Disease Control and Prevention (CDC). She has written *The HPV Vaccine Controversy: Sex, Cancer, God and Politics; A Guide for Parents, Women, Men, and Teenagers* (Praeger, 2008).

**Jennie Jacobs Kronenfeld,** PhD, is professor in the sociology program in the School of Social and Family Dynamics, Arizona State University, Phoenix. Research interests include medical sociology and aging and the life course, with special emphasis on health policy, health care use, and health behavior. She is the author of *Medicare* (Greenwood, 2011) and serves as editor of the research annual *Research in the Sociology of Health and Health Care.*

**Paul G. LaCava** is an assistant professor of special education at Rhode Island College in Providence, RI. He earned his graduate degrees at the University of Kansas and currently teaches undergraduate and graduate courses in special education, research, and autism spectrum disorders.

**Margaret M. Lotz** earned a PhD in cell and molecular biology from Duke University and completed a postdoctoral fellowship at Harvard Medical School. She works as a clinical research coordinator, data manager, and analyst for clinical cancer trials in cancer biomarkers. She is coauthor, along with Marsha A. Moses and Susan Elaine Pories, of *Cancer,* in the Biography of Disease Series (Greenwood, 2009).

**W. Bernard Lukenbill,** PhD, is professor emeritus in the School of Information at the University of Texas at Austin. He received his degree from Indiana

University, and his published works include *Health Information in a Changing World: Practical Approaches for Teachers, Schools, and School Librarians* (2010).

**Lois N. Magner** is professor emeritus at Purdue University and author of *A History of Infectious Diseases and the Microbial World* (Praeger, 2009).

**Donna M. Malvey,** PhD, is associate professor of health services administration at the University of Central Florida, Orlando. She has an MHSA degree from George Washington University and a PhD in administration–health services from the University of Alabama at Birmingham. She is a coauthor, with Myron D. Fottler, of *The Retail Revolution in Healthcare* (Praeger, 2010.

**Lisa Barrett Mann,** M.S.Ed., specializes in working with children and youth with Asperger Syndrome and other autism spectrum disorders.

**Julie McDowell** is a science and health care journalist based in Washington, DC. She is the author, editor, or coauthor of several books in the sciences, including *The Nervous System and Sense Organs* (Greenwood, 2004), *The Lymphatic System* (with Michael Windelspecht, Greenwood, 2004), and *The Encyclopedia of Human Body Systems* (2010). She holds an MA in nonfiction writing from Johns Hopkins University in Baltimore, Maryland.

**Laura McLaughlin** received her master's degree in public health, MPH, from the University of Virginia, Charlottesville, in 2011. She is employed in the health care consulting field in Washington, DC.

**Michele Morrone** holds a PhD in environmental planning from Ohio State University and an MS in forest resources from the University of New Hampshire. At Ohio University, she is associate professor of environmental health, the director of environmental studies, and associate director of academic affairs at the Voinovich School. She previously served as the chief of the Office of Environmental Education at Ohio EPA and is the author of *Poisons on Our Plates: The Real Food Safety Problem in the United States* (Praeger, 2008).

**Marsha A. Moses** is a professor at Harvard Medical School and is the director of the vascular biology program at Children's Hospital in Boston. She has published extensively in the field of cancer research and holds some 70 patents, both issued and pending. The focus of her research is the regulation of tumor growth and progression and angiogenesis. She is coauthor, along with Margaret M. Lotz and Susan Elaine Pories, of *Cancer,* in the Biography of Disease Series (Greenwood, 2009).

**Samantha Murray,** PhD, is a lecturer in cultural studies in the Department of Media, Music, Communication and Cultural Studies at Macquarie University in Sydney, Australia. Her published work includes *The 'Fat' Female Body* (2008), and she has contributed to the *Cultural Encyclopedia of the Body* (Greenwood, 2008).

**Richard L. Myers** is professor of environmental science at Alaska Pacific University in Anchorage. He received his PhD from Florida Institute of Technology and his MS from the University of Alaska, Fairbanks. His published work includes *The 100 Most Important Chemical Compounds: A Reference Guide* (Greenwood, 2007).

**Brenda Smith Myles,** PhD, is an associate professor at the University of Kansas who writes and speaks internationally on Asperger Syndrome and autism. She co=-authored *Autism Spectrum Disorders: A Handbook for Parents and Professionals* (Praeger, 2007).

**Dianne L. Needham** is a professional journalist who writes about health, medicine, and science. A former communications specialist for the National Institutes of Health, with extensive experience as a communications practitioner and writer in the public and private sectors, she holds a master's degree in political economy.

**David E. Newton** is the author of more than 400 textbooks, encyclopedias, resource books, research manuals, laboratory manuals, trade books, and other educational materials. He taught mathematics, chemistry, and physical science; was professor of chemistry and physics at Salem State College in Massachusetts; and was adjunct professor in the College of Professional Studies at the University of San Francisco.

**Frank John Ninivaggi,** MD, is an associate attending physician at Yale-New Haven Hospital; assistant clinical professor of child psychiatry at Yale University School of Medicine, Yale Child Study Center; and a member of the Yale-New Haven Community Medical Group. He is also staff psychiatrist at Hall-Brooke Hospital in Westport, Connecticut, and the medical director for the Devereux Glenholme School in Washington, Connecticut. He is the author of *Ayurveda: A Comprehensive Guide to Traditional Indian Medicine for the West* (2007).

**Stephenie Overman** is a full-time freelance writer who specializes in workplace and health care issues. She is editor of *Staffing Management* magazine and was editor of *Executive Talent* magazine. She has written for a variety of publications, including the *Los Angeles Business Journal, Daily Labor Report, Bulletin to Management, Employee Relations Weekly, HR Magazine,* and *Independent Business.* She has a master's degree in labor studies from the University of the District of Columbia. She is the author of *Next-Generation Wellness at Work* (Praeger, 2009).

**Howard Padwa,** PhD, works as a researcher in Los Angeles. He studied at the University of Delaware, the London School of Economics, and L'Ecole des Hautes Etudes en Sciences Sociales in Paris before earning his PhD at UCLA. He, with Jason Cunningham, is the coauthor of *Addiction: A Reference Encyclopedia* (ABC-CLIO, 2010).

**Melissa Palmer** is an internationally renowned hepatologist and the author of the best-selling book *Dr. Melissa Palmer's Guide to Hepatitis and Liver Disease.* She maintains one of the largest private medical practices devoted to liver disease in the United States. Dr. Palmer graduated from Columbia University and was trained in liver disease at the Mount Sinai School of Medicine in New York City.

**Kelsey Parris** is an independent scholar in New Orleans.

**David Petechuk** is an independent scholar. He has written on numerous topics, including genetics and cloning, and has worked with scientists and faculty in areas such as transplantation and psychiatry.

**Susan E. Pories** is the co-editor of *The Soul of a Doctor* (2006) and coauthor of *Cancer: Biography of a Disease* (2009). She is a surgeon at the Beth Israel Deaconess Medical Center and the Mount Auburn Hospital and an assistant professor of Surgery at Harvard Medical School.

**Gretchen M. Reevy,** PhD, is a lecturer in the psychology department at California State University–East Bay, Hayward. She is the author of the *Encyclopedia of Emotion* (ABC-Clio/Greenwood, 2010), co-editor of *Personality, Stress and Coping: Implications for Education* (2011), and *The Praeger Handbook on Stress and Coping* (Praeger, 2007).

**Brian Regal,** PhD, FLS, is assistant professor for the history of science at Kean University. His books include *Pseudoscience: A Critical Encyclopedia* (2009) and *Icons of Evolution* (2008).

**Alice C. Richer,** RD, MBA, is a dietitian who specializes in sports nutrition, food allergies, and general nutrition. She received her MBA from Boston College and undergraduate BS in food and nutrition from University of Rhode Island. Richer is the author of *Understanding the Antioxidant Controversy* (2007), with Paul Milbury, and *Food Allergies* (2009).

**Meryl Rosofsky** is adjunct professor in the department of nutrition, food studies, and public health at New York University and writes about food and culture.

**Kathy Sexton-Radek,** PhD, CBSM, is a licensed clinical psychologist in private practice and professor of psychology at Elmhurst College, in Elmhurst, Illinois. Her most recent publication is *Combating Your Sleep Problems* (2008).

**Leslie Shafer** is a writer who has studied environmental science, with public works and advocacy experience. She is especially interested in environmental health issues.

**Andrew F. Smith** is a freelance writer and speaker on culinary matters. He teaches culinary history and professional food writing at the New School in Manhattan, serves as general editor of the Food Series at the University of Illinois Press, and is general editor for the Edible Series at Reaktion Press in the United Kingdom. He is also editor-in-chief of the *Oxford Encyclopedia on Food and Drink in America* (2004) and the *Oxford Companion to American Food and Drink* (2009).

**William C. Smith** is director of programming at the Jefferson Parish Public Library in New Orleans.

**Kara Stefan** is a freelance writer specializing in the financial services and insurance industries. She has extensive experience writing about mutual funds, annuities, group/individual retirement plans, investment portfolio and retirement income strategies, personal finance/budgeting, credit/debt, life insurance, mortgages, bank deposit products, loans, real estate, health care insurance, and wellness programs.

**William C. Summers** is professor of molecular biophysics and biochemistry and of history of science and medicine at Yale University. His books include *Felix d'Herelle and the Origins of Molecular Biology* (1999), and he edited the *Encyclopedia of Microbiology, Second Edition* (2000).

**Terri Cooper Swanson,** MS, Ed, is the autism certificate program coordinator at Pittsburg State University and coauthor of *Autism Spectrum Disorders: A Handbook for Professionals* (2007).

**David S. Teitler,** LAc, is a licensed acupuncturist and Chinese medicine herbalist in Colorado who specializes in the treatment of respiratory conditions.

**Mary Jo Thomas** is an independent scholar who writes about health issues and other topics.

**Dr. Amy Wachholtz** is an assistant professor of psychiatry at the University of Massachusetts Medical School and director of health psychology at UMass Memorial Medical Center. She is currently a health psychologist on the Psychosomatic Medicine Consult Service at UMass Memorial Medical Center in Worcester, Massachusetts.

**Amanda Wheat,** MS, West Virginia University, Morgantown, is a doctoral candidate there in clinical psychology, with clinical and research interests in health psychology and behavior medicine.

**Elizabeth M. Williams** is president of the Southern Food and Beverage Museum in New Orleans and writes about legal aspects of food policy.

**Michael Windelspecht** is associate professor of biology at Appalachian State University. He is the author of two books in Greenwood's Groundbreaking Scientific Experiments, Inventions, and Discoveries through the Ages series (2001) and editor of Greenwood's Human Body Systems series (2004).

# *Index*

Automated external defibrillator, 189, 658

Ayurveda, 91–96; health and disease concepts in, 92–93; universal causes of disease in, 93–96

Azidothymidine (AZT), 2, 465, 867

Back pain, 97–101

Bacteria, 101–5; antibiotic-resistant, 63–67, 244–45, 577–79, 772; bacterial sex, 105; classification of, 102–3; common cold and, 214–16; culture of, 103; irradiation and, 504–5, 508–9; mutually beneficial relationships with other organisms, 103–4; spore form of, 104; spread of, 104–5, 376; virus and, 215, 242–43. *See also* Dental health; Food-borne illness; Probiotics; *specific bacteria*

Balfour, William, 345

Banner, Lois, 279–80

Banting, William, 268–69, 280

Bariatric surgery, 105–8; celebrities and, 106, 107; complications from, 106, 107; FDA on, 107; types of, 105, 107, 273–74

Barrier methods of contraception, 119–20, 121

Bartell, Susan S., 630

Bartlett, Dawn, 426

Bartlett, Rylea, 426

Barto, Julie, 703

Basal metabolism, 108–9

Basic four (foods), 109–12, 587

Basic Seven food guide, 111, 262, 587

Bastyr University (Seattle), 693

Battle Creek Sanitarium, 409, 519

Bay Area Laboratory Co-Operative, 775

Beard, George, 782

Bechler, Steve, 323–24

Beck, Aaron, 249, 251

Beck, Charles, 659, 858

Becklenberg, Mary Ann, 50

Becquerel, Antoine-Henri, 505

Behavioral addiction, 14–15, 17. *See also* Eating disorders

Behavioral therapy, 689. *See also* Cognitive-behavioral therapy

Belief.net, 533

Benbrook, Charles, 639

Benjamin, Reginal, 586

Bennett, Robert M., 346

Benzene, 536

Benzodiazepine Rohypnol, 296

Bereavement, 412

Berg, Paul, 243

Beriberi, 110, 624, 841, 843

Bernheim, Hippolyte, 474

Berries, 1–2, 70, 131–34

Beta-alanine, 55

Beta-amyloid protein, 48

Beta blockers, 130

Beta-carotene, 69, 70

Beyond Pesticides, 596

BFIFC. *See* Bureau of Foods Irradiated Food Committee

Bill and Melinda Gates Foundation, 8, 879

Binary fission, 101, 105

Binge-eating disorder, 149–50, 300, 302–4

Biodiversity, 392, 550, 638, 817

Biodots, 113

Bioengineered foods, 41

Biofeedback, 99, 112–14

Biological clock, 496

Biological effects, 313

Biological living, 519

Biological warfare, 650

Biomedical Research Training Amendments (1978), 589

Biotechnology, 56, 394

Biotin (B7), 104, 265, 612, 842

Biotoxin, 308

Biphasic reactions, 43

Bipolar disorder, 114–17, 247

Birth control, 117–26; abortion and, 124; emergency contraception, 125; history of, 119–20; new contraceptive technologies, 123–24; permanent contraception, 124–25; traditional methods of, 120–22

Birth defects, 233, 265, 842

Bisexual orientation, 385

Black Death, 649

Blackout, 35

Blagojevich, Rod, 323

Blindness, 548, 841

407; Type 2, 36, 53, 80, 181, 182, 185, 253–57, 406, 407, 451–52; WHO on, 253

Diabetes Control and Complications Trial, 257

*Diagnostic and Statistical Manual of Mental Disorders* (*DSM,* APA): on addiction, 16–17; on ADHD, 84; on Asperger syndrome, 72, 88; on autism, 86; on bipolar disorder, 115–16; on depression, 246–47; on eating disorders, 299–301; on GID, 389; on SAD, 732; on substance abuse, 294–95, 492

Dialysis, 533

Diaphragm (contraceptive), 120, 121, 122

Dias, J., 801

Diet: balanced, 53, 55, 69; cancer and, 173–74, 830; high-fat, 128. *See also specific diets*

*Diet and Die* (Malmberg), 283

*Diet and Health: Implications for Reducing Chronic Disease Risk* (National Research Council), 259

*Diet and Health, With Key to the Calories* (Peters), 269, 283

*Dietary Goals for the American People,* 259. *See also* Dietary Guidelines for Americans

*Dietary Goals for the United States* (Senate Select Committee on Nutrition and Human Needs), 111

Dietary Guidelines Advisory Committee, 258, 260, 840–41

Dietary Guidelines for Americans (USDA), 258–61, 629; on fats, 832; SMI and, 729, 730; on sugar-sweetened drinks, 184; 2010 release, 111, 587, 840; on variety of foods, 278, 840

Dietary modification trial, of WHI, 869, 870

Dietary Reference Intakes (DRI), 261–62, 700, 831

Dietary Supplement and Nonprescription Drug Consumer Protection Act (2006), 266

Dietary Supplement Current Good Manufacturing Practices and Interim Final Rule (2007), 682

Dietary Supplement Health and Education Act (1994), 53, 262, 809, 844

Dietary supplements, 262–68; amino acids as, 53–56; athletes and, 55; for back pain, 100; definition of, 262; Dirty Dozen, 516, 517; FDA on, 54, 263, 265–67, 538–39, 682; government legislation on, 262–64; herbs as, 263, 266–67, 809–10; labels for, 53–54, 262–63; popular, 264–66; problems with, 263, 266–67; as unnecessary, 259; web-based resources for, 267. *See also* Vitamins; *specific supplements*

Diet drinks, 283

Dieting, 268–74; açaí berry and, 1; American Dietetic Association on, 81, 276, 454, 522; American Medical Association on, 81, 283; body image and, 136; celebrities and, 270, 271; control, loss of pleasure and, 272–73; fad diets, 55–56, 269–70, 278–85, 885; gender and, 271–72; low-carbohydrate diets, 56, 79–81, 180, 522; low-glycemic index diets, 407–8; NIH on, 106; online resources for, 274–77; origins of modern, 268–69; yo-yo, 630, 713, 885–87. *See also* Weight control; *specific diets*

Diet pills, 266, 269, 324

Digestion-resistant starch, 343

Digestive cures, 282

Dill, D.B., 664

Dimas, Stavros, 392

Dinitrophenol, 269, 282–83

Dioxin, 536

Dirty Dozen: dietary supplements, 516, 517; of foods with most pesticide, 636

Discoid lupus erythematosus (DLE), 541

*Discover,* 641–42

Disease model of addiction, 19

Diseases and disorders: diseases of mouth, 227–30; drug-resistant, 650; TCM on causes of, 804, 805–6. *See also specific diseases and disorders*

Dissociation, 475

Diuretics (water pills), 130

Division of Perinatal Systems and Women's Health, 422

DLE. *See* Discoid lupus erythematosus
DNA. *See* Deoxyribonucleic acid
DNA ligase, 243, 244
DNR. *See* Do Not Resuscitate
Döbereiner, Johann Wolfgang, 152
Doctors in the media, 285–87
Doll, Richard, 162
Do Not Resuscitate (DNR), 532
Donovan, Robert, 389
Dopamine, 15, 22, 291–94, 754
*Doshas,* 92, 95
Dream Interview Method, 289
Dream therapy, 287–91; interpretation of dreams, 290–91; therapeutic use of dreams, 288–90; value of dreams, 287–88
Dressing Room Project, 136–37
DRI. *See* Dietary Reference Intakes
Drinking. *See* Alcohol
Driver, Deamonte, 227
Drug Enforcement Agency, 563
Drugs: for hypertension treatment, 130; off-label use and economics of, 359; pharmacy compounding of, 359. *See also* Food and Drug Administration; *specific drugs*
Drugs, recreational, 291–98; consequences for possessing and selling, 296; control status of, 292; detection of, 296; dopamine and, 15, 291–94; medical problems from, 2, 4, 5–9, 18, 295; multidrug experience and cocktail effect with, 296; street names for, 293; teen brain and, 17–18; treatment for, 297; withdrawal, 15. *See also specific drugs*
Druker, Stephen M., 396
Drywall, 312–13
Duesberg, Peter, 7
Du Rand, Johnnette, 769
Durkheim, Emile, 790
DV. *See* Daily value of nutrients
Dyspepsia, 411
Dysthymic disorder, 247–48

*E. coli* bacteria, 244–45, 360–61, 365, 483
*E. coli* infection, 305–6, 363, 368, 371–72
EAR. *See* Estimated average requirements

Early Head Start Program, 421, 424
*Eat and Grow Thin* (Thompson, V.), 283
Eating disorders, 60–61, 149–50, 271, 299–305; characteristics of, 299–300; *DSM* on, 299–301; FAQs about, 302–4; medical problems from, 301, 302–3; NIMH on, 60, 150, 299–300, 302–4; prevalence of, 300–302; substance abuse and, 301; vegetarians and, 833–34. *See also* Anorexia nervosa; Binge-eating disorder; Body image; Bulimia nervosa
*Eating for Life* (Phillips), 276
Economic Opportunity Act (1964), 420
Economic Research Service, 333, 367, 727, 856
Ecstasy. *See* MDMA
ECT. *See* Electroconvulsive therapy
Edible Schoolyard project, 306–8, 854, 856–57
eDiets.com, 276
Edington, D.W., 871
EDTA. *See* Ethylenediamine tetraacetic acid
Edward I (king of England), 30
Edwards, H.T., 664
"The Effects of Stress Management and a Low-Cholesterol Diet on Heart Disease" (Ornish), 642
Eggs. *See* Poultry and eggs
Ehrenberg, Carl Gustave von, 102–3
Ehrlich, Paul, 745
Eight Principles, TCM, 807
Eijkman, Christian, 843
Eisenhower, Dwight, 505, 673, 818
Electrocardiogram test (EKG), 441
Electroconvulsive therapy (ECT), 252
Electrolytes, 548, 762, 852
Electromagnetic fields, 313
Electromyogram, 191
Ellis, Albert, 708
Emergency Planning and Community Right-to-Know Act, 319
Emerging Women Projects, 136–37
Emerson, Ralph Waldo, 280, 410
Emotion-focused therapy, 691
Emotions and influences, TCM, 805–6
EMS. *See* Eosinophilia myalgia syndrome
Enamel fluorosis, 236

Group therapy, 691
Guided imagery, 414–18; history of,
 416–17; new applications for, 417
Guillain-Barre syndrome, 199, 360
Gulf of Mexico oil spill (2010), 501
Gupta, Sanjay, 285, 286
Gyllenhaal, Jake, 308, 857

HAART. *See* Highly Active Antiretroviral
 Therapy
HACCP. *See* Hazard Analysis and Critical
 Control Point program
Hahnemann, Samuel, 458
Hales, Stephen, 126
Halloran, Jean, 371
Harris, C.N.D., 801
Harris, T.O., 782
Harrison Narcotics Act (1914), 758
*Harvard Health Letter,* 339
Harvey, Arthur, 596–97
Harvey, William, 280
Hatch Act (1887), 815
Haug, Jon Birger, 579
Hay, William, 269
Hayashi, Chujiro, 704
Hay diet, 269
Hayflick, Leonard, 169
Hayflick number or limit, 169
Hazard, 308
Hazard Analysis and Critical Control
 Point (HACCP) program, 196,
 371–72
HCG. *See* Human chorionic gonadotropin
HDL. *See* High-density lipoproteins
Headache, 12, 154, 803–4
Head Start and Healthy Start, 419–25
Head Start Reauthorization Act (1994),
 421
Head trauma, 51
*The Healing Factor: Vitamin C against Disease*
 (Stone), 655, 845
Health and medical tourism, 425–31; ethi-
 cal criticisms of, 429–30; future of,
 430–31; losers in, 428–29; who travels
 abroad and reasons why, 426–28
Health care: costs of Alzheimer's disease,
 51; disparities in, 77; doctors in the
 media, 285–87; universal coverage,

427, 429, 430. *See also* Psychosomatic
 health care
Healthcare Financing Administration,
 225, 642
Health Care without Harm, 697
Health Forest Initiative, 817
Health insurance, 431–37; basic facts and
 terms for, 432–33; coverage and costs
 of, 434–35; for dental health, 234–35;
 history of, 433–34; ideal height-and-
 weight charts, 282; on international
 medical care, 430; managed care,
 554–56; number of people with, 435;
 reform legislation on, 435–37
Health maintenance organizations
 (HMOs), 554, 555
Health Omnibus Program Extension
 (1988), 590
Health Research Extension Act (1985),
 589
Health Resources and Services Administration (HRSA), 419, 424, 866
Health Savings Account (HSA), 437–40
Healthstyles 2000 national mail survey,
 147
*The Health Consequences of Smoking—Nicotine
 Addiction* (Koop), 756
The Health Project, 872
Health Tracking Household Survey
 (2007), 716
Healthy, Hunger-Free Kids Act (2010),
 599
*Healthy People: The Surgeon General's Report
 on Health Promotion and Disease Preven-
 tion* (Department of Health, Educa-
 tion and Welfare), 111
Healthy People 2020 initiative, 311
Healthy Schools Campaign, 602
Healthy Start. *See* Head Start and Healthy
 Start
Healthy Weight Commitment Founda-
 tion, 601
Healthy Youth! Program, 660
Heart attack, 188–89, 442–43
Heartburn and acid indigestion, 58,
 165
Heart disease: CDC on, 209; cholesterol
 and, 206, 208–9; dental health and,